In *UNBLEMISHED* you'll learn:

- Acne is not your fault.
- You don't need to change your diet to improve your skin.
- Acne can be treated properly using over-the-counter medications.
- You can take charge of your skin using 3 simple steps.
- And most important, you *can* get rid of your acne forever!

"Rodan and Fields have created an acne treatment that is genius. There's no reason to use anything else."

—Patricia Wexler, M.D., attending physician
at Beth Israel Medical Center

STOP BREAKOUTS!
FIGHT ACNE!
TRANSFORM YOUR LIFE!

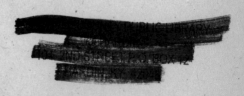

APR 0 4 2007

Unblemished

stop breakouts! fight acne!
transform your life!
reclaim your self-esteem
with the proven 3-step program
using over-the-counter
medications

Katie Rodan, M.D., and Kathy Fields, M.D.

the creators of Proactiv® Solution, America's number one acne-care system,
and Rodan & Fields CALM®

foreword by Vanessa Williams

ATRIA BOOKS   new york   london   toronto   sydney

*To our wonderful patients, for teaching us more about dermatology
than all the textbooks, lectures, and medical seminars combined.
And to our loyal customers, whose thoughtful letters, emails,
and phone calls have been our inspiration.*

This work is not intended to be a substitute for professional medical advice, diagnosis, or treatment. Always seek the advice of your physician or other qualified health professional with any questions you may have regarding any specific medical condition. The authors and publisher expressly disclaim responsibility for any adverse effects arising from the use or application of the information contained in this book. The results of the suggested treatments are based on the observations of the authors and on the scientific literature. The information and authors' comments about acne treatment and references to specific products are not approved or endorsed by any of the manufacturers of the products mentioned herein.

The names of the actual companies and products mentioned herein are the trademarks of their respective owners.

ATRIA BOOKS
1230 Avenue of the Americas
New York, NY 10020

Copyright © 2004 by Rodan & Fields Inc.
Foreword copyright © 2004 by Vanessa Williams
Illustrations copyright © 2004 by Tami J. Tolpa

All rights reserved, including the right to reproduce this book or portions thereof in any form whatsoever. For information address Atria Books, 1230 Avenue of the Americas, New York, NY 10020

ISBN: 0-7434-8204-2
      0-7434-8205-0 (Pbk)

First Atria Books hardcover edition March 2004

10   9   8   7   6   5   4   3   2   1

ATRIA BOOKS is a trademark of Simon & Schuster, Inc.

For information regarding special discounts for bulk purchases, please contact Simon & Schuster Special Sales at 1-800-456-6798 or business@simonandschuster.com

Manufactured in the United States of America

acknowledgments

We would like to thank the following people for their generous love, support, and brilliant advice. Without them, this book, our products, and clear skin that millions have enjoyed would never have happened.

Our husbands: Amnon Rodan, a converted "believer" to our vision, who gave up his day job and used his genius, experience, and chutzpa to help get us out of the kitchen and onto the store shelves, all while cracking the whip so we could finish this book. Garry Rayant, whose dental philosophy of prevention inspired our therapeutic skin-care approach.

Our kids: Elana and Daniela Rodan, and Richard and Mark Rayant, for keeping us humble, grounded, and rich in love.

Our middle-of-the-night "rescue machines," aka our in-house advisers: Katie's dad, Judge Harry Pregerson; her brother, Judge Dean Pregerson; Uncle Gil Glazer; and dearest friend Melanie Cook for their strategy, biased support, and clear thinking when the chips were down.

Our friends at Guthy-Renker and Lieberman Productions: Bill Guthy, Greg Renker, Karen Barner, Stacy Tanner, and Lenny Lieberman, for their marketing genius, which allowed our products to become a household name.

Our friends at Estée Lauder: Leonard and William Lauder, Fred Langhammer, Dan Brestle, Diane Ackley, and Pauline Brown, for taking us to the next step.

Our brilliant pen woman, Karen Moline, and our wise editor, Tracy Behar, with whom we closely worked to correct our grammar, improve our punctuation, clarify our text, and help us "omit needless words." We are forever grateful to Judith Curr, our publisher; Karen Mender, deputy publisher; and Anne Harris, publicist at Atria Books.

Our in-house PR team: Tina Thomson, Nicole Benoist, and Marianne Diorio, for helping spread the word about our products and this book.

Our creative team: Mark, George, James, Shaun, and Matt, for their beautiful and artistic input.

Our hairdresser, David Lassman, who knows all but tells none, for giving us his "drag tips for straight chicks," and for allowing us to use his salon for weekly meetings around the shampoo bowl.

And special gratitude to the rest of our families: Connie, Ken, Dan, Blanche and Gene Fields, Bernadine, Sharon Pregerson, and Diane Glazer; our attorney, Steve Cooper; our agents, Barbara Lowenstein and Madeleine Morel; and our favorite "uncles" Ken and Irwin. We are indebted to all of you.

Our mentors: Dr. Gene Farber and Allan Kurtzman. We hope you are looking down upon us from heaven, pleased with the results of your guidance.

contents

foreword

acne is the pits—literally—for nearly fifty million Americans. Whether they're fourteen or forty, acne can leave its sufferers hurt, ashamed, and cringing with embarrassment, rushing from one pimple panic to the next without finding any lasting solutions.

I know, because I was one of those sufferers.

Acne doesn't care who you are or how famous. It's all acne, and it's all miserable. I had my first breakout at age sixteen, then struggled with acne for years. I saw several dermatologists, was given endless prescriptions of antibiotics, took Accutane as well (while being terrified by its potential side effects), and got countless facials, scrubs, treatments—you name it, I endured it. Yet nothing worked.

As the years went by, I found myself continually frustrated and confused by the continuing myths and misinformation about acne perpetuated by the media. Did I wash my face the wrong way? Was I using the wrong products? Did I put on too much or too little? Will that expensive new cream really work? What about that chocolate truffle I ate yesterday? Will my face ever get better?

And then I discovered Proactiv Solution when my teenage daughter started breaking out. Believe me, the last thing I wanted was for her to suffer as I had. Although I was wary of any products sold on infomercials, frankly, we both had nothing to lose. So we started using Proactiv Solution—together—and our acne went away. For the first time in my adult life, I no longer had to worry about my skin. It was an unbelievable feeling.

Since then, I've met and worked with Katie and Kathy, and they've explained to me why their system is so unique—and uniquely simple. They're both doctors so they understand what causes acne. They've spent years working with chemists to better understand what ingredients when combined will work successfully together to stop acne in its tracks. They've learned how to achieve maximum results using minimal ingredients. And, like me, they've both suffered from acne, so they understand its devastating effects on their patients.

It's not easy to admit to the world that I suffered from acne, but I'm so glad I found hope—and can now share that hope. Acne can't yet be cured, but it *can* be treated.

Once you've mastered their approach, you will no longer have to accept your genetic destiny. You no longer have to be scarred and hurt—physically and emotionally. You can unplug your pores, remove the bacteria, shrink the swelling, and zap those zits. This book will show you how easy it is to have the healthy and glowing skin you deserve—for life.

introduction

"Clear skin is the most universally desirable feature in sex appeal."

—Desmond Morris, *The Human Animal*

We survived the three-year Stanford dermatology residency program in 1987 after four years of medical school and four more years of post-graduate medical training. We were loaded with massive amounts of knowledge and were ready for anything: skin diseases, such as mycosis fungoidosis, drug reactions, wounds, moles, and cancers. The last thing we thought we'd see all day, every day, was acne. That's because we'd been taught in our residency that only a scant 3 percent of adults in America have acne.

But something strange was happening. After being flooded with acne patients our first year in private practice, we jokingly decided that *all* 3 percent of those adults happened to live in the Bay Area and had come to our offices.

We soon learned it was no joke. Part of the problem was that our patients did not want to identify with *acne*. Instead, this is what we'd hear:

"I get bumps when I get my period."

"I get blemishes only once in a while, but it's not acne."

"I'm really stressed out. These are my stress bumps."

"My new moisturizer made me break out."

"Oh, that pimple will go away. Can you check this mole?"

"That's just a pimple—I don't have *acne!*"

These patients honestly didn't realize that those pesky period bumps or blemishes were acne. You know why? Because no one told them they were.

And because acne is a four-letter word. As in U–G–L–Y.

Call it a condition, call it occasional, even call it a disease (which is what it is)—whatever the name, it's still acne and it's still ugly. It's one of the most emotionally charged skin diseases known to mankind—it is, in fact, the number one skin disease in the world—and no one wants to live with it.

If you *do* have acne, what does that mean? Will you have it forever? How can you make it go away? Why haven't you grown out of it? That nice lady at the makeup counter in the department store told you if only you stopped eating chocolate and used the right products, you could get rid of it forever. If only she were right!

The vast majority of acne sufferers have no idea what causes their problem. They're devastated and desperate. Many don't go to dermatologists because they're embarrassed and think they'll grow out of it, praying, hoping some miracle will make it just go away. Sometimes they can't afford regular doctor visits. Or they have gone to different doctors in the past and didn't get the results they'd hoped for. Others are too shy to ask someone they know for a recommendation, so they continue to scour drugstore and department store shelves for some new product that might finally work.

We're here to tell you that there is *no* magic potion to permanently cure the complex condition of acne. Acne is caused by too much oil clogging the pores, an overgrowth of bacteria, and the body's response, which is inflammation and swelling. It is triggered by hormones and genetics, promoted by stress, and affected by the environment. No fad diets or even Accutane can permanently cure acne. But you can arm yourself with something more potent: knowledge. Once you learn the basics, you'll realize that acne *is* treatable, controllable, and preventable. You don't have to live with it anymore. We both lived with it, and we were both miserable. That's one of the reasons why we're determined to take the UGLY out of acne and help everyone face the world with clear, glowing skin.

katie's story

I grew up in Woodland Hills, California, a suburb of Los Angeles, and when the pimples first appeared in my teen years, I was longing to get rid of them. I'd sit mortified with embarrassment in the dermatologist's waiting room, praying I wouldn't run into any of my classmates. I'd put the stinky, yellow prescription-strength sulfur cream on my pimples at night. The medicine stained my pillowcase, but I was determined to endure any kind of punishment, bad smell, or whatever to have clear skin. My brother always had perfect skin, but his gorgeous girlfriend didn't, so we'd sit in my bathroom, mixing creams and lotions to make our faces better. We even drank a horrible-tasting brewer's yeast concoction after reading it was the answer for acne! And one time we even tried applying her dad's fungus cream—that's how desperate we were. Trust me, nothing worked. I used to think that if I stayed in school forever, I'd have zits forever. All that stress did not help my genetic destiny, which was acne.

When I was in my first year of medical school, I realized my calling was to be a dermatologist. I had been deeply affected psychologically by my acne and I was determined to fix the problem. Then I met Kathy.

kathy's story

I grew up in Waukegan, Illinois, a suburb of Chicago. I had what I called "one-sies." One big juicy pimple here, another one there. I never went to a dermatologist. Instead I used Oxy and Stri-Dex pads, and they helped me in my teen years. I thought I was lucky.

But then in my twenties my acne came back with a vengeance, my pesky monthly reminder. When I was in dermatology residency, I used to wonder, who'd want to come to me for treatment for their acne if I couldn't cure my own? Then I met Katie.

creating proactiv solution

We like to tease each other that Proactiv Solution was invented because Kathy was looking for a date.

Actually, we'd become friends while studying for our medical board exams at Stanford University, when we were stressed beyond belief. After we passed our exams and set up our practices, we bonded even more. By then Katie had two little girls and single Kathy would hang out at her house in San Francisco, letting Katie fix her up with her eligible bachelor friends.

One day, Katie said, "I had an acne patient today, in her twenties, who brought in the products she was using: a little jar of Lancôme cleanser and a red bottle of Oxy. She's a typical adult who is confused about how to treat her acne and take care of her complexion, so she's applying the strongest spot-kill therapy formulated and marketed to teenagers, and then she's using her pretty Lancôme cleanser because it makes her feel better—*not* like a teenager."

We started talking in earnest about effective over-the-counter treatments for all those thousands of acne patients we were seeing. You see, at Stanford acne was a seldom-seen disease among patients in the clinic. In the hallowed halls of a prestigious academic center, acne was almost disregarded as too trivial, and there was little instruction given regarding its treatment. At one lecture the professor asked us if we knew the difference between acne and rosacea. We still remember that lecture—because we *didn't* know the difference! We were too busy learning about other skin conditions, diseases, and syndromes, most of which we'll never see or treat in our lifetimes. For our teachers, and for the medical establishment, acne was no more important than a small pebble in the Grand Canyon.

As we continued our discussion about acne treatments, we remembered the mantra of the wonderful chairman of our department, Dr. Gene Farber: "Find a hobby in dermatology. Otherwise you'll go out into practice, treating acne, warts, and eczema day after day. You'll be bored, and you'll be miserable with your career." Then he would give us examples of Stanford dermatology graduates who found their hobbies in such diverse fields as psychiatric dermatology, psoriasis day-care centers, or Moh's skin cancer surgery.

So there we were in 1987, the only women in our practices (all of our doctor colleagues were men), and the women patients flocked to us because we understood what they were going through. Plus, we love makeup, skin-care products, and pampering, and we'd never tell any of our patients to stop wearing their makeup or stop going for facials if it made them feel better.

Bingo! There was our hobby: acne. We decided to make our own acne products for all those women who had outgrown the teenage creams, washes, and lotions.

We had no idea what a challenge this would become. We never thought it would turn into Proactiv Solution, the bestselling acne system in America. We never thought we'd end up running a business while continuing to practice medicine. Our initial goal was to create a conceal-and-heal kind of product, something to put on pimples to treat them while covering them up at the same time. A camouflage spot-kill that smelled nice, not like the nasty sulfur we'd used as teens.

As we learned and studied more about acne, we tested our ideas at dinner parties and our prototype products on our friends and relatives. We'd meet with local chemists, who could help us create the formulas then give us outrageous bids we couldn't afford. We felt trapped in a maze, stumbling around, needing advice badly. We'd run in one direction and get hit on the head. Then we'd run in another. But the advantage of having a twosome is that we would keep each other going, never losing our enthusiasm and vision.

For five long years, from 1988 to 1993, we saw even more patients and refined our concept and products, figuring out what medicines worked best. Some of it was just dumb luck . . . but we also had good instincts. We'd been writing prescriptions for creams that were harsh and nasty. The treatments available those years were often worse than the acne itself. At follow-up appointments our patients would bring back their tubes, and we'd see they'd barely used them. Compliance was a major problem. So after careful research, we decided to go with the lowest possible strength of our favorite tried-and-true acne medication—benzoyl peroxide. This way, patients could use it daily over their whole face. We worried for months whether our new concept and products would irritate our patients' skin or be ineffective.

But our products worked, and then we had one of those "Eureka!" moments when we realized we turned all of our training on its head. You see, all the other products before Proactiv Solution were *reactive*. They were spot treatments: "Apply to affected areas only." In other words: Treat *only* the pimple. React *only* to the pimple. It was the one medicine/one zit approach. But this approach didn't make any sense, because by the time that pimple erupts on your skin, as you'll see in chapter 1, it has already been percolating below the surface for weeks. Spot-treatment might dry the pimple up a day or two faster, but it can't get to the root of the complicated problem of acne. By treating the full face daily, continuously, with a combination of medications, acne can be stopped at the source. It can be prevented.

Figuring out this concept and turning it into reality was an incredible journey. We knew only a few basic business principles. We were cautious about every expenditure, from product formulation to package design, because every single step was paid for out of our own checkbooks. In some ways frugality was a blessing, because it made us very resourceful and we carefully thought our ideas through before acting on them. In the end it took us longer, but that was okay, because the end result had to be right.

We were also amazingly lucky to have wonderful friends who wanted to help. One is a woman named Judi Roffman, who worked in market research. She told us we needed to do focus-group testing, and she'd help us recruit people. So we packaged our formulas into trial sizes and recruited adult women who'd already seen a dermatologist, already tried medicines, and had to own up to the fact that they had acne. At that point we were focused on treating adult acne, because we knew this was a vast, misunderstood group of patients that no single product was addressing.

We found women for this focus group, had them use our products for a month, then brought them into a conference room where we sat behind a one-way window so we could watch and hear them. We devoured M&Ms out of sheer nervousness while listening to the women discuss the pluses and minuses of our products.

This group was very useful for two reasons. First, although all of these women had been recruited because they had visible acne, in the group situation, *not one* would openly admit it. Because acne is U–G–L–Y. They had blemishes, they had monthly breakouts, but they most definitely did not have "acne."

But they did. From this we learned that identification with acne was taboo!

The second useful finding was that although they liked how well the products worked, they didn't like how they smelled. We'd made the mistake of making them fragrance-free. The products didn't feel as if they were designed for grown-ups, and our testers felt like teenagers again. In our effort to be dermatologically correct, we'd gone too far. We needed to go right back to our original concept of the luxuriousness of Lancôme plus the medicating power of Oxy.

Rod Mora, a businessman friend of Katie's, agreed. "Expand the concept," he urged us. "Beauty is the big segment. We all want beauty creams, and you're selling zit cream. Can you get into the beauty category?" And we said, "Well, no, we're treating acne." And he said, "Wait, let's turn it. Flip the tortilla and look at it from the underside."

In other words, instead of women needing one product for medicating and another product for skin care (like moisturizer or cleanser), we could make dual-function products. And so, we made medicated skin care. We worked with brilliant chemists who created formulas with special delivery vehicles that didn't burn or irritate skin and that allowed the medicine to penetrate into the pores to remove the acne-causing bacteria. We also proved the products' efficacy on our willing friends and patients who tested them. These products were low strength, safe to use every day, and a pleasure to apply. They smelled and felt nice, and, oh, by the way, they also stopped that pesky acne problem no one admitted they had.

Next we had to choose a name, because we needed something slightly more sophisticated than "Zits-Away." Something with "Derma" in it, we thought. Or something that sounded French. We needed help, so we became the first clients of Courtney Reeser, a creative genius who was a former director of a huge ad agency. After spending many hours with us to understand our unique product concept, he said, "I've got the name for you. It's so perfect. It's proactive."

We said, *"Huh?"* We needed convincing. It wasn't Dermage or Dermanique or Ondine. We wanted beauty. We wanted cobalt-blue jars. We wanted a beautiful French name.

"Be *proactive*. It's an enduring word," he insisted. "Treat preventively. Treat before the breakout happens. Treat the whole face. Take control."

He was right, and Ondine flew out the window.

The more we thought about it, the more we realized what a perfect word "proactive" is. Because acne is a chronic condition, it makes people feel helpless. Once you take a stance and become proactive, you're no longer its victim. You're in control now; acne's not controlling you. When you prevent the process of acne, you never have to be reactive to it again.

marketing proactiv solution

We then had to become proactive ourselves and figure out a way to sell Proactiv Solution. We couldn't just walk into Walgreen's and say, "Here you go. Our product belongs on your shelf." We'd spent years studying the market and realized that the selling of beauty products was a multibillion-dollar industry. Acne products were a tiny $250 million market in comparison. No one thought teenagers would spend serious money on skin care. (Boy, that's sure changed!) Plus everybody was trained to spot-treat only, so the public would have to be entirely reeducated about our novel concept of treating the whole face with different medications every day, akin to brushing their teeth. It seemed like an overwhelming proposition. We were already up to our eyeballs in debt. So after a series of meetings, we worked our way up to the top management of Neutrogena in 1993, hoping they'd want to license our formulas.

They listened carefully, then Allan Kurtzman, the CEO, told us to make an infomercial.

We just about fell off our chairs. We thought infomercials were offbeat or second-class and we were being insulted. But then he explained that if his company put another Neutrogena product on the drugstore shelves, how would customers know what it was? What would entice them to choose ours from the myriad other creams and lotions? How would consumers be taught to use our new products as a system? There was so much confusion and competition already. . . .

And he was right. We didn't believe it at the time, though, especially when Lloyd Coteson, the president of Neutrogena, said, "Are you ready to dance with the devil? You may never be able to walk down the dermatology corridors again because you're about to cross the line from academia and enter the commercial world."

Back then, you see, few dermatologists sold any products. We were going to be perceived as pariahs by our peers. We were going to be selling out. We were *scared*.

But then we met with the folks at Guthy-Renker Corporation, creators of the best infomercials in the world—which contrary to our uninformed bias at the time *aren't* second-class—and they helped convince us that infomercials were the way to go. The infomercial was a thirty-minute opportunity to teach and explain acne, debunk myths, and show before-and-after results on real people who used Proactiv Solution. Frankly, because some infomercials had a bad reputation, many people had low expectations for how Proactiv Solution was going to work. Even though we validated Proactiv Solution's results on 300 people before rolling out the infomercial in October 1995, we were still worried. We had no idea how well our product would perform on a larger population. Would people like Proactiv Solution? Was our full-face method right? Would this be one huge mistake for us?

But it was that money-back guarantee that made people take the leap of faith to buy Proactiv Solution. Plus we insisted on immediate delivery—not the standard four- to six-week wait. People with acne were suffering today; they didn't want to wait six long weeks before receiving their product. Proactiv Solution was a need, not a want. It wasn't an asparagus steamer or an ab-buster. *It was something that was going to change their lives.*

Early on some customers told us that in a moment of weakness they bought Proactiv Solution then left it unopened for weeks. They felt embarrassed at buying something through an infomercial. Eventually desperation drove them to try it, and lo and behold, it worked! Not only did it work but it exceeded the promises they'd heard in the infomercial. Proactiv Solution took care of the zits they had today *and* prevented the next cycle of breakouts, so a few weeks later, when women were due for those six monthly zits on their chins, they got only one. The month after that, they had none. They didn't need makeup anymore. Their pores were smaller. Their skin was glowing. Friends were commenting—and they were reordering. Because acne is visible, people would literally watch as fellow students or coworkers became positively transformed, physically and emotionally. Suddenly, bottles of Proactiv Solution began showing up in dormitory bathrooms, health club lockers, and suitcases opened in airport security lines. Word of mouth was contagious. Sales grew rapidly.

We soon realized that infomercials were a terrific way to sell acne products after all. For women, it's like buying their first tampon, which usually left them embarrassed, hoping that nobody was looking in their basket. The same mortification happens to acne sufferers. No one wants to be seen shopping in the drugstore aisle buying pimple creams, especially adult women who hide their condition behind layers of makeup. Buying and reordering from an 800 number gave privacy and anonymity to all of our customers without the humiliation of the whole world knowing about their acne problem.

And, more important, the real-people testimonials in the infomercials helped educate millions of viewers that acne is a chronic and complicated condition that isn't their fault. Rich or poor, a supermodel like Stephanie Seymour or a mail carrier, the infomercials featured real people with whom our viewers could identify. These testimonials took the stigma away and helped viewers realize they were not alone. We understood the pain, shame, and embarrassment. We made it okay to talk about acne. The information was empowering.

In January 1999, an article in *Allure* magazine entitled "Phenomenon" was published. It was a tell-all story, proclaiming that an infomercial product, Proactiv Solution, really worked. In the article, Dr. Patricia Wexler, one of

America's leading dermatologists, substantiated this with her own story. When we first met Pat at a dermatology conference, she'd told us that she'd treated her daughter with Retin-A, with Accutane, with oral antibiotics, and with every benzoyl peroxide product in the world. Nothing worked, and she worried that people would see her daughter's acne and wonder, "Your mom is this famous dermatologist, and look how bad your skin is! She can't even fix you." She was ecstatically relieved when Proactiv Solution cleared her daughter's skin. Dr. Wexler has been recommending it to her acne patients ever since.

be proactive

When people ask us to describe exactly what we do, the answer is simple: We're not about making good skin better. We're about making problem skin healthy and beautiful.

Twelve years ago, when we were researching the acne market, somebody said to us, "There's no money in acne. Forget about it. Make a wrinkle cream, because you could make millions."

We said, "We don't want to make a wrinkle cream. You know why? Because they don't work. Because there's always going to be a wrinkle cream of the month and we want to be here for the next hundred years. The only way to last in the marketplace is to deliver an honest product that truly does what it says it's going to do."

We're not a trend. We're not a fad. We're not about to chase after the latest hype. Benzoyl peroxide, for example, is the key ingredient in our acne products because it's effective. There's never been any bacterial resistance to it. It's been around for fifty years, and it's safe. There's a lot to be said for the tried and true, especially when we incorporated it into a completely different kind of formulation than all those that preceded Proactiv.

By combining skin care with medicine, we brought acne out of the closet. No medical student is taught anymore that only 3 percent of adults have acne.

We see ourselves as driven doctors on a mission to improve skin. We are absolutely *passionate* about treating acne. While it is nice to make wrinkles 27 percent less noticeable, we are more interested in restoring your self-esteem to 100 percent. We're trained to prevent and heal disease. And whatever you call it, acne *is* a disease.

We see the practice of dermatology as the practice of the art of medicine. Sometimes when we were mixing and testing our potions we laughed that we were more like witch doctors than medical doctors. We also look at dermatology as the only specialty in medicine that treats the outside as well as the inside. We're determined to lend an empathetic ear to our patients and customers, and do our best to clear their skin in order to enhance self-esteem and improve quality of life. We know that you can have one pimple and feel as bad as someone with a face full of pimples. If it hurts, it hurts. It's not the quantity of pimples that matters to us, it's the *quality* of your skin and its impact on your life.

This book provides sound, practical advice based on science, not on myth. In it, we will teach you everything we know about acne so you can make informed decisions about how to take care of your own skin. At the same time, we hope that you'll see the lessons we learned in trying to get Proactiv Solution launched—how we believed in what we'd created and how we stayed focused in our determination to help people—as wonderful life lessons, too.

It's time to be proactive. This one word links us and our philosophy to the products we're so proud of. It's a good metaphor for life, too. We hope you'll use this book as a comprehensive resource. With it, you'll be able to treat your skin differently from the way you've treated it in the past. You're already halfway there because you're committing to being proactive about acne.

Learning to take care of your skin is not difficult or expensive. While the process of acne is complex, treating, controlling, and preventing it can be simple. Having clear skin is priceless, so take control. Be proactive. You *can* change the face of acne—and you *can* change your life.

WWW.UNBLEMISHED.COM

Information and education about acne are constantly evolving. In order to keep you up to date on new acne treatments and procedures, visit our site at www.unblemished.com. It includes photographs and diagrams not found in this book.

chapter one
skin under siege

"My little nephew, who's only two, turned to me and said, 'Auntie, can I connect the dots on your face?' He didn't know what he was saying, but I was totally humiliated. I used to wake up crying because I'd feel a new lump on my face every morning."

—Amanda, age thirty-one

No matter what your skin color or type, whether you're eight, eighteen, thirty-eight, or sixty-eight, you can get acne. You may have one pimple or a hundred, but the process is the same. *Acne vulgaris* is the most common and often the most debilitating skin disease that exists. Over 90 percent of all people on earth suffer from it at one point or another. So even if you didn't get it as a teenager, chances are extremely high that you'll experience it later in life. It's a rare human indeed who manages to get through life without a single zit!

Before we explore acne in detail, let's learn a little bit about the organ it affects: the skin.

all about skin

Even when it is covered with acne, your skin is still a marvelous organ. It reflects who you are and how you feel, and it keeps you safe. It has an almost magical ability to repair itself, and we certainly almost always take it for granted. (Except, of course, when plagued by acne.) Constantly replenishing itself, the skin covers a whopping twenty square feet and constitutes 15 percent of our total body weight. In the three layers of one square inch of skin you'll find:

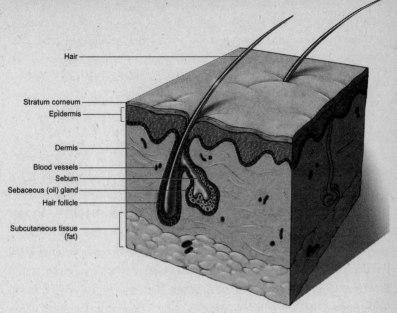

Hair

Stratum corneum
Epidermis

Dermis

Blood vessels
Sebum
Sebaceous (oil) gland
Hair follicle

Subcutaneous tissue
(fat)

Normal skin

- 19 yards of blood vessels
- 65 hairs
- 78 yards of nerves
- 100 sebaceous glands
- 650 sweat glands
- 1,300 nerve endings
- 20,000 sensory cells
- 129,040 pores
- 9,500,000 cells

Epidermis—Top Layer

The first living layer of the skin is the epidermis. This microscopically thin layer
is seven to ten cells thick and in a young adult completely renews itself every
twenty-eight days. Nearly 95 percent of the epidermis is composed of new cells
called keratinocytes. The remaining 5 percent is made up of the cells that produce melanin, the substance that gives skin its color, and the all-important
Langerhan cells, which work with the immune system to help fight infections.

As keratinocyte cells age, they flatten out and eventually lose their nucleus, becoming horn cells. These horn cells create the stratum corneum, the outermost layer of skin. Even though the stratum corneum consists of dead, overlapping horn cells, like shingles on a roof, it serves a vital function as our first line of immunological defense between the outside world and our bodies.

The renewal rate of the epidermis diminishes with age. As a result, the stratum corneum becomes thicker and the pores pack up with dead skin cells, which makes them look larger.

Dermis—Middle Layer

Most of the skin's volume is found here. The dermis is composed of collagen and elastin fibers; nerve endings that sense temperature and pressure; blood vessels supplying nutrients to keep everything replenished and renewed; sweat glands, which function to cool you down, and erector pili muscles, which contract, causing you to shiver and making your hairs "stand up" (these functions keep you at a stable 98.6 degrees Fahrenheit); hair follicles; and those pesky oil glands, which produce the sebum that keeps skin soft, pliable, and waterproof. However pesky they are, you can't live without those oil glands (although when your acne is bad, you certainly wish you could!).

Subcutaneous—Bottom Layer

Here lie lots of fat cells. These fat cells are good fat cells. Without them, you'd lack insulation and protection for your fragile organs. Also rooted in these fat cells are most of your hair follicles. The hair follicle and the attached sebaceous, or oil, gland share the space known as the pilosebaceous gland (*pilo* means hair and *sebaceous* refers to the sebaceous, or oil, gland). The pore is the passageway from the base of the hair follicle to the surface of the skin. Sebum, an oily substance composed of free fatty acids, cholesterol, triglycerides, and wax, is released from the sebaceous, or oil, gland into the pore and travels to the skin's surface to keep it pliable and protected. Without sebum, your skin would look as dry as dust.

what kind of skin do you have?

From a dermatologist's viewpoint, contrary to all those surveys published in women's magazines, just about everybody has combination skin. Human bodies are constructed with the greatest density of oil glands in the T-zone—the nose, cheeks, chin, and forehead—so that even if you have dry spots, you will most likely also have oily spots.

The texture, pore size, and oiliness/dryness of your skin is in large part determined by your genes and regulated by your hormones. There's nothing you can do about your body's natural inclination to be dry or oily. You can, however, do something about how the environment in which you live affects your skin. For example, it's easy enough to humidify (or dehumidify) the air inside your home.

Equally important is the fact that your skin changes as your body ages. You can have oily skin as a teenager and dry skin as an adult. Be aware that as these changes take place, your skin care needs change, too. We often see women still using the same products after age thirty, which may not be the optimal treatment plan for their skin.

What if your skin is mostly dry?

You can still have dry skin even when it's covered with acne. If you look at the surface layer of the dead cells in the epidermis (the stratum corneum), they're superhydrated in high-humidity environments and desiccated in dry ones. Drinking gallons of water won't necessarily plump up your skin in Arizona—you'll just be spending much more time in the bathroom. And as you age, circulation naturally slows down, hormones dwindle, oil production diminishes, and the surface dead cell layer thickens and fissures, allowing water loss from the skin. The result is that your skin won't be as moist as it was when you were younger. Some medications also dry out skin, most notably Accutane.

Using humectant agents (moisturizers) can help relieve dry skin. So can humidifiers. Air conditioners and forced-air heating systems tend to zap the moisture out of the air, so be judicious with their use.

What if your skin is mostly oily?

"My skin's too oily—make it stop!" We hear that all the time from our patients. Unfortunately, there's no little faucet we can turn off or on to decrease or increase oil flow. Oil production constantly changes. For instance, one month your skin might be oily the week before your period; the next month it might not. And, you may have oily skin and terrible acne or oily skin and no acne. Oily skin is not a life sentence for acne or even necessarily a symptom of acne.

Living in a hot, humid climate will stimulate oil gland production. Exercise, stress, and androgenic (masculinizing) hormones, such as testosterone or DHEA-S, will also increase oil flow.

Oily skin generally needs no moisturizers except on the eyelids. Oil absorbers; loose, oil-free powders; and medicated, clay-based masks will help absorb excess oil. However, frequent facial washing (in excess of two to three times a day) may eventually result in *increased* oil production, because when the surface of the skin is excessively stripped of lubrication, the oil glands' response to perceived dryness is to produce additional oil.

Why Is Dryness/Oiliness So Important?

Knowing that the layer of dead cells (the stratum corneum) in the epidermis is crucial to healthy skin, we became interested in trying to stabilize, protect, and repair the barrier function it provides. Any assault to this top layer increases the skin's susceptibility to infection and environmental irritants. This can produce a range of skin conditions, from impetigo to herpes eczema to contact allergic dermatitis.

One enduring myth about acne is that the best form of treatment is to strip all the oil off your skin. Drying the skin's surface with ingredients like rubbing alcohol leaves the skin parched and irritated, with greater susceptibility to infection while failing to treat the acne process. Perhaps you've even tried to clean your skin with harsh scrub soaps that contain apricot or walnut pits, which can tear your defenseless cells. You look raw and red. Your skin peels. It itches. It doesn't heal properly, and your acne doesn't go away. As a result, your acne may take longer to heal and leave scars behind.

In chapter 5, you'll see how an acne treatment program can be gentle yet effective, maintaining a healthy balance of dryness and oiliness in the epidermis.

Do You Really Have Sensitive Skin?

Many of our patients tell us that they have sensitive skin. In truth, the vast majority of people do *not* have sensitive skin even though they *think* they do.

The clinical definition of sensitive skin is skin that has a noticeable reaction with product application. It turns red, itches, tingles, or burns. Or all four.

There are two causes of sensitive skin: environmental and genetic. Environmental factors causing sensitive skin are usually product-derived. Most people tend to use more than one product on their face, and in each of the products there are often ten to twenty different ingredients. The more products you layer on, the more ingredients you are exposed to, and the more likely you are to create a sensitive skin response. When you strip your skin of its barrier function, irritated skin often follows.

Then there is the genetic factor. Twenty percent of babies develop eczema, also called atopic dermatitis, within the first six months of life. Atopic dermatitis is often accompanied by allergies, asthma, and hay fever. By the time children are twelve, most outgrow atopic dermatitis. However, because the skin of people with atopic dermatitis may remain somewhat immunologically compromised, the risk of developing skin sensitivity is greater. Patients with a history of atopic dermatitis in childhood are especially prone to eyelid dermatitis, hand eczema, and keratosis pilaris (tiny red bumps on the back of arms) as teenagers or adults. These patients may also be intolerant of some topical acne preparations.

Many people with rosacea, another genetic condition, have sensitive, reactive skin. For more information on skin sensitivity, see chapter 13.

TEST YOURSELF FOR SENSITIVITY

It's easy to do what we call a use test. Simply take your new product and dab a little bit on the side of your neck, under your ear, twice a day for several days. (Obviously, if you're testing a cleanser, be sure to rinse it off with lukewarm water.) This part of your neck tends to be more sensitive, so if you don't have a reaction within a day or two, you're probably fine.

Don't forget to start slowly with any medicated products. Many people want to literally scrub acne off their faces. It's better not to jump in and start blasting away with new medicine. More is *not* better. With a new product, start out once a day or once every other day at first. Continue this way for one to two weeks. Increase usage to twice daily once you find you can tolerate it.

what is acne?

Acne is *complicated*. Many factors are involved in its creation. It is, however, most influenced by genetics and hormones. These hormones, known as androgens, stimulate a four-step process in the skin.

Step 1   Abnormal keratinization in the pore leading to a plug (clogged pores)

Step 2   Overproduction of oil (sebum)

Step 3   Overgrowth of *p. acnes* bacteria

Step 4   Inflammation (swelling) as a reaction to the bacteria and its by-products

The bump that appears on your face is actually the final step in a process that began two weeks before. Even though that painful bump on your face looks bad and feels worse, the *real* damage is happening underneath the skin. The secret to controlling acne is to get down deep in the pore—to stop the acne process before bumps are visible on the skin's surface.

Step 1: Clogged Pores

Normally, skin cells are in a continuous, gradual state of renewal. As the old cells die, they mix with your skin's natural oil and are sloughed off, making room for fresh, new skin every thirty days.

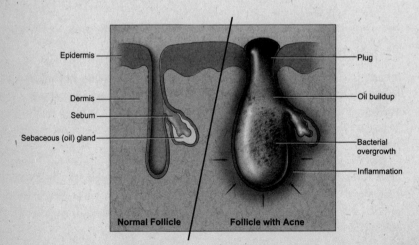

Normal follicle versus follicle with acne

But sloughing doesn't always happen as it should. Sometimes the dead skin cells don't shed evenly or cell turnover slows down (as it does when we age, for example). When this happens, skin cells become "sticky." These sticky cells combined with oil clog your pores. A plug called a *comedo* (*comedones* is the plural) is formed inside the hair follicle. It's like a cork in a bottle. The cork-like plug traps oil and bacteria in the follicle.

Step 2: Overproduction of Oil (sebum)

Hormones, known as androgens, stimulate oil production in the sebaceous glands, which are attached to your hair follicles. Normally, the oil (sebum) flows freely to the surface of your skin. But if your hormones tell your sebaceous glands to get moving, they'll churn out sticky oil, which results in potentially clogged pores and a wonderful environment for bacteria to grow.

Step 3: Bacterial Attack

Once your pores are clogged, an anaerobic bacteria naturally growing on your skin called *Propionibacterium acnes* (*p. acnes* for short) proliferates and starts feeding on the trapped oil. It likes the oxygen-free atmosphere deep in the pore. The overgrowth of *p. acnes* digests the entrapped sebum, breaking down the oil molecules into smaller particles. When a tiny bit of these broken-down oil molecules leaks outside the follicle, your body is going to respond.

Step 4: Inflammation

The body's response to the bacterial invaders and the oil by-products is a swarming army of red and white blood cells sent to contain the infection, attempting to wall off the follicle. The end result? Intense swelling and inflammation experienced as pimples, bumps, pain, and suffering. Otherwise known as acne.

Different Kinds of Comedones

Though all acne starts the same way, the lesions may look different on your skin.

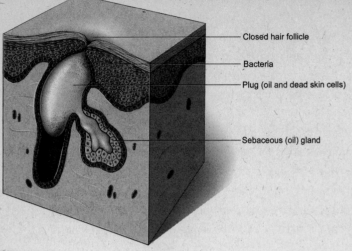

Whitehead

Whiteheads

If the plug stays below the surface of the skin, it's called a closed comedo, or a whitehead. The white debris is composed of trapped sebum and dead white blood cells.

Blackheads

If the plug enlarges and widens the pore, it's called an open comedo, or a blackhead. Blackheads are not caused by trapped dirt, even though that's what they look like, and you can't wash them away. The black spots are from a buildup of melanin, the dark pigment in your skin, and oxidized oil.

Different Kinds of Pimples

(For more photographic examples, go to www.unblemished.com.) Acne can be noninflammatory or inflammatory. Noninflammatory acne consists of blackheads and whiteheads. Inflammatory acne occurs from an immune response to the bacteria and plug. The degree of inflammation determines the different kinds of pimples, the severity of acne, and ultimately the potential to scar.

The different kinds of pimples are:

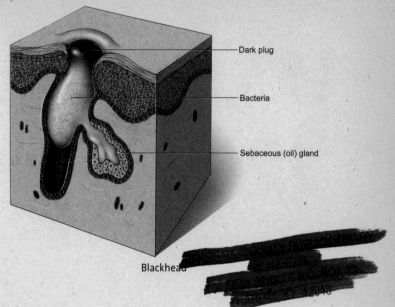

Dark plug

Bacteria

Sebaceous (oil) gland

Blackhead

Papules

Papules are small, pink, domed bumps. They are tender to the touch.

Pustules

Pustules are small, round, pus-filled lesions. They are swollen and appear red at the base, with a yellowish or whitish center.

Nodules and Cysts

Nodules and cysts are large, deep, and painful bumps filled initially with blood, then with pus. Nodules can linger under the skin's surface for weeks or even months and hurt so badly you aren't even tempted to squeeze them. Persistent nodules can harden into deep cysts. Both nodules and cysts may leave deep scars.

Different Grades of Acne

(For more photographic examples, go to www.unblemished.com.) Most people think of acne as juicy, red, nasty bumps. Yet blackheads, whiteheads, papules, pustules, nodules, and cysts are all part of the acne spectrum. Dermatologists have a grading system that helps determine the correct course of

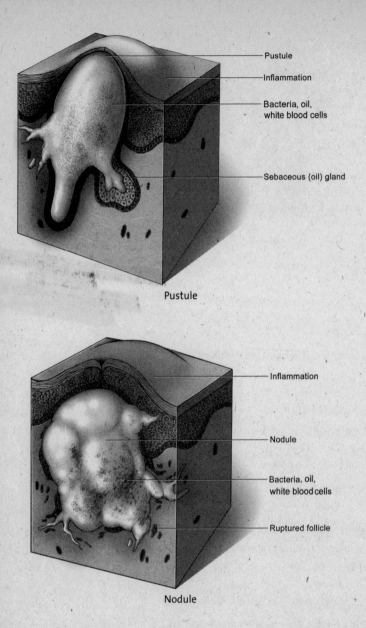

Pustule

Nodule

action. The number one priority of a dermatologist is to prevent permanent scarring, so moderate-to-severe category is managed most aggressively.

A dermatologist's second priority is to clear your acne so you look and feel

DOES ACNE HAPPEN ONLY ON THE FACE?

Unfortunately, no, acne does not happen only on the face. Acne is a disease of the pilosebaceous gland. The greatest density of pilosebaceous glands is found on the face, the ears, neck, chest, back, scalp, and shoulders. There are far fewer pilosebaceous glands in the lower arms and legs, and there are none on your palms or the soles of your feet, so you're guaranteed never to get acne there.

Patients with severe acne can develop nodules of fantastic size and in the most unusual locations, such as inside the ear canal. These can be terribly painful. There is also a condition called *Acne Conglobata*, which is a rare and serious form of inflammatory acne that develops primarily on the face, back, and chest. In addition to pustules and nodules, there may be severe bacterial infection and draining sinus tracts under the skin, which always lead to scarring. If you have symptoms of *Acne Conglobata*, you should contact a dermatologist immediately.

For more information about acne on the body, see chapter 14.

better about yourself. In mild cases, permanent scars are not a worry, so there is more leeway in trying different topical products.

Due to fluctuations in hormones and other factors, the grading of your acne can change as you age—over months, years, or even your lifetime. For example, a thirteen-year-old boy might have mild acne. If left untreated, by the time he's sixteen, his acne may become severe. Our grading system gives an instant checklist for appropriate treatment.

what causes acne?

Acne is not your fault. Acne is not caused by the food you eat or how often you wash your face. It's caused by a *complex combination* of factors on two sides of the equation.

The first side is genetic, and it is totally beyond your control. Those with a family history of moderate-to-severe acne are at greatest risk, and the onset is often in the early teen years. You can no more change your genetic destiny than you can permanently change the color of your eyes. The other side of the equation is what we call cofactors or promoters, which can exacerbate preexisting acne. We will explore both the genetic factors and cofactors that cause acne.

THE RODAN AND FIELDS GRADING SYSTEM

Mild Acne

Comedones*	Papules	Pustules	Nodules/ Cysts	Scar	No. of Areas Involved
several–many	very few	very few	none	no	1 location only

Mild-to-Moderate Acne

Comedones*	Papules	Pustules	Nodules/ Cysts	Scar	No. of Areas Involved
several– numerous	few–several	few–several	occasional	no	1 to 3

Moderate-to-Severe Acne

Comedones*	Papules	Pustules	Nodules/ Cysts	Scar	No. of Areas Involved
scattered	numerous	numerous	many	often	1 to 3

* whiteheads and blackheads

Genetic Factors

Genetics

Genetic factors include: how easily the *p. acnes* bacteria proliferate on your skin; how much your body is inclined to produce a swelling response to the bacteria; how much oil your body produces; how easily your pores get plugged; and how quickly your skin cells turn over. These contributing factors to acne are all determined by your genetic makeup. In addition, if both parents had significant acne, your risk for developing acne is very high.

Hormones—Female

How a woman's hormones are regulated changes throughout her lifetime. Fluctuations in estrogen levels (and also androgen levels) can cause acne. As a result, many women experience acne monthly, in sync with their menstrual cycles. Also, the flood of hormones released by the body during and after pregnancy can cause acne. When estrogen levels become more erratic during perimenopause and menopause, acne can appear once again.

WHY IS MY ACNE SO BAD WHEN MY SISTER DOESN'T HAVE ANY?

I am eighteen and an identical twin. My sister and I did everything alike—food, exercise, school—but my sister's skin was clear and gorgeous while I had really bad acne, which made it even more heartbreaking for me. I went to dermatologists, and what they gave me left my skin peeling and red. My father was really upset seeing what one daughter was going through. I was crying all the time, upset all the time with my terrible skin, when my sister's was fine. People in school would compare us: "Who's the pretty twin? Who's not?" And I obviously knew which one I was.

—*Susannah, age eighteen*

Susannah's heartbreak is a perfect example of genetic unpredictability, even in identical twins. One person in a family may get tiny, little pimples that last only a day while another gets five-pounders that last a month and scar to boot.

Everybody has an intrinsic inflammatory response. This is caused by your immune response to any event, such as an insect bite or a drug new to your system. For example, with an insect bite one person may have a small, itchy bump while in another the bite may cause significant swelling. With acne, the immune response to the bacteria differs from person to person. One person may have only blackheads while another responds to the bacteria with explosive red and tender nodules. This inflammatory response cannot be controlled by diet. While genetically programmed, it is hormonally and environmentally influenced. For example, African Americans have a vigorous response to the *p. acnes* bacteria, but because of their dark skin, the red, inflammatory response is difficult to see. Unfortunately, after the pimple has healed, a highly visible brown spot (postinflammatory hyperpigmentation) often remains on the skin, a leftover reaction to the inflammation. Often the brown spot is worse than the acne itself. (We'll discuss this further in the section on postinflammatory hyperpigmentation on page 34.)

Having a unique genetic predisposition to acne can be comforting, even if your acne is raging out of control, because it firmly asserts that your acne is not your fault, any more than your height or crooked teeth are your fault. An orthodontist can fix your teeth. We can help suppress your genetic predisposition to acne.

Hormones—Male

During puberty, everyone begins to produce hormones called androgens. Androgens cause the sebaceous glands to enlarge, which is a natural part of the body's development. The rate at which you produce sebum, or oil, within the sebaceous glands is affected by your hormone balance, which is often in flux, especially in women. When androgens stimulate sebaceous glands, too much sticky oil and too little shedding of the dead skin cells occur, causing that plug. *Wham!*—here comes the acne. This explains why 90 to 95 percent of teens have some form of acne.

Cofactors/Promoters of Acne (in descending order of importance)

stress
environment
medications
mechanical irritation
cosmetics and occlusive sunscreens
diet

Stress

You need only look at the faces of college students cramming for exams to see how stress can affect acne. Stress hormones, specifically cortisol, are released by the body and trigger increased oil production by the sebaceous glands. Stress also delays wound healing, so the breakouts last longer.

Environment

Outside factors, such as pollution, exposure to oil or grease in the workplace, dry air in your house, and high humidity outdoors, have an effect on your skin and can contribute to acne. Sun exposure and sunburn can cause acne to flare up. Even flying, by disrupting the body's circadian rhythm (naturally occurring sleep cycles), can stimulate an acne outbreak, to say nothing of what the dry air on airplanes does to your skin.

Medications

Over-the-counter as well as prescription medications may have side effects that can affect the body's chemistry and hormones, leading to an outbreak of acne. (See table, Prescription Drugs That Can Cause Acne, page 28.)

Mechanical Irritation

Excessive rubbing or irritation to the skin, such as holding the telephone too close to your chin or sweating in a football or bicycle helmet, leads to acne. Anything that chronically rubs on a certain part of your body—a baseball hat worn backward with the strap pressing on your forehead, athletic shoulder pads, or even the strap of a purse across your shoulder—can promote acne.

Cosmetics and Occlusive Sunscreens

Some cosmetics, including moisturizers and makeup, or other products, such as occlusive (thick, blocking) sunscreens, can irritate your skin and cause acne because of their comedogenic, or pore-clogging, ingredients. Beauty treatments, such as waxing, often irritate the skin and may contribute to acne.

Diet

We don't believe that sugar, fat, or caffeine directly cause acne. Nor do we believe that eating greasy french fries or potato chips causes oily skin and breakouts. Current research shows that sugars contribute to internal inflammation throughout the body. Yet while acne is a disease of inflammation around hair follicles, it occurs even if you don't consume sugars and starches.

Remember, a pimple is weeks in the making, therefore the pimple you see today cannot be a direct result of the chocolate sundae you ate yesterday. That said, some people may be hypersensitive to certain foods. For example, foods containing excessive amounts of iodides, such as salt, seafood, and seaweed, are linked to acne. If you know that a specific food tends to worsen your acne, it's best to avoid it. To help you test whether your acne is food-related, keep a food diary to see if flares of acne correspond to dietary changes in the previous weeks.

PRESCRIPTION DRUGS THAT CAN CAUSE ACNE

Antiepileptic Drugs

hydantoin derivatives	phenobarbitol	trimethadione

Halogens

bromides	chlorides	halothane	iodides

Hormones

androgenic hormones, if given to women	corticosteroids		
corticotrophin (ACTH)	Depoprovera	DHEA	oral contraceptives

Others

Antabuse	dantrolene	lithium salts	maprotiline
psoralens	quinine	rifampin	thiouracil and thiourea

Tuberculostatic Drugs

ethambutol	ethionamide	isoniazid

acne myths and misinformation

Now that you know what really causes acne, let's put to rest all the myths and misinformation about it.

Acne Is Your Fault

False. Acne is not and never will be your fault. Acne is caused by a combination of factors. These include genetics, hormones, bacteria, overabundance of oil, the plugging of skin pores, your unique immune response to the *p. acnes* bacteria, stress, environmental factors, medications, excessive rubbing or irritation, cosmetics, and even traveling. It is *not* caused by how you wash your face (or with what) or by any of the foods you eat. Some people never break out; some never stop.

Acne Can Be Cured

False. There is not yet a cure for acne. It's a complicated condition. Even the prescription drug Accutane, the strongest oral medication for acne, does not provide a permanent cure. But you can help prevent and control mild to moderate acne blemishes once you start following our program.

If You Leave Your Acne Alone, You'll Outgrow It

False. Don't wait. It's so important to start treating breakouts early. Untreated, acne can get worse. For example, comedones (blackheads and whiteheads) can evolve into pustules and pimples. If it does get worse, it can leave scars—physically on your face and emotionally in your heart for a lifetime.

Acne Is Just a Little Problem. Don't Overreact. Stop Worrying About It

False. Almost everyone who has acne is embarrassed by it—if not mortified and depressed. Acne not only lowers self-esteem, it often affects social behavior. It's hard to have a social life if you don't want to leave the house. Acne can even affect job performance, especially if you feel inhibited about being seen and judged by your peers.

Spot Treatments Will Cure Acne

False. Spot treatments may help dry up a newly visible pimple, but that pimple started forming weeks before you were aware of its existence. Instead of spot treatments, it's wise to preventively treat all acne-prone skin on a daily basis so breakouts can't get started in the first place. Think of treating acne as you think of brushing your teeth: Do it every day and prevent a problem.

Acne Is Caused by Eating Greasy Foods, Chocolate, or Caffeine

False. Medical studies have found that diet—including chocolate, pizza, potato chips, and french fries—rarely affects acne.

However, if certain foods consistently make you break out with acne, it's common sense to try to avoid them. For example, for some who are supersensitive, eating foods with a high iodine content, such as shellfish, dried fish, and seaweed, may cause flare-ups, which may explain why the Japanese, who usually have a terrific, balanced, low-fat diet, still get acne. Some other studies theorize that the hormones in chicken, beef, and dairy products may precipitate early adolescent acne, but the jury's still out on that subject. If you're concerned, substitute other sources of protein and calcium for these products or try hormone-free, organic versions of them.

Sugar Causes Acne

False. An article entitled "Acne Vulgaris: A Disease of Western Civilization" was published in the *Archives of Dermatology* in December 2002. The writers concluded that there's an astonishing difference between Western and non-Western societies in terms of how much acne people get—a difference that can't be due just to what's in the gene pool. They blamed acne on excess consumption of sugar in Western countries. However, critics of this study noted that the authors looked only at a small, genetically distinct tribe of natives in Papua, New Guinea, to represent non-Western societies. This tribe has a much later onset of puberty than other societies around the world, which means their hormones associated with acne kick in later in life. It is therefore not a representative group.

Finding out what causes acne onset will be a tremendous help in acne treatment all over the globe. But to blame acne on sugar alone disregards scientific research and clinical observation. It's been our experience that eliminating all sugar or fat in a diet doesn't eliminate acne. We do advocate a healthy diet filled with complex carbohydrates, such as vegetables, fruit, whole grains, and low-fat protein. We believe refined sugars and excessive fat should be kept to a minimum to maintain a healthy body weight. Unfortunately, however, making changes in your diet alone will not stop acne. So don't beat yourself up because you just had a chocolate brownie; it is not going to create pimples weeks down the road.

Drinking Tons of Water Will Flush the Acne Away

False. Drinking six to eight glasses of water each day is healthy for your body. But not even the priciest designer-bottle spring water can flush away acne. There's simply no proof that water can clean the skin from the inside out. Furthermore, while dehydration may temporarily make your skin look lifeless, it won't lead to breakouts.

Sun Exposure Will Heal Your Acne

False. Small amounts of sun exposure may appear to be helping your acne at first; the blue band of visible light helps to sterilize the *p. acnes* bacteria. Breakouts temporarily dry up and your new tan helps camouflage angry, red blemishes. But prolonged sun exposure eventually increases the plugging of your pores, producing blackheads, whiteheads, and small pimples. Plus the very real danger of skin cancer, to say nothing of premature wrinkling, cannot be overstated. Exposing your skin to the sun without sunscreen will never be a good idea. Its risks outweigh its very minimal benefits.

Acne Is Seasonal

False. Some people claim their acne is seasonal, worse, perhaps, in summer. While temperature and humidity may increase the oil production of your skin, for most there aren't seasons for acne. It's a year-round problem.

Sunscreen Causes Acne

False. A good noncomedogenic sunscreen will not cause acne. However, a heavy, occlusive sunscreen will attract and hold on to heat in your follicles, flaring inflammation and causing numerous small red bumps to form. This reaction is not true acne but a condition called miliaria.

Find an oil-free, noncomodegenic sunscreen formulated for acne-prone skin. The risk of skin cancer is simply too great to do without it. This is true for people of all ages and all races. Reapply it frequently if you are sweating in the heat or after you go swimming.

Also remember that acne medicines, such as benzoyl peroxide, Retin-A, and salicylic acid, may increase your skin's sensitivity to sun exposure. This is even more reason never to leave the house without first applying sunscreen.

Acne Comes from Not Washing Your Face Enough

False. Acne is not caused by dirt or uncleanliness. In fact, if you overwash your face or strip it with rubbing alcohol in an effort to feel clean, you can produce irritation. While face washing does remove surface oil, there is evidence that too frequent washing may stimulate oil production. Washing twice a day is more than enough to remove bacteria and aid in exfoliation.

Acne Is Caused by Oily Skin

False. It is possible—and often common—to have both dry skin and acne. You can also have both oily skin and no acne. Pores will become plugged and acne will form whether your skin is dry or oily.

Using the Right Cosmetics Will Cure My Acne

False. Some eager salespeople at the cosmetics counters may say anything to entice you into trying their line of new potions and creams. Buyer, beware!

If I Have Acne, I Can't Use a Moisturizer

False. Many people think that if they have acne, they can't use moisturizers. Actually, noncomedogenic moisturizers, the kind that don't cause clogged pores, are a must to hydrate parched, dry skin.

Acne Is Contagious

False. Acne is a noncommunicable disease. Even if you run your hands over the face of someone with the worst case of acne you've ever seen, you won't get any pimples as a result. You can no more catch acne than you can catch cancer.

Accutane Is the Miracle Cure for Acne

False. Accutane is the most successful drug used to treat acne, but it should be used only for severe cases, not mild ones. It works by shrinking oil glands for one to two (sometimes three) years, and it normalizes the cells lining the pore so plugging does not occur. A significant percentage of people who use Accutane need a second or third course of the drug, and most require topical skin treatments long term to keep their acne at bay. Accutane also has significant side effects, which require careful monitoring by your dermatologist.

For more information about Accutane, see page 53 in chapter 2.

Hair in Your Face or Hats on Your Head Cause Acne

False. Hair and hats by themselves can't cause acne. But using the wrong kinds of products on your hair or too much of them can exacerbate acne. We call this condition mousse abuse. Comedogenic, acne-triggering hair products, whether mousse, gel, pomade, or oil, can occlude (plug) pores near the hairline, creating fine blackheads and whiteheads. People who wear hats to hide their acne may inadvertently cause excess perspiration and irritation, triggering acne breakouts.

Blue Light Therapy Can Cure Acne

False. Blue light therapy is an interesting approach to the treatment of acne, but it's not a cure. Blue light is part of the rainbow of visible light (410 nanometers wavelength) emitted from a light source from a machine in a doctor's office. It works by sterilizing the skin for a short period of time, removing acne bacteria and *temporarily* improving acne when used in conjunction with traditional topical acne medications. As more dermatologists use blue light therapy, we'll get a better idea of how well it works or whether its expense and frequent visits will disappoint patients in the long run. Studies are ongoing, but it's simply too soon to tell.

We will discuss blue light therapy and radio-frequency treatments on page 60 in chapter 2.

acne scars

One of the most important reasons to be proactive about treating acne is the risk of scarring. The long-term effects of acne, both physical and emotional, can last much longer than breakouts, sometimes forever.

Most Acne Scars Aren't True Scars

Luckily, 90 percent of what many people view as scars aren't true scars. They are the pink or brown pigmentation spots that follow a healed pimple. The medical term for these spots is postinflammatory hyperpigmentation.

When a blemish heals, the normal process is for a flat red-to-pink spot (called a macule) to form, followed by a flat brown mark, then total fading. The red-to-pink spot can take two to three months to turn brown, and it can take anywhere from six months to a year before it generally fades away. It's a long time to wait. People of color tend to find the brown spots more disfiguring than the actual pimples that caused them in the first place. The good news is that postinflammatory hyperpigmentation is a treatable side effect of acne. Bleaching agents effectively get rid of brown spots and are safe and easy to use.

What Is a True Scar?

(For more photographic examples, go to www.unblemished.com.) A scar by definition is a permanent, deep-seated change in the skin. It is a visible reminder of injury and tissue repair. After an injury, white blood cells and an array of inflammatory molecules help fight infection and heal damaged tissue. But not all the damaged tissue can be restored. You cannot erase a true scar, not even with a laser. You can modify it, you can soften it, sometimes you can replace one kind of scar with another that is more easily camouflaged, but you'll never be able to go back to the clear skin you had before that pesky pimple.

As with acne, some people are simply more likely to scar, especially those with a family history of severe, scarring acne. Sometimes acne scars stay exactly the same for decades; others diminish with time. Unfortunately, those with the most severe forms of inflammatory acne, with deep nodular lesions, are also most likely to have scarring problems. True scars signify that your acne is moderate to severe. You need immediate professional help from a dermatologist.

There are two kinds of true acne scars: those caused by increased tissue formation and those caused by tissue loss.

Keloids

Increased tissue formation scars are called keloids. For those who are geneti-cally susceptible, the body doesn't heal pimples properly but instead pro-duces excess collagen, which forms into lumpy, fibrous, red-brown nodules, often linear in shape. Keloids aren't painful but can feel almost rock-hard. One tiny pimple can suddenly trigger the body to go haywire and create a ram-bunctious overcompensation response, forming a keloid. Although African Americans tend to be the most prone to keloids, we've seen them in people of all races, and of all ages. Keloids are most common on the chest, back, shoul-ders, and jawline in people under age forty.

Keloids can be very difficult to treat. Cutting them out usually causes them to grow back larger. Instead, we try cortisone injections to flatten them or to help reduce redness. See a dermatologist the minute you start to see keloids form.

Scars caused by tissue loss are more common and take many forms:

Dell scars are shallow, sunken depressions in the skin with fairly smooth edges, making your skin appear to have waves or ripples.

Ragged-edged scars have sunken depressions with ragged, uneven edges.

Ice-pick scars are usually found on cheeks. They're small, deep holes with jagged edges and steep sides. They can evolve over time into **depressed fi-brotic scars,** which also have sharp edges and steep sides but are larger and firmer at the base.

Atrophic macules are soft marks with a depressed base. Blood vessels just below the surface of the scar may make them appear purplish when they are recent, but this discoloration usually fades to pale ivory.

Follicular macular atrophy is more likely to occur when acne has ap-peared on the chest or back. These small, soft white lesions resemble white-heads but are true scars and may persist for months, years, or remain perma-nently.

For more information on treating scars, see page 62 in chapter 2.

Scar Prevention

Firefighters always say that the best way to stay safe in a fire is to prevent it from happening. The same is true with acne scars. Stop the acne and you'll stop the scars before they've had a chance to form.

Another method to prevent acne scars is to stop picking! The more inflammation you prevent, the less likely you are to scar. Unfortunately, pimples are an invitation to pick. But picking and squeezing—with fingernails, pins, you name it—can cause permanent damage. Picking not only worsens the pimple you're attacking; it makes the surrounding skin even more irritated and swollen, triggering new eruptions. A severe form of picking, called *Acne excoriée des jeunes filles,* often leaves incurable, disfiguring gouged-out scars and holes in the face. (For more information, see the section on compulsive picking on page 83 in chapter 3.)

Another common complaint from adult women is the sudden proliferation of chin hairs along with acne nodules. This invites aggressive tweezing and digging at the hair that worsens the acne and may lead to scarring. If you can afford it, laser hair removal or the prescription hair-growth retardant, Vaniqa, can be very successful. Take away the reason to pick and you'll stop picking.

A pimple that's bothering you today will go away faster if you let it be. If you pick and poke and prod and squeeze it, you may be reminded of that pimple forever.

Acne in the Media and on the Internet

We're thrilled that more and more information about acne (and rosacea; see chapter 13) is being published so everyone can better understand this disease. However, we're concerned about all the myths and misinformation available to anyone who surfs the Internet. There are many wonderful websites filled with facts to help you learn about skin and acne, but there are also many run by frauds and the disgruntled. Chat rooms can be great, especially for teenagers who see them as safe places to vent and talk about what products worked and which ones they liked and didn't like. But there are also chat rooms devoted to Accutane and other controversial drugs, for example, that can be filled with people who may have had bad experiences and therefore assume that the drug is harmful for everyone and should be banned. When this happens, we lose the opportunity to treat and heal—as well as comfort—people who are convinced, through reading and believing misinformation on the Internet, that we can't help them.

So search the Internet all you like, but be smart about what you read. Use it for the helpful psychological support it can provide, but read the medical information on personal websites with a grain of salt. If it sounds too good to be true—like an amazing herbal cure for acne—it probably is.

chapter two
acne treatment

Only about 7 percent of teenagers with acne see a dermatologist—and even fewer adults do. The vast majority of acne sufferers never go to a doctor for advice and treatment. Instead, they self-treat. Sadly, many of those who do see a physician do not always comply with the prescribed treatment or don't get the results they'd hoped for.

As you know, myths and misinformation about acne abound, especially when it comes to self-treatment. We've heard some astonishing stories from our patients about what they were advised to do. They are so desperate they're willing to try just about anything. Perhaps you've tried some of the following home remedies for acne yourself.

HOME REMEDIES FOR ACNE (WHICH WE DO *NOT* RECOMMEND!)

antifungus creams	baking soda paste	cornstarch
dishwashing liquid	egg whites	hydrogen peroxide
lemon juice	milk of magnesia	mud from the garden
Preparation H	raw garlic	rubbing alcohol
toothpaste	urine from a newborn baby	vinegar
Windex (remember the film *My Big Fat Greek Wedding?*)		

---

over-the-counter treatments

Once you realize that those home remedies don't work, you usually turn next to your local drugstore shelves, scanning the vast array of topical over-the-counter acne products and wondering if something will work. These products include cleansers, lotions, creams, gels, medicated pads, cover-ups, spot treatments, pore strips, and masks. Some work well. Others have no active ingredients. Many are extremely harsh or contain ingredients in high concentrations that irritate your skin, so your skin actually looks worse.

The ultimate goal of acne treatment and prevention is to:

1. Unplug pores
2. Remove bacteria
3. Reduce inflammation (swelling)

This can be achieved by using a combination of over-the-counter products with active ingredients designed to unplug pores, remove bacteria, and lessen inflammation. No single medication can do it all. Using a combination of medications works on these three steps of the problem. Full-face, daily treatment is the key to halt acne in its tracks and prevent future breakouts.

FDA-Approved Over-the-Counter Acne Drugs

The only FDA-approved active ingredients to fight acne without a prescription are:

- benzoyl peroxide
- resorcinol
- salicylic acid
- sulfur

The above over-the-counter topical medicines are regulated by the FDA, which issues specific guidelines about which drugs are acceptable for acne treatment and in what concentration, how they're to be used, and where they're manufactured. The combination of drugs is also regulated: It's not legal for a company to make a drug claim by combining different active ingredients, such as benzoyl peroxide and salicylic acid, in one product.

Products containing one of these ingredients in an approved concentration may claim acne treatment and prevention on the product label and in accompanying educational literature. No acne therapeutic claims can be made for products lacking either benzoyl peroxide, resorcinol, salicylic acid, or sulfur.

Benzoyl Peroxide

Benzoyl peroxide is an antimicrobial by definition. It's the world's best acne "bug" remover, attacking the *p. acnes* bacteria very effectively. There's also evidence that it may penetrate the oil in the plug, may control excess sebum production, and lessen skin inflammation. In the forty years it's been used, there is not a single documented case of bacterial resistance to benzoyl peroxide, which is why it's our favorite acne-fighter. If it works for you in the beginning, it will continue to work, because your bacteria can't become immune to it.

Benzoyl peroxide comes in strengths of 2.5 percent, 5 percent, and 10 percent. We recommend using the lowest possible concentration, as it is less likely to irritate skin while still highly effective. In fact, medical studies demonstrate that a 2.5 percent benzoyl peroxide product is equally as effective in removing the *p. acnes* bacteria as a 10 percent product with less potential irritation.

Benzoyl peroxide has been available over the counter since 1962. Older formulations employed larger crystals that could burn or irritate the skin. Recent formulations use highly milled benzoyl peroxide, allowing it to penetrate better into the pore with much less irritation. An irritation reaction appears as many small pink bumps. A true allergy to benzoyl peroxide is rare, occurring in 1 to 3 percent of the population. The allergy develops within a few days to weeks of use; the area turns red, swells, and is bumpy, itchy, and occasionally weepy. These allergic reactions will stop by themselves once use of benzoyl peroxide is discontinued. A 1 percent hydrocortisone cream, available over the counter, will hasten the resolution of the allergic reaction. If complete clearing of the allergy fails to occur within three days, see a dermatologist for stronger medication.

Benzoyl peroxide is a category C drug, meaning it has not been tested on pregnant or nursing women. It has also not been tested on children under age twelve.

Resorcinol

Resorcinol is an exfoliator, which loosens and softens plugged pores. It is often used with sulfur. The technical term for resorcinol's exfoliating properties is *keratolytic*.

Salicylic Acid

Salicylic acid is a beta hydroxy acid derived from willow tree bark. It is kera-tolytic, which means it works as an exfoliator to loosen and soften plugged pores.

Sulfur

Sulfur is a keratolytic agent. It may also have an antibacterial effect, by inhibiting the growth of *p. acnes* bacteria, and it may also help reduce redness and swelling by decreasing the formation of free fatty acids. Some people are highly allergic to oral sulfa drugs (like Bactrim or Septra) but tolerate topical sulfur just fine.

Cosmeceutical Agents

Other, less effective ingredients without FDA approval have been docu-mented in professional literature as potentially effective for use in controlling

---

WHAT OVER-THE-COUNTER ACNE DRUGS AND COSMECEUTICAL AGENTS DO

Drugs

benzoyl peroxide	Primarily removes *p. acnes* bacteria, with some mild ability to help unplug pores, control oil production, and reduce inflammation
resorcinol	Unplugs pores
salicylic acid	Unplugs pores
sulfur	Unplugs pores; may help to reduce inflammation and remove *p. acnes* bacteria

Cosmeceuticals

glycolic acid (an AHA)	May help unplug pores
green tea	May help reduce inflammation
niacinamide	May help reduce inflammation
retinol	May unplug pores and reduce inflammation
Vitamin F	May regulate oil production

Is Acid Going to Hurt Me?

When you hear the word "acid" in relation to acne treatment, your first reaction is most likely one of fear that it's going to harm your face. But the type of acids used to treat acne aren't the normal kind that will eat your skin off. Acids derived from fruit juice, sour milk, fermented grapes, vegetables, and other plants can help control acne and also help reverse signs of aging. These chemicals are called alpha keto-carboxylic acids or alpha hydroxy acids. Salicylic acid, glycolic acid, lactic acid, and malic acid work by exfoliating the skin. They help slough off the dead skin that collects inside pores, contributing to the plug that starts the acne process. These acids help increase cell renewal. Both actions are important in successfully treating acne.

acne, even though they are not allowed to be labeled as such. These are considered cosmeceuticals, because they are cosmetic agents with potential pharmaceutical activity. They include:

- alpha hydroxy acids (AHA)
- green tea
- niacinamide
- retinol
- Vitamin F (linoleic/linolenic acid)

Products containing cosmeceuticals and no FDA-approved acne medication use euphemisms such as "pore clearing," "blemish fighting," or "skin calming" to imply acne treatment without violating FDA guidelines.

Formulas Matter!

Why will one salicylic acid or benzoyl peroxide–containing product feel good and control your acne, but another product with the same active ingredient(s) irritate or fail to work? While ingredients listed on a product label may look strikingly similar, the formulas and the resulting product efficacy are often vastly different. Far more than an ingredient list, the effectiveness of a formula on your skin depends upon the manufacturing techniques, the precise percentages, penetrability and origin of each ingredient, and the final pH. Therefore, when buying any product, beware of imitators and knock-offs claiming to work as well as an original.

the risks of self-medicating

Over-the-counter topicals are generally safe. The worst that can happen is either irritation or an allergic reaction, in which case you'll become red or have a rash that might need treatment. However, discontinuing use usually allows the irritation or allergic reaction to go away on its own.

Remember that all FDA-approved drugs have a finite shelf life. The expiration date should be clearly labeled. Expired drugs lose their potency and may become contaminated, so throw them out on the expiration date.

Below is a table of common over-the-counter topical drugs for acne that are FDA-approved, easy to use, and effective. You can safely use them as directed.

COMMON OVER-THE-COUNTER TOPICAL DRUGS FOR ACNE

Drug	Formulation	Over-the-Counter Brand
benzoyl peroxide	cream, gel, lotion, soap	Proactiv Solution, Rodan & Fields CALM, Clearasil, Fostex, PanOxyl, Dryox, Persa-Gel
salicylic acid	cleanser, gel, lotion	Proactiv Solution, Rodan & Fields CALM, PROPApH, Stri-Dex, Oxy Night Watch, Clearasil Clearstick Maximum Strength
sulfur (or sulphur)	cleanser, lotion, mask	Proactiv Solution, Rodan & Fields CALM, Sulpho-Lac Acne Medication, Liquimat, Therac Lotion, Sulmasque
sulfur and/or resorcinol	lotion	Proactiv Solution, Rodan & Fields CALM, Sulforcin Lotion, Rezamid Lotion, Acnomel Cream

When it comes to self-medicating, we're most concerned when consumers look for magic bullets in the so-called safe arena of herbals and alternative products. Because they are not regulated by the FDA, there is no guarantee that their ingredients are safe or potent in the promised dosage. Topically applied herbal agents are generally safe, but their effectiveness is unproven. In

PORES AND PORE STRIPS

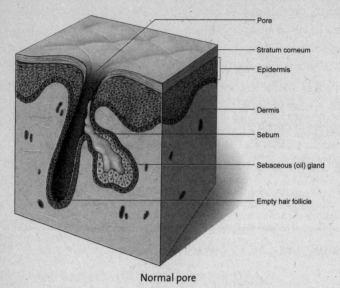

Pore

Stratum corneum

Epidermis

Dermis

Sebum

Sebaceous (oil) gland

Empty hair follicle

Normal pore

A pore is the passageway from the base of your hair follicle, with its attached oil gland, to the surface of your skin. Unfortunately, pore size is genetically determined, and pores tend to get bigger as we age. So pore strips, which are allegedly designed to get rid of blackheads and shrink pore size, *can't* permanently change the size of your pores.

Nor can they get rid of blackheads. That yucky gray stuff you see on the pore strip after you've ripped it off your skin is not a mass of blackheads. It's normal oil filling your pores. Some oil is good. It hydrates your skin. Yank it off and guess what? It's back in the morning. Temporarily removing surface oil, whether by pore strips, exfoliants, peels, or microdermabrasion, can make your pores look smaller, but it's only temporary.

We've seen patients suffering from pore-strip irritation because they are overdoing it. Use pore strips occasionally if you like. However, the most effective prescriptions for treating and preventing blackheads, as well as minimizing pore size, are the tretinoins: Differin, Retin-A, or Tazorac. With these, after an initial peeling and drying of the skin, improvement of pores is seen in three to four months.

If you prefer to avoid the tretinoins, Proactiv Solution has a pore strip medicated with salicylic acid to help unblock clogged pores. We've also invented a patented blackhead extractor, Rodan & Fields CLEAN, to remove blackheads. You can use our device, or ask your dermatologist to perform blackhead extractions for you.

WHAT CAN ACNE MASKS DO?

Masks for acne can provide healing, soothing relief. They're designed to cool the skin, provide medication, reduce redness, and absorb oil. Acne masks are usually clay-based, and medicated with either sulfur or salicylic acid for soothing, cooling, and unplugging. Kaolin clay is used to draw out excess oil.

Hydrating masks or exfoliating masks (for wrinkles) are generally not recommended for acne. Some may even irritate and exacerbate pimples. Papaya masks in particular can be great for those who don't have acne but can cause more facial redness and irritation in those who do.

---

addition, oral herbal supplements may interfere with prescription medications and have the potential to cause debilitating side effects. Remember that all natural is not always better.

when should you go to a dermatologist?

The overwhelming majority of people with acne have mild to moderate acne. Our system, as you'll see in chapter 5, is designed to help you. You should see dramatic results within six to eight weeks, if not sooner.

If you've used a combination therapy—benzoyl peroxide, salicylic acid, and sulfur—over your entire face at least once or twice daily for six weeks and

---

BE SMART WHEN STARTING ANY NEW ACNE REGIME

Whenever you start a new acne regime, we recommend that you avoid trying new cosmetics, such as moisturizers or makeup, at the same time. Some ingredients might interfere with the acne medicine. Other creams or moisturizers, for instance, may be inherently comedogenic and cause pimples. Be sure all other products you put on your face have not expired. Also avoid using other products when you're exercising or sweating a lot.

Remember to avoid picking, which always makes acne worse. And if you're going through a divorce, moving, or coping with family traumas—in other words, you're super-stressed—give your new acne program additional time to work.

have not seen any changes and are still getting new acne, you need treatment from a dermatologist.

We dermatologists can't change your genetic predisposition to acne, but we can prescribe oral drugs, topical creams, and antibiotics. These medications are more potent than over-the-counter products. For women, we can use hormones, such as birth control pills. We can monitor progress and tweak programs until we find the perfect one for you. We can prescribe Accutane, the most potent drug in the antiacne arsenal for severe, stubborn cases of acne. We can extract blackheads and zap emergency zits with cortisone injections. We can perform salicylic acid or glycolic acid peels or microdermabrasion to help exfoliation. Most important, we can provide a sympathetic ear. We know how much pain your acne causes. We're determined to help you.

If you have any acne scars, *run* to a dermatologist. Acne scars can be disfiguring for life. They must be treated by a professional.

how to choose a dermatologist

There are only about 9,000 dermatologists in America. Most people go to one only when they have problems, such as skin cancer, psoriasis, moles, or cosmetic skin aging concerns.

Since the average person with acne is either self-treating or getting advice from his or her regular doctors—pediatricians, gynecologists, and general practitioners, none of whom are specifically trained in acne treatment—he or she may not be receiving the most advanced and successful treatments. These doctors may be relying on information learned in medical school or from drug company representatives. In addition, these doctors are busy treating a wide variety of health complaints so treating acne may not be their number one concern.

When seeking treatment for your acne, we always recommend that you see a dermatologist. The best way to choose a dermatologist whose style suits your personality is by word of mouth or a recommendation from your primary physician or other trusted medical professional. If you have no personal reference, visit the American Academy of Dermatology website at www.aad.com to find a local doctor.

questions to ask before choosing a dermatologist

We suggest you call a new dermatologist's office first and ask some simple questions that can help narrow your search. Good doctors encourage communication with their patients and will be happy to have their staffs answer the following questions:

- Does the doctor treat acne?
- Is the doctor board-certified by the American Academy of Dermatology?
- Does the doctor perform such treatments as acne surgery?
- If the practice is closed to new patients, when can you call back to see if the practice is reopened? Can this doctor recommend any other doctors in the area? (A doctor fresh out of dermatology residency, for instance, might be more available.)

information to bring to the dermatologist

A patient recently came in with a list of questions and her background information, then flushed beet red. "I'm embarrassed," she said, staring down at the paper. "I'm sure doctors hate this."

On the contrary, we love patients like this. They're organized, conscientious, and serious about treatment. Bringing in a list is an excellent use of time. You'll have all your questions answered from the start, and the doctor will have more time to discuss treatment alternatives and specifics.

Here's what to include on your list:

- Whether you've seen another doctor or dermatologist for acne;
- If so, what treatment was used, and how successful was it? Did you have side effects from any medications you used? Include any current prescription medications prescribed for acne, such as birth control pills;
- Any other medications currently prescribed by a doctor for other medical conditions, such as seizures;
- Herbal or vitamin supplements you are currently taking;
- Any performance-enhancing supplements;
- Products you've tried and liked;
- Products you've tried and hated;
- Makeup and your current skin-care regimen, including moisturizers, toners, sunscreens, and eye makeup remover;

- What sports you play;
- What your lifestyle is like;
- What big events you have coming up, such as exams, a wedding, or a job change;
- Anything that triggers your acne;
- How acne has affected your emotional and social life;
- Whether you frequently pick at your pimples.

This list will help your doctor plan the right course of treatment. And if that initial course of action fails, he or she will have a backup plan. Your doctor should remind you to call if there are any side effects from the medications, and your first follow-up appointment should be within four to six weeks.

dermatologist treatments

Dermatologists have many different methods for treating acne. These are the standard treatments, usually prescribed in some combination:

- antibiotics—oral
- antibiotics—topical
- hormones
- isotretinoin (Accutane)
- peels
- retinoids

GOING TO THE DERMATOLOGIST CAN BE INTIMIDATING

Going to any new doctor, for whatever condition, is scary. It's embarrassing to undress, tell your story to a nurse, tell it again to a doctor, and perhaps be in the room with your parents. Acne patients who have been teased tend to be understandably hypersensitive. Plus acne creates such a sense of shame that talking about it is often excruciating. To have someone touching and looking closely at your face can be extremely difficult. And sometimes patients are afraid that we *can't* help them.

Once you do find a doctor who specifically treats acne, having your background information prepared and in hand at the doctor's office can save you much embarrassment (see page 47). Remember, we've seen it all before. We're here to help you.

antibiotics—oral

Oral antibiotics work by removing the *p. acnes* bacteria and decreasing inflammation. One of the biggest hurdles facing modern medicine, however, is the overprescription of antibiotics. The result is a growing resistance to these drugs, which means that diseases that once could have been wiped out with a course of antibiotics may now have dire potential.

We are not advising avoidance or discontinuation of antibiotics. Yes, they are overprescribed, but sometimes they are prescribed for the right reason. For example, some patients, especially those with moderate to severe acne, need antibiotics. We prescribe antiobiotics we feel are safe and effective, such as doxycycline and minocycline, both easily absorbed forms of tetracycline. Tetracycline has been prescribed for decades to reduce acne inflammation. It is easy to tolerate and has few side effects, although tetracycline resistance is emerging. Erythromycin, on the other hand, has been so overprescribed that 50 percent of people are resistant to it. Still, erythromycin and tetracycline have value for moderate to severe acne because of their anti-inflammatory potential.

Other oral antibiotics include sulfa drugs, such as Bactrim and Septra. They are effective orally but can cause worrisome reactions, such as serious skin allergies and bone marrow suppression. Clindamycin taken orally has been used for over forty years and is a second-line antibiotic, prescribed when the tetracyclines or erythromycin medications fail. The most significant, though rare, adverse reaction associated with clindamycin is pseudomembranous colitis, which is a bloody diarrhea that requires treatment by a gastroenterologist.

For those on antibiotics, we always set a timetable. The average course of treatment is about one to six months. We schedule an appointment for a month to six weeks after the antibiotics are prescribed to assess a patient's response. Because we're seeing them only at one point in time, we always ask how their skin has looked in the previous weeks. If a patient is happy with his or her progress and hasn't had any side effects, we continue the treatment until the skin is clear. The patient will be using topical medications concurrently, yet we may add Differin or Retin-A, to see if either can aid in further improvement or address other problems, such as postinflammatory pigmentation. The next appointment comes in another six to eight weeks. If the patient has been responding well, we'll lower or stop the oral antibiotic dose and continue topical treatment.

THE MOST COMMONLY PRESCRIBED ORAL ANTIBIOTICS FOR ACNE (IN ALPHABETICAL ORDER)

Antibiotic	Side Effects	Contraindications
clindamycin	colitis	history of previous allergy, pregnancy, breast-feeding*
doxycycline	sun sensitivity, intestinal upset, discolored teeth	"
erythromycin	intestinal upset	"
minocycline	headaches, pseudotumor cerebri, lupus-like reaction, hives, sun sensitivity, discolored teeth	"
tetracycline	sun sensitivity, intestinal upset, discolored teeth	"
trimethoprim-sulfamethoxazole	sun sensitivity, allergies, bone marrow suppression	"

* This contraindication is applicable to every antibiotic on this list.

There is no miracle antibiotic cure for acne. You're used to taking an antibiotic when you have bronchitis and witness your cough quickly resolve. Unfortunately, acne is not the same kind of condition. You didn't get it overnight, and it's not going to go away overnight. If patients don't improve, we might change to a different antibiotic. For female patients, birth control pills and spironolactone (Aldactone) are another option. Finally, if these treatments aren't successful and we think the acne is severe enough and prone to scarring, we move to Accutane. It's far better to have five months of Accutane treatment than months or years on antibiotics that will never cure you.

Some patients flatly refuse to take oral antibiotics, and we respect that. After years of working with what's become the Rodan and Fields Approach, we've seen how well a combination of topical medicines can work to fight acne, as long as you treat the full face on a daily basis. Prescription oral antibiotics don't always work better than topical treatments. We know this from millions of our Proactiv Solution customers.

TAKE CARE OF YOUR PRESCRIPTIONS

Medications, whether prescription or over-the-counter, should *not* be stored in a hot, damp room. They should be stored in a cool, dry place. If you store medicine in your bathroom, use the medicine cabinet. It's there for a reason: to protect your medications from sunlight, moisture, and heat. Don't place your prescriptions in front of a window where sunlight will beat down upon them.

antibiotics—topical

Topical antibiotics, such as azelaic acid, clindamycin, erythromycin, and sodium sulfacetamide, remove bacteria. Topical erythromycin loses effectiveness within a few months because bacterial resistance quickly develops. Clindamycin remains a favorite topical antibiotic, but bacterial resistance is also becoming a growing problem. Benzoyl peroxide and erythromycin (Benzamycin) and benzoyl peroxide and clindamycin (Benzaclin or Duac) are formulas combining both medications; they may work better than either drug being used alone. Azelaic acid, a newer agent for acne, is mildly effective

THE MOST COMMONLY PRESCRIBED TOPICAL ANTIBIOTICS FOR ACNE (IN ALPHABETICAL ORDER)

Antibiotic	Side Effects	Contraindications*
azelaic acid cream	dryness, irritation	allergy, breast-feeding, pregnancy
clindamycin gel, solution, or lotion	dryness, colitis	"
clindamycin plus benzoyl peroxide (Benzaclin or Duac)	dryness, irritation	"
erythromycin gel or solution	dryness, irritation	"
erythromycin plus benzoyl peroxide (Benzamycin)	dryness, irritation	"
sodium sulfacetamide	dryness, irritation	"

These drugs are category C, meaning they have not been tested in pregnant and nursing mothers.

against the *p. acnes* bacteria and has some ability to decrease plugging and reduce inflammation. Benzoyl peroxide and glycolic acid (Triaz) is an antimicrobial, which also helps exfoliate. Sodium sulfacetamide is an older antibacterial agent making a comeback for acne and rosacea. Metronidazole (MetroLotion) is FDA-approved for rosacea and may have value in fighting the symptoms of acne.

hormones

Beginning at puberty, androgenic, or masculinizing, hormones play a key role in acne development and persistence. In women the stimulation comes from the androgenic hormones testosterone, DHEA-S (dihydropriandronsterone sulfate), and progesterone, manufactured by the ovaries and the adrenal glands. In men the stimulation comes from testosterone and dihydroxtestosterone, made in the testes.

During puberty, these hormones cause acne in a three-step process. They enlarge the size of the sebaceous glands, they stimulate oil production, and they affect the keratinization of pores, creating plugs.

Hormone manipulation to treat acne in men is, unfortunately, biologically unsafe. With women, however, it is possible though tricky. The usual prescription is birth control pills, which contain a combination of estrogen and progesterone. Acne can become better or worse with this treatment—each woman's response will be different. There are many low-dose estrogen birth control pills that have been proven effective for the improvement of acne; they include OrthoTri-Cyclin, Orthocept, and Yasmin. A minimum of three months on the pill is required to assess effectiveness. Spironolactone is a mild diuretic and, like birth control pills, is also an antiandrogen. It can help manage female acne, especially when taken in combination with birth control pills.

Note: Women who have persistent, severe acne, thinning hair, and obesity should rule out the possibility of polycystic ovarian syndrome before undertaking any type of treatment for acne.

Note: DHEA-S has androgen hormone-like effects, and if taken as a supplement can make acne worse, so we do not recommend its use even though it is available in health food stores.

For more information about hormone therapy for women, see chapters 7, 9, and 10.

isotretinoin (accutane)

Isotretinoin is the generic term for Accutane. Accutane is a synthetic Vitamin A derivative that creates a potentially long-lasting change in the cells lining the pore. This change allows cells to slough off naturally, without clumping and plugging the pore, the first step in the development of acne. With Accutane, pores no longer become plugged, so oil can flow freely to the skin's surface. Plus, the quantity of oil is decreased as Accutane temporarily reregulates the sebaceous (oil) gland to produce less. Accutane's benefits may last years and in some cases are permanent. (For photographic examples, go to www.unblemished.com.)

Accutane is the most important drug to date in the arsenal of medications used to treat severe and persistent nodular, cystic acne. Available since 1984, it has provided dramatic improvement in the majority of the twelve million patients treated with it. These patients would have had few options otherwise. Of the more than five thousand patients we have treated during the past twenty years with Accutane, we found that about 60 percent needed only one course of treatment. About 30 percent needed a second course. After a second course, only 10 percent of patients failed to permanently respond and have required a third course of the drug.

Although Accutane can be very powerful in treating severe acne, it works by reducing oil production, so the downside is that your skin will become very dry and your lips chapped. You must be closely monitored when taking it, as Accutane can have other side effects, though the overwhelming majority of patients will not experience them. These include nosebleeds and muscle and joint soreness; the latter can be treated with a nonsteroidal anti-inflammatory medication, such as ibuprofen. Accutane is known to cause birth defects in a developing fetus if a pregnant woman takes it. Therefore, women must use appropriate birth control methods for one month before therapy begins, during the entire course of therapy, and for at least three months after therapy stops. Accutane does not, however, affect future pregnancies.

Truly serious side effects from Accutane, such as liver and pancreas damage, depression, and brain swelling are *extremely* rare and can be reversed when the medication is stopped. The relationship between Accutane and depression or suicide is still being investigated. Keep in mind that suicides reported in Accutane-treated patients have been rare and that there may have been other precipitating factors. For many patients, acne itself is a depressing problem to have. By removing this stigmatizing problem—whether by Accutane or by other therapeutic options—we have seen countless lives transformed and depression lifted. (For more information about Accutane's side effects, see sidebar.)

If you have severe acne that has not responded to other treatments, you are a candidate for a five-to-six-month course of Accutane. Your prescription dose of Accutane will be tailored to your weight and should always be taken with a meal, because it's better absorbed with food. In addition, your response to Accutane, side effects (if any), and dosage will be carefully monitored by your doctor every month. You will have mandatory blood tests, including liver profile studies, a complete blood count, and cholesterol and triglyceride levels to detect any significant abnormalities, such as liver inflammation and a dangerously high triglyceride level, which could inflame the pancreas (pancreatitis); a decreased white blood cell count; or a seriously lowered red blood cell count. A serum pregnancy test is drawn on all fertile females monthly.

Unfortunately, Accutane suffers a terrible rap. Not only is it being overprescribed for mild acne but some people with severe acne—for whom it can be most helpful—won't take it for fear of side effects. That's a tragedy for everyone. No one should end up with permanent scarring because of a lack of correct information about Accutane's risks.

If you're afraid of Accutane, you need to talk to your doctor. Don't be embarrassed to express your concerns. When patients tell us they're terrified of Accutane and worry about the side effects, we tell them the majority are most likely to have dry skin and chapped lips. That's it. Also remember that acne changes throughout most people's lives. Accutane can make a significant long-term impact, but it's not always a cure. It will, however, improve your acne by decreasing the inflammatory component. You'll have no bumps, or you'll have smaller bumps instead of larger cysts, which can be helped by topical medications in the long run. The Rodan and Fields Approach has been helpful

POSSIBLE SIDE EFFECTS OF ACCUTANE*

Minor Side Effects
chapping of the lips
dry mouth, nose, or skin
inflammation of the mucous membrane of the eye
itching
muscle aches
nosebleeds
photosensitivity
reduced night vision

Serious Side Effects
abnormal liver enzymes
birth defects in developing fetus
brain swelling
depression
falling red and white blood cell count
increased cholesterol and triglyceride levels
mood changes
pancreatitis
persistent headaches

* All of these side effects, except birth defects, usually go away after the medication is stopped. Patients who experience side effects while using Accutane should tell their doctor. The doctor may be able to reduce the dose so that the side effects are decreased or stopped.

for maintaining clear skin for people after they have been treated with Accutane.

peels

Dermatologists can perform peels with salicylic acid or glycolic acid. Microdermabrasion is a sanding/vacuuming procedure of the skin. Both can aid exfoliation, help minimize scarring, and increase the penetration and potency of daily topical medications.

retinoids

Retinoids stop the formation of microcomedones—the precursors of pimples. Retinoids, such as Avita, Differin, Retin-A, and Tazorac, are great for unplugging pores. They normalize the cells that line the pore, which allows dead cells to slough off evenly and regularly rather than getting sticky and clumping together to clog the pore. Retinoids may also have a direct anti-inflammatory effect, stopping the formation of pimples. For this reason, they are often the key starting agent for acne treatment. They work best with benzoyl peroxide and a topical antibiotic, listed on page 51.

All of the retinoids can cause dryness, redness, chapping, irritation, flaking, and sometimes an initial worsening of your acne. In the first months of treatment, as acne impurities are brought to the surface, there is often an initial flare of acne. Don't worry—your acne should improve over the next two to three months.

Stick to your program. Forget about a quick fix. And pace yourself. It's especially important not to overdo it with retinoids, as they can leave you looking like a boiled lobster. Start using them nightly once a week, then increase gradually to two or three nights a week as tolerated. Avoid the immediate eye and mouth area. Your face and neck will be more sensitive; chest and back less so.

Don't be afraid to try retinoids simply because you're worried about possible irritation. There are many different strengths and formulations. Cream formulations are less drying than gel or lotion bases. If your skin is sensitive, start with low-strength (0.025 percent) Differin Cream or Retin-A 0.04 Micro Gel.

Also note that it is imperative to protect yourself from the sun when using a retinoid. Skin treated with retinoids may be more susceptible to sunburn. Sunlight can also deactivate the beneficial effects of a retinoid. We recommend using sunscreens with the active ingredients zinc oxide or avobenzone, such as Neutrogena Ultra Sheer Dry-Touch Sunblock SPF 45, Ombrelle Sunscreen Lotion SPF 30, Proactiv Solution Daily Protection Plus SPF 15, Proactiv Solution Oil Free Moisture SPF 15, or Rodan & Fields COMPOUNDS Protect SPF 15, to protect your skin while using retinoids. Zinc oxide and avobenzone provide the best protection against the two main wavelengths of sunlight that destroy the skin—UVA and UVB. Your skin will be shortchanged if your sun-

THE MOST COMMONLY PRESCRIBED RETINOIDS FOR ACNE

Drug	Concentration	Side Effects
Avita Cream	0.025	dryness, irritation common, increased sun sensitivity. Not to be used during pregnancy or while nursing
Differin Cream	0.10	"
Differin Gel	0.10	"
Differin Solution	0.10	"
Retin-A Micro Gel	0.04	"
Retin-A Micro Gel	0.10	"
Tazorac Cream	0.05	"
Tazorac Cream	0.10	"
Tazorac Gel	0.05	"
Tazorac Gel	0.10	"

screen lacks either of these two active ingredients. People with jobs that require them to work outdoors, such as construction workers or lifeguards, should take extra precautions if they are using retinoids and use a high SPF sunscreen and wear a broad-rimmed hat.

compliance

Acne treatment is often a lifelong program. Think prevention. Apply or take your medications daily. If you do not comply with the directions, your treatment is likely to fail. Use your medications properly—don't use them on Monday and forget on Tuesday, or use them once a day sometimes and twice a day other times. Be consistent. Most of all, be proactive.

If you're experiencing irritation or have any other problems, it's up to you to call your dermatologist and ask for help so that your program can be tailored to your needs. Stopping treatment partway through because you don't like it or can't be bothered is not going to help. Acne will not go away by itself.

TREATMENT FOR DIFFERENT GRADES OF ACNE

Mild (Noninflammatory/comedonal—mostly blackheads and whiteheads)

benzoyl peroxide—topical	primarily removes *p. acnes* bacteria, with possibly some mild ability to help unplug pores, control oil, and reduce inflammation
retinoids—topical	unplug pores, reduce inflammation
salicylic acid—topical	unplugs pores

Mild to Moderate (papulopustular—numerous pimples)

antibiotics—topical	reduce inflammation, remove bacteria
azelaic acid—topical	reduces inflammation, removes bacteria
benzoyl peroxide—topical	primarily removes *p. acnes* bacteria, with possibly some mild ability to help unplug pores, control oil, and reduce inflammation
contraceptives—oral (women only)	regulate hormones
retinoids—topical	unplug pores, reduce inflammation
spironolactone*—oral (women only)	antiandrogen
sodium sulfacetamide	removes bacteria
sulfur—topical	keratolytic; may reduce inflammation and remove bacteria

* Prescribed in conjunction with oral contraceptives

Moderate to Severe (numerous papulopustular and/or nodular/cystic)
There are four different treatment combinations:

(1)

antibiotics—oral—moderate-to-high-dose	remove bacteria, reduce inflammation
benzoyl peroxide—topical	primarily removes *p. acnes* bacteria, with possibly some mild ability to help unplug pores, control oil, and reduce inflammation
retinoids—topical	unplug pores, reduce inflammation

(2)

antibiotics—topical	remove bacteria, reduce inflammation
contraceptives—oral (women only)	regulate hormones

CODE_BLOCK_0acne treatment   59

| retinoids—topical | unplug pores, reduce inflammation |
| spironolactone*—oral (women only) | antiandrogen |

Prescribed in conjunction with oral contraceptives

(3)

antibiotics—oral—high-dose	remove bacteria, reduce inflammation
contraceptives—oral (women only)	regulate hormones
retinoids—topical	unplug pores
spironolactone*—oral (women only)	antiandrogen

Prescribed in conjunction with oral contraceptives

(4)

| Accutane | reduces oil production, unplugs pores, reduces inflammation, stops growth of bacteria |
| contraceptives—oral (women only) | regulate hormones |

when to expect results—be a proactive patient

Under a dermatologist's treatment you should expect to see results within a minimum of four to six weeks. Some people need at least six to eight weeks. Be patient.

Sometimes acne fluctuates. If you've been using a certain product, such as an oral or topical antibiotic, and your acne suddenly worsens, you may wonder if this product is no longer effective. Discuss this with your dermatologist. Perhaps your hormones have shifted or you're under major stress or perhaps you've developed a resistance to the antibiotic. If so, you may require more aggressive therapy to bring your acne back under control.

We encourage you to become a proactive patient. If you're unclear about the order of applying medicines or which medicine is to be used in the morning, which in the evening, ask your doctor to write a schedule for you to take home and follow. This will help simplify your treatment routine and bring about quicker results. Equally important, be sure to do your own skin analysis when you look in the mirror, and adjust your treatment according to what you see. For example, if your skin is dry and chapped, don't reapply more Retin-A that evening; it will merely serve to exacerbate the condition of your already

BUYING PRODUCTS FROM DERMATOLOGISTS

Some dermatologists sell their own lines of products, and many are effective. Doctors can instruct laboratories to create unique creams and other products in varying strengths and formulations that aren't available over the counter or by prescription.

Before you buy these products, however, ask your dermatologist why they are better than commercially available products. Very few products are actually created by the dermatologists who sell them. Reputable companies make them, then sell them to doctors, who add their private label. You should never feel any obligation to buy something from your dermatologist, especially if your insurance may help cover the cost of a comparable prescription.

irritated skin. It's okay to take a brief drug holiday now and then. If need be, call your doctor and discuss it.

blue light therapy, radio-frequency treatments, and laser treatments

Full of promise, yet still to be proven and completely tested, blue light therapy and radio-frequency treatments are far from mainstream acne therapy.

What exactly is blue light therapy? In the prism of visible light, the blue end, at 410 nanometers wavelength, may remove the *p. acnes* bacteria by destroying the bacterial cell membrane. Blue light is *not* UVA, UVB, or UVC, the radiation from the sun that penetrates through the atmosphere and can cause cancer.

Despite the hype, blue light therapy is not perfect, with hit-and-miss results. It works temporarily to sterilize the skin and helps clear mild-to-moderate papules, pustules, and some nodules. It does not clear comedones (blackheads and whiteheads) or cysts. It's best when combined with other topical agents, such as Proactiv Solution or Rodan & Fields CALM.

Blue light therapy requires twice-weekly appointments, each lasting fifteen minutes, for a minimum of four weeks. As a result, some acne may go into remission for four to six months. Yet acne will reoccur unless you maintain follow-up blue light treatments and use a daily topical medicated program. It's a good last step to try before taking oral medication.

Another new trend in the fight against acne is a radio-frequency treatment called Thermage. It provides heat energy, which penetrates deeply into the skin, heating oil glands, tightening collagen, and shrinking scars. This painful treatment avoids burning the surface of the skin as it heats underlying tissue, so there is no surface wound. Preliminary studies showed that one to two treatments with radio frequency gave a positive response in clearing acne in a small group of patients. Thermage may also improve acne scarring. How long the results will last is unknown at this time. We're not yet fans of this treatment because we have concerns about long-term harm—radio waves can penetrate deeply into fat, bone, muscle, nerves, and arteries, which makes this treatment potentially risky. We don't yet know if the sebaceous glands are permanently destroyed, or what side effects may appear many years from now.

Nonablative (noncutting) lasers are also being used to temporarily treat acne. There are many painless, nonwounding lasers, some used with a topical photosensitizing agent, Levulan, that may temporarily shrink oil glands and sterilize the skin. The treatments are expensive, many sessions are required, and efficacy is unproven. It's best to discuss these options with your dermatologist to avoid being misled by hype in the media.

acne surgery

Acne surgery is medical jargon for blackhead removal and injection of cysts. These are simple procedures done in the dermatologist's office or with an esthetician. They are usually quick and painless and help you achieve clearer skin within a few days. (For photographic examples, go to www.unblemished. com.)

It's important to remove deep-seated blackheads properly and completely, with either a vacuum suction device or comedone extractor. Blackheads on your skin will either remain looking ugly for months to years, or erupt into a larger pimple. Removing them properly helps clear your acne. We developed a patented instrument, Rodan & Fields CLEAN, to gently extract blackheads using vacuum suction and downward firm pressure. With Rodan & Fields CLEAN, you can extract your own blackheads at home.

Dermatologists can also inject cysts and nodules with a very dilute solution of cortisone, a potent anti-inflammatory. It quickly shrinks the tissues, working rapidly for those big juicy, often subterranean and painful cysts. Because the injection needle is extremely fine, it shouldn't hurt at all. Cortisone injection is especially helpful if your face erupts (with one pimple or dozens) before a big event, such as a wedding. It's the quick fix for movie stars and prom queens to clear an unsightly pimple overnight. But it's important to have it done properly and carefully with a dilute solution, because there is a potential side effect, a little dent in the skin, called steroid atrophy. It takes many months to resolve.

acne's aftermath—treatments for scars

Acne scars can be more upsetting than the pimples and cysts from which they originated. Yet as you read in the previous chapter, most acne scars are not true scars, which means they aren't permanent. These postpimple marks are pink, red, or brown spots that will eventually fade.

Pink or red marks usually take three to four months to heal and can be covered by makeup (see page 346 in chapter 17). Darker brown marks or postinflammatory hyperpigmentation can last six months to a year or longer. Postinflammatory hyperpigmentation is caused by the melanin pigment in the dermis found in cells called melanophages, scavengerlike cells that remain behind to clean up the pus and mess caused by papules and pustules. The challenge for medicine treating postinflammatory hyperpigmentation is penetration to the depth of the upper dermis, where melanophages are located. The darker your skin, the darker the spots and the longer you'll tend to suffer from postinflammatory hyperpigmentation.

Yet there's no need to despair over these marks. They can be treated painlessly and effectively with skin lighteners containing hydroquinone, which gets rid of the abnormal color packets without affecting normal skin color. In other words, you don't have to worry about bleaching your skin to a lighter color. We created our Rodan & Fields RADIANT regimen line to target hyperpigmentation. It can also be improved with Proactiv Solution Skin Lightening Lotion, Esoterica, or Porcelana products.

Superficial scarring, such as small, shallow depressions, may be improved with topical retinoids, such as retinol, which is available over the counter, and with prescription medications, such as Renova and Retin-A. If caught early, depressed, shallow dell scars may respond to microdermabrasion, which helps stimulate collagen production. A minimum of six to eight treatments performed at weekly intervals is typically required.

More serious scars and their treatments include:

Dell scars are shallow, sunken depressions in the skin, with fairly smooth edges, and **ragged-edge scars** have sunken depressions with ragged, uneven edges. Several treatments with microdermabrasion can soften ragged-edge scars a bit. Laser resurfacing (with CO_2 lasers) or radio-frequency (Thermage) treatments are promising for long-term improvement. Areas of sunken depression may be filled with materials such as bovine or human collagen, Hyalform Gel (hyaluronic acid), or Restylane. Permanent fillers, such as Artecoll and silicone, are making a comeback. They can be used to spackle inside the sunken areas and even them out. Be aware that if an adverse reaction, such as an allergy or migration of material occurs with a permanent filler, your only recourse is to have the area excised, which will leave an even larger scar.

Ice-pick scars are usually found on cheeks. They're small, deep holes with jagged edges and steep sides and can resemble gigantic pores. They can evolve over time into **depressed fibrotic scars,** which also have sharp edges and steep sides but are larger and firmer at the base. These scars are difficult to treat. They require surgery, either cutting out the hole and sewing the sides together or transplanting skin from behind the ear to fill in the excised hole and finally lasering the entire area so it blends with the surrounding skin.

Sinus tracts are seen in severe scarring cystic acne, leaving spaghettilike tracks or tunnels under the skin that connect one sebaceous gland to another. These tracks under the skin pull down and tether the skin. Extensive surgery to remove these sinus tracts may lead to further scarring and increase the likelihood that new cysts will form in these damaged areas.

Acne scars on the body are more difficult to treat than scars on the face. There is a higher density of blood vessels supplying blood to the face than elsewhere on the rest of the body so wound healing on the face is usually excellent. Body scars are tricky for another reason, too. There are fewer pilosebaceous glands on nonfacial skin, and that skin is very thick. Because it is the migration of cells from the pilosebaceous glands that heals injury, the fewer these units, the poorer the healing. If any doctor or aesthetician says he or she can easily fix acne scars on the chest or back, be wary. We wish it could easily be done, but it can't.

There are some treatments that can be effective for body scars. If body scars are red, we can use pulse-dye laser or other vascular lasers to remove the red component. If the scars are brown, we can aggressively use lightening agents. Depressed scars can be lifted with filler materials, and ice pick scars on the body can be excised as on the face.

As you can see, there are numerous options available to treat the marks and scars that acne leaves behind. Left alone, with time, scars will improve and become less noticeable, blending into the rest of your face. Working with a cosmetically oriented dermatologist or plastic surgeon to correct the most noticeable scars will do a great deal to help your appearance and self-esteem. But remember, prevention of scarring is your ultimate goal, and there is no reason to avoid acne treatment from a dermatologist when so many options are available.

chapter three
acne's psychological aftermath

"I think the most hurtful thing that I experienced while I suffered with acne was that people automatically assumed I had acne because my diet and hygiene were poor. Instead of asking, they automatically offered me their 'solution' to my acne—which of course wasn't any solution at all. The hurt just didn't go away."

—Hilary, age twenty-nine

"Only people who have acne know the pain I go through—emotionally and physically."

—Brendan, age seventeen

No matter how splendid your personality or how nice your clothes, an automatic assessment is made about anyone with blemishes. You will be judged simply because your skin is not clear. "There is no single disease that causes more psychic trauma, more maladjustment between parents and children, more general insecurity and feelings of inferiority, and greater sums of psychic suffering than does acne vulgaris." This observation was made in an article by Dr. M. Sulzberger and Dr. S. Zaidems that is well-known to dermatologists, "Psychogenic Factors in Dermatological Disorders." It was published in *The Medical Clinician of North America* in 1948, and it is more true than ever nearly sixty years later.

Acne sufferers have every right to be upset. Acne is not a life-threatening disease in itself, but it's definitely life-*diminishing*. We firmly believe that the emotional quality of your life is as important as the physical quality; the two are inextricably intertwined. Yet because the root causes of acne are usually misunderstood, the lingering pain of its emotional fallout is even more likely to be misunderstood as well. After all, many people still believe that somehow acne is *their* fault, which usually exacerbates their worries and suffering.

Nor is anyone helped by the stigma surrounding acne. Stigma from the disease itself and stigma from not being able to confront it and discuss it. Stigma causes shame and self-consciousness, which causes further retreat from life. No matter where you go or what you do to conceal it, every time you look in the mirror, acne is there to remind you of just how dreadful it makes you feel.

"Acne teaches us to look for flaws," said Dr. Gayle Robinson, former president of the American Counseling Association. "It so focuses you on what's wrong that you develop a perspective of yourself as looking for flaws. That becomes habitual, a way of viewing yourself."

Acne's psychological effects are too often dismissed or discounted. We believe that acknowledging the pain caused by acne is one of the first steps in effective treatment. This can't happen without effective communication. "Acne's impact on the psyche is underestimated by parents, the general public, and sometimes even by physicians," according to Dr. John Koo, a dermatologist, psychiatrist, and the director of the psychodermatology clinic at the University of California at San Francisco Medical Center. "There is a tendency to trivialize all skin concerns in general. This ties in with the general myth that skin diseases are only skin deep. So the comment becomes, 'Aren't you glad you *only* have a skin disease? It would be *much* more horrible if you had diabetes, or arthritis, or asthma, or epilepsy.' But for those with acne, it is *not* more horrible. People with acne suffer as much as people with other diseases," he says.

In fact, some acne sufferers can be as upset and depressed by mild cases of acne, with only one pimple occurring once a month, as they can be by severe acne with the potential to scar. "We found that the cosmetic impact of even mild acne can cause a profound emotional burden for some young people," reported Dr. Madhulika Gupta, a professor in the department of psychiatry at the University of Western Ontario, Canada, when she conducted a study for the *British Journal of Dermatology* in 1998. This was confirmed by another survey sponsored by the American Medical Association, which showed that teens with acne are likely to have lowered self-confidence and poor self-image and to refrain from participating in social activities. Sixty-seven percent of those surveyed said their acne was mild; 30 percent said it was moderate; and only 3 percent said it was severe. No matter how many pimples appeared, all those who were surveyed suffered.

Many with acne also become anxious. Several controlled studies have shown that, justifiably, the worse the acne, the greater the anxiety. One study, which included a survey of 2,000 members of the Acne Support Group in Britain, found that 75 percent felt depressed, 40 percent felt anxious, and 15 percent felt suicidal.

These are feelings that must be acknowledged, not discounted. If a new patient drives across town, goes through the hassle of parking, and waits in our offices for her appointment, even if she has only a few pimples, we know she's upset. This is not an issue of vanity; it's an issue of self-respect. It's about treating a disease. Any condition that obstructs a person's relationship to the outside world, even if it's only a few blemishes, matters a lot. We're determined to take that person's need and disease seriously, assess the situation, and together devise the best treatment plan to fix it.

The desperate need for an acne patient's psychological pain to be acknowledged was emphasized when a new patient came to us in 1998. She told us that she'd begged her regular doctor, a general practitioner, for a referral to a dermatologist when her acne raged out of control. "You're married," he told her with a shrug. "What do you care what your skin looks like?" No acne sufferer should have his or her pain disregarded this way.

WHAT PEOPLE WITH ACNE HEAR ALL THE TIME

"She's really beautiful . . . except for her skin."

"Oh, do you have a rash?"

"Are you going to go out of the house without anything on your face?"

"How come your skin's so bumpy, Mommy?"

"What's that red thing on your face?"

"Are you eating junk food?"

"Don't you ever wash your face?"

"Why do you wear so much makeup?"

"Mommy, you look like a clown."

acne's emotional effects

Dr. Koo has helped us categorize acne's interrelated emotional effects. For teens the effects can be crippling, causing changes in their social life, academic achievement, and emotional development. For adults, social lives and job status can suffer greatly.

Our patients have no shortage of stories about the toll acne has taken on their lives, and we're quoting them verbatim here. Remember that you are not alone in your struggle with acne.

Psychological Factors

Impaired Self-image, Self-esteem, and Self-confidence

The first thing that nearly all the people we've ever talked to about acne have told us is that their self-esteem and self-confidence plummeted as soon as the pimples arrived. The more pimples, the lower the self-confidence.

> "My *exterior* affects my *interior*. Acne has kept me from being *me*, basically. I consider myself to be very attractive, and I take good care of myself, but acne lowers my self-esteem and leaves me with no self-confidence."

> "When you feel ugly because your skin looks ugly and infected, it puts a damper on a lot of the choices you make in your life."

> "Modeling agencies told me the only thing I had to do was clear up my skin, that I had what it takes to be a model but I had to 'take care of myself.' They didn't know how much it hurt me to hear this. They didn't understand that it wasn't my fault, it was genetic. Yet I still thought there was something wrong with me inside, that I would never make it. I used to cry every single night."

> "My acne got so bad that nothing would cover it, not even makeup. I was so ashamed of my complexion that I hid it all the time, either with my hands over my face or my hair down. I couldn't face the world."

Problems with Body Image

People with acne often see themselves as damaged goods and grow to loathe their bodies. We've noticed that our patients tend to consistently rate their acne as more severe than it is, in part because these patients have to deal with the devastation they feel whenever they leave the house.

> "Each and every morning I would wake up and have 'fear of the mirror syndrome.' I'd expect to feel and see these rock-hard marbles on my face and be reminded once again of the pain and leprosy I've felt for so many years. How could I expect others to look at me?"

> "People tend to talk *at* me instead of *to* me. Like they're talking to my pimples, not me. I always felt like it was my fault that people looked at me like that. Their stares seemed to say, 'What's wrong with you? Don't you know you have this on your face? Can't you take care of it? Can't you get rid of it?' "

> "I grew my hair really long to hide my face behind my hair, and that made it worse, because if you hide your face a lot, you're more prone to picking your acne and creating scars."

> "I used to cover it all up with makeup, which would make it look worse. I remember hiding in the bathroom stalls at school and just not wanting to go to class until the bell rang. Once in class, I had a mirror in my pocket to make sure I looked all right. I used to stay home when I had really bad breakouts because I didn't want to go out and have everyone stare at me."

Embarrassment Leading to Social Withdrawal

Parents of teenagers are often as devastated by their teens' acne as their teens are when they see their kids become shells of their former joyous selves. Teens with acne who had been outgoing and social can turn into withdrawn and reclusive loners who refuse to participate in activities they once loved. Adults also hide the shame acne causes them through social withdrawal.

> "I wouldn't even go out of the house without having makeup on. I used to joke with my friends and say that I wouldn't even take the garbage out without having makeup on because my face was that bad."

> "My thirteen-year-old daughter would get bellyaches when she got upset about her acne. She would be really sick, and she missed a lot of school last year as a result. Also, she wouldn't want to go anywhere with me, not out in public at all."

"I didn't get to experience all the things I should have experienced as a youth because of my skin problems. I had bumps. I had pimples everywhere. I didn't go to my prom. At graduation, I was trying to hide in the corner. It was horrible. I was scared to talk to people, to go to work. I didn't want anybody to see me. I was never in any photographs."

"My son was so introverted that he didn't want to look at anybody, talk to anybody, or go out to the store or anywhere where he'd see people. He'd just stay in his room."

"I missed a lot in life by having acne. You feel like you're not worthy of going to events that could have major impact on your life."

"I would sit on the train, and I was afraid to look up because I'd be thinking that people were staring at the way I looked. Sometimes I would just wish I could tear my whole face away. I used to pray every morning when I got up, 'God, what am I doing wrong to my face? Help me!' "

"The turning point for me was earlier this month when I went to pump gas. It was just a quick errand so I ran out with no makeup on—usually I always cover my face with makeup even though you can still see the redness and lumpiness underneath. The gas station attendant is used to seeing me with makeup. He looked at me and covered his mouth like he was surprised and asked, 'What happened to your face? Do you have a rash?' I couldn't bring myself to admit to him that I have acne, and I told him, 'Yeah, I have an allergic rash.' I was so embarrassed. I drove home in tears."

Depression

Professor Bill Cunliffe, a leading authority on acne and coauthor of a report published in the *British Journal of Dermatology* in 1986, did one of the first studies on severe depression from acne and facial scarring, which he and his colleagues claimed could lead to suicide. "Our message is that acne causes a lot of psychological and social effects, with low self-esteem, job discrimination, employment problems, and interpersonal problems, and that there are people who will take their own lives as a consequence," Dr. Cunliffe reported. The average age of the acne suicide victims was twenty.

The overwhelming majority of people with acne *never* have depression so severe that it leads to suicidal thoughts, but their feelings of sadness and loneliness nevertheless need to be addressed and treated.

"I guess it really hit when I turned sixteen. It even got so bad that when I had my senior pictures taken and I saw the proofs, I got sick. Everybody else was looking at theirs going, 'Oh, man, look how good they are,' and showing them to everybody. I left school, sat in my car, and cried. I would not let anyone see them, not even my family. It wasn't until I had them retouched that I ended up showing them to anybody, and a friend of my little brother said, 'You have clear skin in this picture. How did that happen 'cause you look like a pizza face?' Of course that hurt my feelings even worse. I thought I would grow out of acne, but I never did. I was so depressed I could barely function."

"I suffered from adult acne for seven years and it was devastating. I never suffered from acne as a teenager, and it truly disturbed my life. I'm around a lot of professional people every day, and having acne made it really tough to go into work and face the people that I had to face."

Anger

Acne patients often turn their anger inward, beating themselves up for something that is, as we know, not their fault. Sometimes this anger gets directed at others, too.

"I would get so mad about my face that I lashed out at anybody who tried to help."

"My brother turned to alcohol for solace because he was so angry and upset about his acne. That only made him angrier. He was like a lost soul."

"I was furious that I was wasting so much money on products that didn't work."

Preoccupation

Becoming obsessed with acne is hard to avoid, especially since we live in a society that places such a premium on appearance.

"Acne used to be the last thing on my mind before I went to bed, and it was in my thoughts all throughout the day. It consumed me and controlled me in a lot of ways."

"I used to lie awake at night worrying that my husband wouldn't find me attractive anymore."

"I looked like a monster and was so surprised my husband even married me. That's the honest truth, because I felt like a monster!"

Confusion/Frustration

Often acne sufferers are confused and frustrated after trying countless over-the-counter products, none of which deliver the intended results. This is exacerbated when they don't know where to go for advice.

"I became very frustrated because I was clean and sober for eleven years, but my skin still looked horrible, with a great deal of scarring from years of me just trying to scratch those things right out of my face."

"First I went to the drugstore, and saw this wall of acne products: dozens of cleansers, masks, and leave-on products. Then I went to the department store, and the salesperson recommended a three-step cleansing program along with makeup and concealers. I tried tons of different products and nothing worked. Everything just dried out my skin. I had no idea who to listen to for advice or where to turn next."

"I learned to live with the embarrassment."

Limitations on Lifestyle

Because acne makes people ashamed to be seen, they often arrange their daily schedules and even make career choices to avoid any exposure that might embarrass them. They also spend countless hours in the bathroom, carefully applying camouflage makeup to hide the blemishes. This is time they wish they could spend on more enjoyable activities.

"Years of having to live with 'the curse' kept me from outdoor activities when I was younger and a modeling career which I was close to having. Because I couldn't bear having to wear thick cover-up makeup and feeling self-conscious, I didn't pursue modeling."

"I am an avid swimmer and surfer, and my acne made it a real problem to go to the beach and into the water. I was always mortified when the makeup washed off and everyone could see what my face really looked like."

Difficulty with Family Members

It's bad enough to be judged by strangers. Those with acne are especially devastated when family members are not sympathetic. We'll discuss this problem in depth on page 78.

"One day my skin was fine, and then in a matter of weeks it was red, bumpy, dry, flaky, and I had these weird surface whiteheads. I was almost twenty-six—too old to get acne, right? Of course I was wrong. My family would make comments like, 'Oh, no more peaches-and-cream complexion.' That was incredibly painful to hear and completely insensitive."

"Even my family, who had seen me without makeup before, would ask me what was wrong with my face and if something had happened to me. They thought something was wrong because of the blemishes. What saddened me the most was my kids saying, 'Do something with those pimples.' They didn't want to be seen with me."

"My brother used to call me all sorts of names."

"I used to take a shower and wear an oversized towel on my head afterward so I could pull down the sides to hide my face. My family called me 'Towel Head' because I insisted on keeping the towel on until I could get my makeup on and cover the blemishes."

Reduced Dating

Acne sufferers often do not want to be seen, much less touched. People who feel unlovable often do not wish to risk any further rejection.

"It's something huge when you can't live a normal life because of your skin. My dating life was completely dead."

"When I was in college I was out on a date with this guy who said, 'You know, you'd be really attractive if you didn't have such bad acne.' I banned the word 'acne' from my house after I got married. My husband couldn't say 'acne' or 'zit,' the only thing he could say was 'blemish' if he had to say anything at all, because it brought up such terrible memories."

"I had moved away from my small hometown to a big city, got a divorce, and was really upset about a lot of things in life. One of the things I faced being newly single was the humiliation of adult acne. I was just so afraid to even meet anybody because I wouldn't know what my face was going to look like or how much makeup I was going to have to put on. I didn't smile very much because it hurt to. I was sitting by myself around New Year's Eve, and I figured, 'I'm making a New Year's resolution that I'm finally going to get some clear skin so I can stop being embarrassed when I meet people.' "

Reduced Participation in Social Activities

If self-esteem is suffering, it's hard to muster the energy and confidence to have a normal, successful, and fun social life.

"I was a complete loner in high school. I was too embarrassed to want to be part of any group. Besides, who would want to be seen with me?"

"The only good thing about my acne is I'm getting great grades, because when my skin is broken out I just sit in my apartment and study. It's so sad, but that's the way I feel. I just don't go out."

"I never wanted to go out because I had to wear makeup, which I hated. Putting on makeup would take so much time away from my kids and the little spare time I had. Even as an adult, I was really ashamed to go on campouts or swimming because everybody would see what my face looked like without makeup. I was so ashamed of how ugly it was—how pimply and red and scarred—and I didn't want to gross others out!"

"As I got older the option of going out with my friends depended on how bad my skin looked. If it was a dark place, I was more comfortable."

Impaired Academic Performance

Many teens with acne are so upset when their acne flares up that they stay home from school, missing valuable classroom time and social activities. Teasing by their peers also leads to anxiety and depression, which makes studying even more difficult.

"I couldn't concentrate on studying because I was always worrying about how bad my acne was."

"If your acne makes you feel worthless, why should you bother studying?"

"My daughter had acne from the time she was eleven. She has attention deficit disorder so her self-esteem was already pretty low. And when the hormones kicked in, that was an issue in itself. But with the acne, she really felt she was ugly and was afraid to go out in public. She became phobic about it, and I had to homeschool her for her seventh grade year."

Increased Unemployment and Career Problems

Studies have shown that acne patients face problems at work, especially in jobs where public contact is a must. "There are all kinds of discrimination against people with acne," Dr. Cunliffe stated. In one of his studies in the United Kingdom, written up in the *British Journal of Dermatology* in 1986, he concluded that unemployment was 45 percent higher among people with acne.

"At work I was promoted to a new position with a lot of responsibilities, including meeting with corporate officers from different companies. About a year later my bosses started taking me out of the field a little bit, saying things like, 'Why don't you stay in the office and catch up on stuff? You can go to the next meeting.' I was no longer just breaking out during my monthly cycle, I was breaking out all the time. Acne truly affected my career."

"Working in the beauty business for twenty years, I always had to look my best, and it took me hours to get ready for work. If my skin looked bad, believe me, my attitude was less than confident. And the person that hurt the most was me."

"People didn't give me as much respect as they could have because they thought I was much younger due to my acne."

"My son had acne so bad that the air force basically told him he couldn't be there."

"I really need clear skin because I've been working as a marine biologist so I get really dirty and wet out on the water. I can't wear makeup all the time to try and cover up my face. It's really horrible."

"Through college I worked with children, and it was very embarrassing. You know, kids don't keep in what they're thinking, and they were asking, 'Why does that lady have lumps all over her face? What's wrong with that lady?' "

"I turned down a promotion because it would have meant more dealing with the public, and I was so self-conscious about my acne that I didn't want to have to talk to strangers."

"My skin was so red and dry that flakes would literally fall off onto my desk. An inconsiderate coworker kept asking why I was doing nothing about it and kept drawing attention to my problem."

acne's emotional toll on teens

Few people survive adolescence unscarred or unscathed. Hormones are raging out of control, bodies are changing, cliques are forming at school, and once-trusted friends are becoming critical overnight. Taunting and teasing about skin—which, in fact, is usually worse than taunting and teasing about weight—go with the territory and have painful consequences. That Britney Spears was at one time called Zitney is no consolation to any young woman with pimples. Teenagers who want nothing more than to be like everyone else can be extremely sensitive to issues of peer acceptance and tend to be overly self-conscious regarding their appearance. It's especially critical to help all teens improve their self-esteem and self-confidence at this stage, because how they feel about themselves now often colors the rest of their lives. Teens tend to be victims of myths and misinformation about acne, so reassuring them that treatment is not only possible but should be highly successful can go a long way toward alleviating emotional upsets.

"Adolescents are at the highest risk for mental disturbances from acne," Dr. Hilary Baldwin, a professor at the State University of New York in Brooklyn, claimed in an article entitled "The Interaction Between Acne Vulgaris and the Psyche," published in *Cutis* magazine in August 2002. "Physical and emotional upheavals, which naturally occur at this time of life, can magnify the consequences of acne lesions. Hormonal volatility, issues relating to body image, sexuality, and dating can blow out of proportion even with relatively minor acne lesions, resulting in long-term emotional and functional consequences. Studies have shown that 30 to 50 percent of adolescents have psychiatric disturbances related to their acne."

"Adolescence is such a tough, sensitive time anyway, and it's especially difficult for teens when the signs of puberty are so starkly evident on their faces," says Dr. Yvonne Thomas, a psychologist in Los Angeles specializing in treating issues related to body image. "It's like having a neon sign flashing 'Look what's wrong with me!'

"To make things worse, kids who are already self-conscious to begin with find themselves at the mercy of their peers, who can be incredibly critical, mean, and uncensored during those teen years," she adds. "How a person looks can permeate into how a person is treated. After all, these kids decide, 'Who wants to be seen with someone who's thought of as a loser, or whose skin is an embarrassment?' "

Many dermatologists are engaged in research to quantitatively prove just how much acne affects teens. A report by the American Academy of Dermatology in March 2001 said that one out of ten teens surveyed nationwide believes that acne is one of the worst things about being a teen—and it makes them like themselves less. An American Medical Association telephone survey across America polled 1,000 acne sufferers, aged twelve to eighteen, about acne's effect on their quality of life. Nearly all of the teens worried about their complexion, with one-third or more indicating that they have felt anxious, embarrassed, or frustrated by their acne. Almost half felt that their complexion affected people's reactions toward them. They also thought that their complexion created an unattractive first impression, either socially or during job interviews, leading to many missed opportunities. Still others claimed that they had few dates either because they were afraid of rejection or because they knew no one would want to ask them out.

Yet there is no need to suffer. Once the acne is treated and controlled, the negative feelings it has engendered no longer have reason to exist. For an example, see Helene's Story—As Told by Her Mother.

family dynamics—"it's all your fault, mom and dad"

Because there is such a stigma about acne, talking about it can be next to impossible. Teenagers suffering through the usual pains and confusion of adolescence are often not communicative about many issues with their parents,

---

HELENE'S STORY—AS TOLD BY HER MOTHER

"My sixteen-year-old daughter is a beautiful person, but the acne became so bad she always wore turtlenecks, long-sleeved tops, and wore her long hair so it covered as much of her face and neck as possible. The acne was so bad on the sides of her neck, her back, her shoulders, and around the edge of her face that it left scarring, and the scarring on her neck was large, red, and pock-marked. We avoided dermatologists because of all the side effects of the drugs. We tried diet changes, vitamins, a Chinese herbalist, acupuncture, and special exercise programs. Finally, my husband and I decided we would take a loan out and send Helene to a plastic surgeon to laser the scars away. It was the most devastating doctor's visit of our lives. The surgeon was very kind and compassionate, and I saw how difficult it was for him to tell Helene that he would not have any success using lasers on her neck, as the damage would be greater than the scars that were already there. Laser surgery was her last hope, and the cry that came up from the depths of her soul cut into both the doctor and me. She felt she had nowhere left to go. We felt especially guilty because my husband and I both had acne as kids and felt responsible for passing it on to her, and now we didn't know what else to do for her.

"Luckily, we next decided to try Proactiv Solution. Three days later, Helene ran into the kitchen in tears, yelling and showing everyone the difference it made. Two months later, she told me she went swimming in a bathing suit and bought a tank top. I cried. It's so hard as a parent to see acne devastate your child's self-esteem and the ability to function completely in the opportunities life gives them.

"Helene has gotten back her life, and we're all ecstatic for her."

---

and parents in response often don't know how to talk to their teens. If parents sound even remotely critical, the result is frequently withdrawal by the teen.

Parents are the best judges of their children's emotional state. Yet because parents sometimes succumb to the same myths about acne that teens do, they can erroneously assume that acne is merely a normal part of being a teen. They think that their kids will simply grow out of it and that their kids should therefore stop complaining. We've had angry parents bring their teens to see us, and we understand that their anger comes from misinformation. We hear things like "He's not washing his face, I can tell." Or "He's not eating right, I'm sure." Or "She's not taking her medicine, just look at her face!" There's a lot of blame, which is unproductive.

"The most important thing for parents to remember is that their kids are not feeling bad for nothing," Dr. Thomas explains. "Acne is happening to them. It's *their reality*. So it must be acknowledged."

The truth is, as you know, acne *is* a normal part of being a teen, but treatment should not be delayed or avoided in the hopes that someone will grow out of it. While waiting for acne to go away, teens can feel tremendously lonely and embarrassed. Worse, they can scar irrevocably.

Parents need to find a manner in which to take charge of the situation without succumbing to anger or blame. (We'll talk about coping and communication between parents and teens beginning on page 87 in chapter 4.) Most parents who watch their kids suffer do so with an innate sense of helplessness that their beloved offspring is in pain. They blame themselves, feeling like bad parents. When their child is no longer making eye contact and holding his head down because he's suffering from a visible disfigurement, it's impossible not to feel responsible. So parents worry that they may be at fault, simply through an accident of genetics or because they don't know about successful acne treatments like ours, and this blame can deepen into shame, then rage. Part of the problem stems from this feeling that they have somehow failed their child.

Moreover, parents are often judged as harshly about their children's acne as their children are. It's a scenario familiar to any parent who has watched his child play team sports—there will always be the hockey dads and soccer moms who take these group activities much too seriously. A little boy is trying his best to hit a home run but strikes out. Instead of shouting encouragement, parents look at the little boy's dad, as if thinking, "Why haven't you spent the time throwing balls to your kid so he's a better player? If you were a *better parent*, your kid would be better. Better at sports. And better at having clear skin."

Feeling such peer pressure can be as upsetting for adults as it is for their kids. Much of this is a projected fear-based reaction. As in, "If sixteen-year-old Jenny's skin is so bad, my sixteen-year-old's skin can suddenly become that bad, too."

High-achieving parents sometimes set unrealistic goals for their children as well. "Perfectionist parents can't stand any flaws in either themselves or their children, whom they perceive to be extensions of themselves," explains Dr. Thomas. "They need to make an effort to separate their children's lives from their own, so that instead of focusing on 'Susie's acne makes me look bad' they can instead deal with 'What is this doing to my child?' "

Once treatment begins, they must accept that acne didn't happen overnight, so successful treatment is not going to happen overnight, either. Nagging won't help. Compliance is a common issue between parents and teens, especially with boys. Although parents recognize that treatment has to be a priority for the teen, sometimes it becomes a power play between the parent and the teen, who wants to assert his or her independence. It is often quite difficult to force teens to do anything, even when it's clearly intended to help the situation. Parents then respond with anger and frustration. When this happens, teens usually feel more ashamed and isolated than ever.

Acne can also create tensions within the entire family. When parents are embarrassed and angry, they tend to lash out. Siblings are usually fond of teasing and name-calling. In addition, younger siblings who see an older sibling suffer understandably worry that the same situation is going to happen to them. Unless the teen's acne is addressed compassionately and without blame, these tensions will continue to escalate, causing hurt to all involved.

acne's emotional toll on adults

Not even movie stars are exempt from the ravages of acne. It was widely reported that the lovely actress Cameron Diaz did not attend the London premiere of *Gangs of New York*, the film in which she starred, because her acne had flared up. "I have a serious pimple problem," she told *Vanity Fair* magazine.

Those with adult-onset acne are dealing with a condition they've never experienced before. Although adults may be more adept at camouflaging the pimples, they often feel stigmatized with what is erroneously perceived as a teenage disease. This is reinforced when they go to the drugstore for over-the-counter help, only to discover that nearly all the products are specifically geared to teen acne. Because adults often don't know where to turn for advice and are too mortified to talk about it with their friends or family, acne can leave them deeply ashamed. They withdraw, often making dramatic changes in every aspect of their lives. Professionally, their job performance can be hindered; personally, their relationships can suffer. We've had female patients who've admitted having problems establishing long-term relationships with men because of acne. They avoided putting themselves into intimate situations because they were terrified that a man might see them without makeup covering up their blemishes.

Adults whose teen acne has cleared up may suffer from residual emotional effects, which they often find too painful to acknowledge. "I've had adult patients who still see themselves as acne sufferers. The torment they endured as teens persists for years, if not decades," Dr. Thomas told us. "They simply can't let go of either the pain or the gnawing insecurities that they are still somehow unlikeable or unlovable because they once had acne. Sometimes these people are very successful professionally and have a happy family life, but inside their confidence is still lacking. Others thwart themselves because they are unable to find the self-confidence that had been shattered due to acne.

"I refer to this as the 'head/heart split,' where a person's thoughts are not congruent with their emotions," Dr. Thomas adds. "People who once had acne may logically know that their pimples are gone and their skin is now flawless, but they constantly berate themselves as still being losers."

This can be particularly difficult for those adults with permanent scarring, as well as for those adults who then watch their children grow and develop acne. With scars, the pimples are gone, but the past is still written on your face. This is a daily reminder of acne pain and can instill a lack of confidence as permanent as the scars themselves. If you have children, you can sometimes unwittingly project your own unforgotten shame onto your children by becoming unreasonably angry at them when their acne worsens. Should that happen, counseling may help defuse some of the rage.

No one should have his or her goals diminished by the shame and embarrassment engendered by acne. And with education and effective treatment, such as the Rodan and Fields Approach, no one has to.

acne and stress

Stress in life is unavoidable; it's part of the human condition. All of us suffer from varying degrees of emotional stress throughout our lives and find that our ability to manage it varies with each new situation. Sometimes stress can actually be a positive force in helping to effect much-needed changes. But for those with acne, stress is one of the cofactors that can exacerbate an already tough situation. On its own, stress cannot cause acne, but it can certainly make it worse. And if you're already feeling overwhelmed, the last thing you need is more pimples!

Why do pimples form when you're stressed? Most likely because of the higher blood levels of androgens and hormones called glucocorticoids secreted by the adrenal glands during periods of psychological stress. Androgens and hormones cause pimples by overstimulating the sebaceous glands.

the vicious cycle of stress

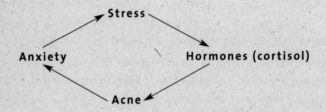

"Disorders characterized by demonstrable physical pathology that can be worsened by emotional stress are termed psychophysiologic disorders," Dr. Koo says. This category can include such conditions as peptic ulcer disease, migraine headaches, and Crohn's disease. According to Dr. Koo, "It is generally accepted that acne probably falls into this category as well since patients frequently complain of acne flares when they experience frustration, stress, or anxiety. For example, college students often report exacerbation of their acne during exam periods. From interviews with 4,576 patients with various dermatological problems, 55.3 percent of those with acne reported a close chronological association between exacerbation of their condition and episodes of emotional stress." Dr. Koo also found that it took only two days after the onset of emotional stress for acne to worsen.

Most studies linking acne flares to stress have been anecdotal, meaning they were not based on controlled scientific studies. However, a study by the department of dermatology at the Stanford University School of Medicine published in the *Archives of Dermatology* in 2003 was undertaken to further prove a link between worsening acne and stress. Their findings were the same as Dr. Koo's. In this study, students with acne were tracked as they studied for exams, and it was found that the subjects who had the greatest increases in stress during exam periods also had the greatest exacerbations of acne severity. "Changes in acne severity correlate highly with increasing stress, suggesting emotional stress from external sources may have a significant influence on acne," the authors claim. Ironically, during this high-stress period, students were so busy worrying about their studies that they were less concerned with their appearance.

We also know that stress slows down wound healing, sometimes by up to 40 percent. Which means that stress can not only worsen acne but can also cause acne to persist longer on your face or body. Just what you need!

"I work full time and am also toward the end of getting my master's degree," Lucy, one of our patients, told us. "On the nights I have class I wear my makeup all day, and I know I'm constantly touching my face while sitting there during class. Plus, I am always stressed. I find I always break out the next day without fail! It's so predictable I actually have to laugh."

Lucy is savvy enough to be able to laugh. And she knows that stress *can* be managed and diminished. For our unique system of stress-busting and therefore acne-busting techniques, see page 98 in the next chapter.

when picking becomes compulsive

Picking goes hand in hand with acne. (For photographic examples, go to www.unblemished.com.) There's a bump on your face, and you want to make it go away. This is a perfectly natural response. Those patients with an innate perfectionist streak can sometimes be the worst pickers, because they find themselves being driven crazy by blemishes.

"I counted the pimples on my face one day and had twenty-four huge cysts that were bulging and full of pus, so I picked and squeezed them," Wendy, age twenty-five, told us. "My family was totally grossed out. I always had a problem with picking. Now that my acne's being treated, I don't have anything to pick, which is amazing! I was sure that the picking would never stop. Now I don't have to worry about it anymore."

Another patient ruled by her need to pick was Samantha, a stunning woman of thirty-five. For her, what started as a little pimple turned into a monster-sized crater leaving untreatable scars. "I had to change a million restaurant reservations because of lighting and change seating arrangements at dinner parties when my skin was bad," she told us. "And I was accused of being completely crazy for picking nonstop in the desperate hope that I could somehow battle this problem. But I kept saying that I wasn't crazy! That if I didn't get pimples I wouldn't pick! People kept looking at me, because I kept picking and digging, hiding in front of the magnifying mirror in the bathroom first thing in the morning, which was a consuming nightmare. I went to every famous facialist in the world and countless dermatologists, and it was interfering with my life to such an extent that it was a primary obsessive-compulsive fixation. But I maintained all along that if there was something that would never allow a blemish to appear, there would be no issue at hand and nothing to battle."

Samantha was suffering from what is called *acne excoriée des jeunes filles*. *Jeune filles* means young girls in French, but we've found that most who have this condition are adult women. "*Acne excoriée* is an example of a more serious interplay between a primary psychiatric disorder and acne," Dr. Koo says. "The frequent end result is severe disfigurement from scarring. It is important to recognize that the diagnosis of *acne excoriée* refers only to the behavioral manifestation of picking acne lesions."

When people can't stop themselves from picking, *acne excoriée* can become an obsessive-compulsive disorder. "Obsessive-compulsive patients are usually aware that they should avoid their picking and that their behavior will cause damage to their skin," Dr. Koo adds. "However, in trying to inhibit their destructive behavior, they instead experience a steady increase in a 'compulsive urge,' which typically makes them restless and ill at ease the longer they resist picking. Eventually, their motivation to stop their behavior is overwhelmed by the intensity of their urge to pick."

Because scarring from *acne excoriée* can be severe, anyone suffering from it should see a therapist for appropriate treatment. Medications, such as certain antidepressants, can help. Dr. Koo has found that hypnosis can help, too. In one study, whenever a patient wanted to pick her face, she was instructed to remember the word "scar" and refrain from picking by saying "scar" instead. She was then able to stop picking.

Acne affects us all psychologically, whether we are among the 90 percent of people who suffer with it at some point in our lives or have loved ones who do. The stories from patients as well as the insights from the experts remind us that we are not alone with our hurt. Recognition of the emotional toll acne takes on our lives is the first step that propels us to take action, and by being proactive and taking action we can fix the visible manifestations of acne in order to heal the more insidious psychological devastation acne can wreak.

chapter four
the healing power of proactive treatment

"Put your best face forward, they say. It's your billboard to the world. Thanks to you I have a much better looking billboard."

—Anita, age thirty-two

the pain and unhappiness caused by acne can and will go away when it is treated properly. All you need to do is be proactive. Treat your acne, and you treat your lowered self-esteem at the same time. "The most significant reduction in anxiety and depression occurs in patients with the greatest dermatological improvement," Dr. John Koo, the director of the psychodermatology clinic at the University of California at San Francisco Medical Center, told us. "There is an improvement in mental state, a decrease in self-consciousness, greater satisfaction with general appearance, and decreased concern about losing weight."

So, stop *reacting* to the world around you, and start *acting* instead. Take control. Be proactive. This way you'll no longer be the victim of acne's ravages. When you change the face of acne, you can literally change your life. This is a tremendously freeing feeling. Becoming proactive will release you from the prison of your pimples.

We always tell our new patients that no matter what state their acne is in now, it will get better. There are many ways to approach the problem, and we'll find the right solution together. We address the outside problem— where the pimples are—with the Rodan and Fields Approach because we know it works. And we address the inside problem—where the hurt can linger—with compassion.

As you know, acne is a complicated condition. It didn't happen overnight, and it won't be successfully treated overnight, either. While your skin is improving, we have many suggestions for different techniques to help you cope with acne and manage both the stress in your life that aggravates your acne and the stress acne itself causes.

parents helping their teens cope with acne

Parents can resist succumbing to blame and yelling at their teens whose pimples are already painful and instead join their teens to create a proactive acne-busting team.

Role Models

Whether they want to admit it or not, teens struggling with adolescence look to their parents as role models for appropriate behavior. As difficult as some teens can be, during these tumultuous years they need their parents' supervision, understanding, and love, as well as clear channels of communication, more than ever.

Parents can work wonders by simply showing their teens that taking care of their own health is and always will be a priority. If parents take good care of their skin, try to exercise regularly, eat a sensible and balanced diet, get enough sleep, and work on family strategies to manage stress, their teens can easily learn by example how to respect and care for their own bodies.

Parents can also instill a healthy sense of self-worth in their teens. Teaching them kindness and to respect all people, no matter what their appearance, are simple values that will last a lifetime. If a teen learns that a person with acne has a disease on his or her skin and that the skin is not a measure of that person's character, that teen will not only treat others better; he or she will be less judgmental about his or her own case of acne.

Most of all, parents should never discount the pain their teens feel. The main focus should always be, "I love my teen, and I will do whatever I can to help." It's important to be extranurturing to counteract the pain caused by acne. Make your home a safe, emotionally secure haven from the slings and arrows thrown at teens by their peers.

Parents who are frustrated, upset, and at their wits' end worrying about their teen's acne often lash out without meaning to. Telling teens, "You'll just have to live with acne"; "Obviously, you're not washing your face enough"; or "I told you to lay off the chocolate" is one of the worst things to do. These statements imply not only that acne is not worth treating medically but that teens can't count on their parents for desperately needed help. Teens may then clam up completely and suffer in silence.

Compliance

An especially difficult situation for parents is when a teen is not compliant with a treatment program. When this happens, parents might need to step back for a while, as hard as this might be to do. We've seen teen patients who willingly begin treatment, then slack off. When they come back for a follow-up appointment, their parents are mad and the teen is sullen, defiant, and depressed. We tell the parents that it might not yet be worthwhile spending their money on acne treatment and that whenever their teen is ready to comply will be the best time to start treatment.

This is exactly what happened with thirteen-year-old Jon. "At first Jon wouldn't do the program," his mother told us. "I did everything and finally just told him, 'When you get tired of looking bumpy, you just let me know.' So when he got tired of it, he started following the directions, and we started seeing results almost immediately. His jaw has almost completely cleared up. And he's going to keep on using it now!"

Another mom has worked out a wonderful method for encouraging compliance. "Now that my own acne is better, my son and I do the Rodan and Fields Approach together every night," she said. "He knows that he doesn't have to go through what I did for years, and it helps him stay on track with his treatment."

Boundaries in the Home

Parents need to set boundaries within the home in terms of the amount of teasing about acne that's tolerated—aside from the normal, inevitable teasing that siblings are going to do anyway! The message should be: "Be sensitive." Family rules can be established to help facilitate this. For example, you may decide that the subject of acne is best discussed in private.

Still, we know how difficult it can be to stop teasing in the house. Which is another reason to treat acne: Take away the reason for teasing, and it will stop. "My little brother and sister used to make fun of me all the time, and they haven't said anything for the past couple of weeks," one teen told us when her acne improved.

"My brother said, 'Yeah, I have to admit you look much better but don't tell anyone I said that,' " another teen girl told us with a laugh. Without the physical reminder of acne, teasing by siblings will quickly subside.

Boundaries Outside the Home

Boundaries should also be established to deal with other relatives who may be misinformed about acne and therefore judgmental. Teens who are hypersensitive about any subject can be devastated when family members are critical. When Aunt Mabel wonders aloud why her niece Janey's face is "such a mess," when in truth Janey has spent hours scrubbing her face raw and then crying in her bedroom, no one feels better.

Parents can also be embarrassed or angered by what they see as meddling, no matter how well-intentioned, especially when relatives, who may not say anything to the person with acne, persist with bothersome questions, such as "What's going on with Michael's face?" Relatives, after all, usually know exactly what buttons to push. As a result, parents, who neither solicited nor wanted any advice, can feel like failures. This can be especially difficult for families when teens have a stubborn case of moderate to severe acne that may need several different courses of treatment, all of which take time.

Parents can ease tensions by remaining calm and not getting defensive. Talking to the Aunt Mabels of the world in a firm yet pleasant voice is a sure-fire method to dissuade further comments or criticism. We suggest rehearsing comments, such as "Yes, Janey is still breaking out, but she is now getting appropriate treatment for a long-standing condition, and this treatment should soon start working. We'd appreciate not discussing it further at this time," so that these comments slip out easily when most needed.

The same statement can be used when anyone makes unwanted remarks. Parents should realize that they have only so much control over what kind of intrusive statements they're going to hear. If parents are cognizant of their own trigger points, especially when cruel and thoughtless taunts make them feel embarrassed about their teens, they can remain calm and avoid being defensive. When parents are firm about not wishing to discuss a painful subject in public, it can be a wonderful lesson for hypersensitive teens, as well as help these teens realize that their parents are on their side.

Learning to Listen

Teens often don't show just how deep their pain truly is, so it's easy for parents to underestimate how much their child is suffering, especially a boy. It can be very difficult to initiate discussions about any topic that engenders immediate defensiveness and shame—especially the subject of acne—particularly with teens, whose favorite sentence seems to be "I don't want to talk about it." When teens say, "I don't want to talk about it," chances are that they *really* do want to talk about it! They're just looking for a comfortable way to start the discussion.

How to Talk to Your Teen About Acne

Parents who want to communicate with their teen about acne need to learn how to *listen*. Here are a few useful tips from Mary Ellen Davis, a teen-counseling expert:

- Be alone with your teen when you want to have a serious talk.
- A great time to talk is when you're together in the car, perhaps driving home from an after-school activity. Or you can suggest doing an activity that your teen particularly likes. When both of you are relaxed and in a place where you won't be disturbed, mention in a casual way that you also had acne as a teen and encourage a discussion. If you didn't have acne, you can easily mention someone close to you who did and acknowledge how this person suffered. The key is to *first* bring up *someone else* who has been treated for or who has suffered from acne, so your child doesn't feel that he or she is being singled out and is about to be criticized.
- Teens are often desperate to talk about certain difficult topics but are afraid to bring them up. If you can listen to appropriate cues, a much-needed conversation can begin. Try throwing out a few casual feelers, such as "I noticed

Jamie's skin has really improved. I wonder what she's using." Or "I noticed you're wearing your hair over your face . . ."

- Try not to bring up touchy topics if your teen is particularly upset about another issue or preoccupied with tests or studies. It's also not a good idea to bring up the subject when your teen has just gotten home from school or you've just gotten home from work.
- When you finally get a teen to open up, listen quietly.
- Repeat what you just heard. Say, "I heard you. You said. . . ." This proves to your teen that you were indeed listening and are not being judgmental.
- Realize and respect the importance of what is being said, even if it sounds trivial at the time. It most likely is *not* trivial.
- Give feedback related exactly and *only* to what your teen is talking about, to show how intently you are listening.
- Parents who are prepared for a discussion about acne can make suggestions, perhaps about seeing a dermatologist or starting a treatment program.

Be Encouraging About Finding Emotional Support

Being a teen suffering from acne can often be excruciatingly painful. Having a good support system in place is crucial. Helping kids feel good about themselves is critical for their emotional well-being.

As part of a good support system, parents must be advocates for their teens. In addition to making an appointment with a dermatologist, parents can go to school counselors, teachers, or principals to ask for help, especially to discuss teasing or bullying. If possible, this is sometimes best done without your teen's knowledge, as he or she can be mortified to find out a parent has talked to a teacher on his or her behalf! If parental trust is an issue, though, be sure to clear this tactic with your teen before you set up an appointment.

"This kind of support system can help teens deal with their acne, one step at a time, to find a solution," Kiki Humrich, a family counselor in San Carlos, California, told us.

In addition, parents can join an online support group for themselves and encourage their teens to join a support group as well. Being able to talk about acne in a sympathetic environment can work wonders. Also, parents can sit down and read the easy instructions for The Rodan and Fields Approach and encourage its regular use. Most of all, they can be reassuring that they're in this together. Since acne affects nearly everyone in the family, parents need to reaffirm that they want to do their utmost to help their teens.

teens helping themselves cope with acne

Teens can be just as proactive about treating their acne as their parents. "When teens tell me 'I still feel ugly,' I tell them they have to live with themselves for the rest of their lives, and they're going to have to look in the mirror at some point," Ms. Davis says. "They can choose to be sad and upset, or they can choose to start feeling good about themselves. It takes work. It might not be fun. But it's got to be done."

Be Compliant and Stick to the Program

The easiest and quickest way for teens to start feeling good about themselves is when they see their faces healing as their acne responds to treatment. It can literally be a miracle when a stubborn case of acne finally goes away—and stays away.

"When I had acne it just didn't feel like I would ever get out of it. After I started Proactiv, it was such a help," fifteen-year-old Justin told us. "I mean, it wasn't just something to put on your face—it was almost like a psychiatrist for me. It made me confident again. It gave me back everything I had before the blemishes came."

Justin realizes that acne will not go away and stay away on its own and that treatment needs to continue. As difficult as it can seem to have to follow a routine every morning and every night, in truth it takes only a few minutes a day. After a few days, it should become a habit as simple and essential as brushing your teeth.

Dealing with Teasing

Being teased and bullied about acne is one of the most difficult things anybody has to endure. It's emotional abuse. Developing a thick skin when your own skin seems thinner than ever is quite a task, one that can seem impossible.

Teens who are constantly tormented by their peers often want to do one thing only: hide in their rooms. One way to cope with teasing while your acne is healing is to force yourself to become more involved in an activity you love, one where what you do is more important than how you look. Focus on your talents and interests. Becoming successful at something that passionately engages you—whether it's music, dance, sports, gardening, community service, or art projects—can help counteract the fear of dealing with strangers (who might be judgmental or cruel about acne) and instead bring you a lifetime of new skills and pleasure.

Don't forget to educate yourself about acne; doing so will help you realize that it's not your fault. And as we often say to our teen acne patients, "That girl in math class with the perfect skin, the one who's been teasing you unmercifully? It's very likely that she'll be sitting in our offices exactly where you are ten years from now, sobbing her eyes out because she's suddenly developed a terrible case of adult acne." And it's true: Just about everyone gets acne at some point in their lives.

Emotional Support Is Key

"We encourage teens to find someone to support them emotionally," adds Ms. Humrich. "Someone of any age who you know will go to the end of the world on your behalf and tell you you're worth it. We live in such a 'lookist' society that having kind people around you with values more profound than skin deep is critical."

Count on your friends and loved ones. Online support groups can also provide much-needed solace from peers. If that isn't enough, professional counseling can help provide a safe haven in which to discuss problems and fears.

All the love and understanding in the world, though, is sometimes not enough for a teen who doesn't know what to do about treating acne. Sonia, who's seventeen, got valuable emotional support from her boyfriend and her family, but that made her feel better only up to a point. "I don't know why my boyfriend finds me attractive because I can't bear to look at myself in the mirror," she told us. "He tells me I'm beautiful. So do my friends, and my mom. I find it impossible to believe them. I still have no self-esteem."

Two months after starting The Rodan and Fields Approach, Sonia is a new person. "I've put my life back together," she said. "I don't have to keep my face down. I can pull my hair back off my face. I know I can because I'm beautiful."

adults helping themselves cope with acne

Acne's effects can linger long into adulthood. Or acne can begin after the teen years are long gone. The key point is to learn to become proactive and create a balanced life to help you cope with what you perceive as flaws. Whatever takes the focus away from acne and its effects will serve to strengthen you—body, mind, and soul.

Treat Your Acne Proactively

If your self-esteem is at an all-time low because of acne, the mere thought of trying a new treatment after so many other treatments may have failed can be difficult, and we certainly understand why. People who have suffered with acne for years have often seen their lives diminish in every respect. When you feel that you are always being judged and when you are not allowed to be yourself because of the state of your skin, it's almost impossible not to feel victimized.

No matter how old you are or how long you have had acne, as soon as blemishes begin to go away, self-esteem is immeasurably improved. "I feel that after a year of using Proactiv Solution, it's the first time in my sixty years that I really feel confident that my skin is going to be okay from week to week, and month to month," a lovely woman named Laura told us. "I never had a serious acne problem, but it was enough to make me uncomfortable. When you're not happy within yourself because you don't feel that you look your best, it just *does* something to you. I think it's particularly nice for more mature women to realize that we have skin problems and something can be done about them."

Emotional Support Is Key for Adults, Too

Adults need a safe haven to talk about acne as much as teenagers do. But even adults who have a built-in support system from spouses, family members, and sympathetic friends and colleagues can still be devastated by acne. "I used to ask my husband 'How can you love me with this face of mine, with all this terrible looking stuff?' And he didn't have much to say other than 'I just love you.' But I could never understand how he could love me," admits forty-year-old Lori.

Often adults, particularly women, are so embarrassed by their skin that

LISTEN TO TEENS

Ironically, acne is one disease where adults can get valuable advice from teenagers, as our patient Carl realized. "I'm a youth pastor," Carl told us. "I work with kids full time, and I've also suffered with adult cystic acne for the last ten years, starting when I was thirty. All of a sudden, I had terrible trouble with my skin. I went through Accutane and several other pretty heavy-duty medications to control it, and it went away for a while but then always came back.

"Then I noticed a couple of kids in my youth group with really bad skin suddenly make a dramatic turnaround—their skin was soft and clear. I asked them what they were using, and they said the Rodan and Fields Approach. I thought, 'What have I got to lose? I might as well give it a shot.' I started the program, and my face completely cleared in ten days. I mean not a zit, not a mark, and even some of the old stuff, which had been discolored and hadn't gone away, disappeared. I'm elated!"

they spend countless hours trying to cover up their blemishes and avoiding situations that might highlight their skin. Counseling and online support groups can be as helpful for these adults as they are for teens. Arming yourself with knowledge is equally beneficial. "I'd been ashamed for a really long time about something that I didn't feel I had any control over," a thirty-five-year-old patient explained. "Once I understood what was going on and was able to take charge of it, I could move forward with a treatment plan."

Successive Approximation

For those who have given up, as many do—especially adults who have resigned themselves to a lifetime of acne—it may be difficult to start a new treatment program. Dr. Yvonne Thomas, a Los Angeles psychologist specializing in body-image issues, suggests a strategy we like to call Successive Approximation, which is in essence a series of small steps toward the complete healing of your acne.

- Don't feel overwhelmed. This problem is not insurmountable. You can conquer it;
- Give yourself rewards every small step of the way;
- Carve out time each day to work on healing your acne.

Taking Time for Yourself

Many adults are so busy juggling work and home responsibilities that they simply don't find the time to take care of themselves. They ignore their acne and tell themselves it can't be helped. Yet a skin-care regimen should quickly become a regular component of your daily routine, as important as eating well, sleeping well, and managing all the hectic aspects of your life. Without it, your skin will suffer—and *you* will suffer. Looking after your skin is not a luxury. It's a necessity.

We hope that the Rodan and Fields Stress-Busting Program, beginning on page 98, can provide useful tips on how you can find the time to make your life happier, healthier, and more productive. As one patient told us, "My life is still full of stress, but thanks to your tips, I feel so much better about dealing with my life that acne just doesn't faze me anymore."

when professional counseling can help

The overwhelming majority of our patients suffering from decreased self-esteem, anxiety, and depression find that their worries and pain go away when their acne is treated properly. Some patients, though, need to be able to talk about these worries. Finding a sympathetic therapist or support group can be tremendously helpful. Counseling can also help educate patients and dispel the myths about acne that cause endless self-blame, encourage compliance with a treatment program to maximize its effectiveness, and set realistic expectations for immediate and future goals.

"It is a fallacy that therapy is only for the 'weak' or the 'crazy,' " Dr. Thomas told us. "I've found that the most healthy and emotionally stable people are the ones with a sense of self-esteem strong enough to admit that they have issues, and they know they can do the work necessary to bring them more happiness and peace within themselves."

Therapy for Teen Acne Sufferers

It may be difficult to convince a teen that counseling can be a good idea, but many teens secretly are relieved once they find a safe haven in which to discuss distress about their acne and other issues. For parents new to the therapeutic process, it may be helpful to interview therapists first to find one sympathetic and encouraging about getting their teen to open up about acne issues. Parents should also acknowledge to their teen that they know these sessions are private.

Therapy for the Parents of Teen Acne Sufferers

Therapy is very useful for parents who have trouble talking to their teens about acne and grow increasingly angry and resentful about acne's presence in their lives. They need to explore where their anger is coming from and, potentially, their sense of shame. It is only natural for the millions of parents who suffered from acne themselves to once again get those terrible feelings of inadequacy and mortification they themselves may not have resolved.

"Parents who are angry at their kids for having acne are often projecting their own defensive subconscious," Dr. Thomas says. "I'd suggest counseling for any parent with an out-of-proportion, angry response to acne. They can learn how to separate their own needs and instinctive responses to criticism from their teen's needs. Parents can replace their teen's fears of being judged with the proper empathetic response. Instead of shouting, 'Why can't you do something about your face?' a parent can calmly say, 'I know you are suffering. What can we do together to fix it?'"

Therapy for Adult Acne Sufferers

For adults who are devastated by pimples, especially those with adult-onset acne, therapy can help diffuse anger and confusion. It can also aid those who no longer have acne but still perceive themselves as losers because they were teased and tormented as teens. Acne sufferers often grow up to be intensely self-critical. "They fear that if someone gets close enough to know 'the real me'—in essence, 'to see me'—they'll 'see' the person they used to be," Dr. Thomas says. "The 'ugly one' or whatever label was pinned on the person with acne."

In addition, we've also found that a very small minority of both teen and adult acne sufferers fall into the category of self-saboteurs. They may be sabotaging their treatment, by noncompliance or sporadic compliance, because they are afraid of success, or because they are depressed and feel hopeless, or because they are used to the negative attention they receive with their acne.

WARNING SIGNS OF DEPRESSION AND SOCIAL PHOBIA

If depression and social phobia in acne sufferers persist, professional counseling should be sought. It should also be considered for cases of severe, compulsive picking, as this can lead to permanent, disfiguring scarring.

Parents should pay careful attention and seek professional advice if there are any marked changes in their teen's behavior. Adults should be able to recognize these warnings in themselves. These changes may include:

- abnormal sleep patterns, either insomnia or hypersomnia (too much sleeping)
- delinquent behavior, such as drinking or drug use
- deterioration in academic or job performance
- eating disorders
- lethargy
- loss of concentration
- mood swings
- spontaneous crying spells
- truancy
- wanting to be left alone
- withdrawal from usual social or work activities

We believe that the greatest success in life sometimes comes from taking the greatest risk—not a dangerous risk but a risk akin to attaining far-reaching goals. Some people just need a little more encouragement to be able to achieve those goals and dreams. Others may suffer from emotional trauma and need professional help to overcome it.

the rodan and fields stress-busting program

If you get up in the morning, look in the mirror, and see a mess on your face, you feel stressed. Your heart rate goes up, and you feel discouraged because you've got something unpleasant to deal with before you've even had your coffee. Acne robs you of the simple pleasure of facing each day without worrying about your appearance.

Stress and acne can become a vicious cycle. Mental picking is like zit picking: Once you start, it can be very difficult to stop, especially when you know that stress triggers flare-ups of blemishes. Then when your acne worsens you're even more stressed out. The key is to be able to break the cycle. And it can be done.

The best way to manage the stress created by acne is to start an effective treatment program. Your sense of control over a previously uncontrollable situation and your sense of relief will be wonderfully palpable. Life can and will change. The next step is to manage the stress in your life that can aggravate your acne by following our stress-busting program!

First, Treat Stress Systematically

We were once given some great advice by a colleague about dealing with life's complicated situations in a systematic manner. This colleague was a surgeon. Early in his surgical career, during a routine operation, he saw his patient bleeding profusely as soon as he put scalpel to skin.

"My first reaction was to think, 'Aargh! Call a doctor!' " he told us with a laugh. "And then I realized, hey, wait a minute, *I am* the doctor! Oh, no, the nurse is looking at me. I better do something and do it right now.

"And then my training kicked in. Instead of panicking, I approached the situation systematically. First, I applied pressure over one area, then I asked my nurse to put the gauze in another place to get it dry. I started in one spot, controlled the bleeding there, then moved on to the next spot. I kept going until the situation was under control. Step by step, until the bleeding stopped."

Signs You're under Stress

- avoidance of problems or people
- binge eating
- biting your nails
- drinking more alcohol
- getting upset by things that normally don't bother you
- losing your appetite
- losing your temper more easily
- picking at your skin
- pulling at your hair
- sleep disturbances

This same approach works effectively for stress. You can learn to manage your stress one step at a time, as proactively as you will learn to manage your acne.

Learning to Let Go

No one can fix all the stress in life. However, people who have a tendency to be either caretakers or ultraresponsible often think they are the only ones who can fix things. Learning to let go of what isn't your responsibility can be a huge relief and an automatic stress-buster.

If you have stressors that are out of your control, such as your commute to work, your mother-in-law's temper, your husband's increased workload, or your boss's bad breath, try to let them go. Easier said than done, we know! But if you learn to let go of what you *can't* control, you can take charge of what you *can* control. What can you realistically change? Certainly not your mother-in-law's temper, but if your job is untenable, you can take action by beginning in earnest the search for a new job.

Once you identify which stressors trigger your acne, paradoxically you can then relax about them. If you have an important exam coming up and you're nervous that your acne is going to flare, well, guess what? The acne is going to subside when the exam is over. At this moment in time, studying is more important than worrying about pimples. Try squeezing a small rubber ball instead of picking your face!

Changing Gears

If you're doing something to fix a problem and it's not working, don't give up. Change gears and try another approach. When we were in the development stage of Proactiv Solution, we often felt like rats in a maze, but every time we came up against another wall, we said, "Fine, okay. Let's try something else. We're not going to give up." No matter how much criticism we heard, we were persistent. We believed in what we were doing, and we weren't going to let naysayers tell us that our idea wasn't worthwhile. If we'd listened to them, we never would have achieved the end results we were after. We would have quit a long time ago!

Treating Stress Proactively

Treating stress proactively means that you develop a strategy to relieve the tough times *before* they happen or *while* they're happening. This will give you a measure of control and comfort, even when your knees are knocking! For example, when you know you're going to be facing a particularly difficult week—let's say you have to give a presentation at work before a roomful of strangers—and you're worried about your acne, use a treatment mask for the five days leading up to that week. Or, if you're taking antibiotics prescribed by your dermatologist, see if you can temporarily increase the dose.

Instant Stress-Busters

We like the idea of having an acne-buddy, someone with whom you can always talk about your skin's appearance, in confidence when you feel down. Other instant stress-busters include:

- setting aside time to relax in a calm, dark, quiet room;
- stretching for a few minutes;
- practicing deep breathing (see How to Breathe Deeply);
- planning a reward for yourself—a massage, a bouquet of flowers, or a luxurious piece of chocolate—once the stressful time is over;
- planning a vacation, even if that vacation may be a year away;
- cutting back on caffeine or other stimulants if they hype you up too much;
- exercising even just a few minutes every day;
- completing a task that provides instant satisfaction, such as cleaning out a desk or kitchen drawer (having your work or kitchen area free of clutter automatically lessens the feelings of being overwhelmed by your surroundings);
- scheduling a pep talk with someone who loves you;
- turning off the TV, especially the late-night news, which can be distressing.

Get Enough Sleep—The Presleep Purge

Adequate, refreshing sleep is crucial to everyone's overall well-being, yet the overwhelming majority of Americans of all ages are chronically sleep-deprived. A recent study showed that getting inadequate sleep can be as

How to Breathe Deeply

Most people breathe improperly, taking shallow breaths through their noses into the top of their lungs. Deep breathing comes from the diaphragm, which is located just above your stomach. If you watch a baby breathe, you'll see how he breathes in naturally from the diaphragm. You can find your diaphragm by placing your hands on your belly, then breathing in deeply. You should feel and see your hands move as the diaphragm expands as you inhale.

To take effective deep breaths:

- inhale through your nose for a count of three
- hold this breath for a count of three
- exhale slowly through your nose for a count of three

Deep breathing usually has an instant calming effect. If you're about to lose your cool, try placing your hands on your belly and consciously deep breathing for several minutes.

We also suggest taking yoga classes or using yoga videos to help you learn new ways to breathe for stress relief.

stressful as not getting any. It's hard to respond properly to any difficult situation when you're too tired to think straight!

Creating sleep rituals can help promote a healthy night's rest. Dr. Thomas has created a unique ritual called the presleep purge. Being able to break the worry cycle can relieve anxiety and break the cycle of obsessive mental picking. And for those who have no trouble falling asleep but find themselves waking up in the middle of the night, practicing the purge then is just as effective.

1. Put a piece of paper and a pen right near your bed. Lie down with the lights off and no distracting noises. Close your eyes. Begin your deep breathing. Continue deep breathing for five minutes to clear your head.

2. Keep deep breathing with your eyes closed. Go over what you're feeling and why. Are you devastated because of your acne? Why? Do you wish you could get rid of it? How? This is your time to acknowledge whatever is bothering you.

3. Open your eyes. Turn the lights on. Immediately write down all the thoughts that just ran through your head. Then take the paper *out* of the bed-

room. Put it somewhere else. Or you can shred it, burn it, or throw it in the trash, if you like.

This purging, combined with the deep breathing, helps you dissociate your troubling thoughts from yourself. By taking them away from where you sleep, you will stop those thoughts from disrupting your much-needed rest.

(For more tips to ensure a healthy night's rest, see page 339 in chapter 16.)

Make a Stress List

A stress list is a terrific way to prioritize what's going on in your life. At a time when no one is going to interrupt you, sit down with several pieces of paper or a nice new notebook or at your computer, and draw up a list of *all* the things that bother you and trigger your stress. Nothing is too small or trivial. Organize this list however you like. Once it's done, rearrange it on a scale ranging from small stressors to supersize stressors. Figure out which are the stressors you can control and which you can't. Then ask yourself "Which of the stressors I can control will I address first?" Some people like to start with the small stressors, then work up to the supersize stressors. Others like to start at the top and work their way down.

Every month reexamine your stress list. See what's changed. Then cross it off the list. Now you can tackle something else more crucial to your life.

Whether you start small or tackle a supersize stressor first, you will quickly realize that ridding yourself of any kind of stress is absolutely empowering.

Keep a Stress Journal

In addition to making a stress list, we've found that the act of regularly writing things down often mitigates stress. Keeping a stress journal gives you a safe place to purge that volcano of stress building up inside you before it has a chance to blow. It gets stress out of your system so you don't keep rehashing it. Your stress collected in journal form can provide a wonderful resource when you are ready to evaluate the stressors in your life.

Your stress journal is intensely personal and private. It is completely uncensored and not for sharing. You can write in your stress journal every day, once a month, or as often as you like. Certainly don't create more stress for yourself by trying to write in it every day if you know you won't write in it consistently. Some people like to jot things down all the time, and some people are just as happy writing sporadically. Having your stress journal available to you when you need it most is what's important. That way, if someone upsets you with a callous remark about your acne, you can pull out your journal and write that person a letter. You're not going to send it, of course. Instead, reread it the next day. Then decide whether you'll keep it, delete it, shred it, or burn it in the sink. If you choose to shred or burn it, enjoy watching your anger dissipate.

Find Time to Exercise

Regular exercise is crucial for everyone's health and well-being. (We'll discuss this more in chapter 16.) It strengthens your cardiovascular system, improves sleep, gives you more energy, and stimulates the chemicals in your brain that give you a sense of contentment. Just be sure to clean your skin completely afterwards, however, as sitting around in sweaty clothing can exacerbate acne.

If your life truly is overfull with responsibilities at the moment, don't create more stress by worrying about finding a consistent time to exercise. Instead, sneak exercise into your schedule. Park your car farther away from the office or the supermarket. Use the stairs instead of the elevator. Attack the weeds in the garden with a vengeance! Remember that every activity that raises your heart rate can improve your health and well-being.

the healing power of successful treatment

We want to end this chapter with comments from people whose lives were transformed once they started using the Rodan and Fields Approach. So many of these comments have a similar theme: "You've given me my life back!" If you or someone you love has acne, we hope you will soon rejoice in a similar transformation. Once you begin to be proactive, you should never have to suffer from acne again.

"Within five days of starting the program, my husband told me that I looked more beautiful than ever. And it almost made me cry because he never even once told me I was beautiful. It was a miracle to hear something like that. I feel happier than ever."

"I'm more focused at school. I've cut twelve inches off my hair, and I've lost a lot of weight. I don't have to hide anymore."

"Now I can finally go out with my teenage daughter and know that she feels good about herself. She's made lots of friends. Her confidence level has been tremendous. I can't even tell you how much that is worth to me. When I consider what the Rodan and Fields Approach has done not only for her face but for her emotionally, I'm just so happy. It's like I got my child back."

"At thirty-seven, I have three children. My kids, not to mention my customers and coworkers, have noticed a difference in my skin and my attitude. I'm so much more productive at work. I look people in the eye now instead of looking at the ground. I know my teenage daughters won't have to go through the anguish and pain I went through. I can't believe I found something that works!"

"I wasn't able to get a modeling contract as a teen because the acne on my face was so bad that they'd have to airbrush every picture ever taken of me, and it just wasn't worth it to my agency. I had the height, the looks, and the rest of the skin on my body was gorgeous. I was devastated and had really given up until I spent the night at the house of a friend who used Proactiv Solution. She had never seen me before without the makeup I wore, which was thick enough to cover the texture of the acne. She said, 'Just try it.' I did, and the next day most of the little bumps were gone. I couldn't believe it.

"After a year and a half I have a modeling contract, and I'm doing very well. When my agent describes me to a potential client, the first thing he says is, 'Her skin is absolutely gorgeous.' Nothing makes me happier than to hear that."

"For the first time in my life since I was a little girl, I am able to wake up and not have to look at my face in the mirror and wonder, 'What kind of strategy do I have to use today with my makeup to hide that spot?' My husband is looking at me differently. He's actually touching my face, which before I always used to wince about because I was afraid he would feel one of my bumps. Now my whole attitude has changed. You've given me my life back at age thirty-four."

"My twenty-nine-year-old brother would never admit to using what he called a 'feminine product,' but after I convinced him to try my Rodan and Fields Approach—which was hard, by the way—the change in his skin was very visible. After two weeks, the marks on his back and shoulders disappeared, and he was just so happy and much more self-confident. Now I can't get him to keep his shirt on!"

"When I was twenty I started getting acne. Worse, I was in school for skin care to get my aesthetician license, and there I was with this horrible face. I would go to class, and everybody would try to talk to me about what I should do and use and this and that, and I would get very upset and defensive.

"After I started using the Rodan and Fields Approach, my acne went away. Now that I'm starting my career, I realize that my acne was a blessing in disguise—because now I can empathize with people who have the same problem. Both the acne and your method for controlling it have helped me very much."

the rodan and fields approach: how it works

When we saw how confused people were about treating their acne, we were determined to take the guesswork out of the process. Acne is caused by too much oil formation leading to clogged pores, an overgrowth of bacteria, and inflammation. It is a complicated condition, but treatment need not be. The most important thing to remember is that our unique Rodan and Fields Approach is a simple, three-step *combination* approach, used on the entire face. It will combat acne when you:

1. **Unplug pores**
2. **Remove bacteria**
3. **Reduce swelling**

We came up with this three-step combination-of-medicines approach after we saw hundreds of patients entering our offices with bags full of their acne products: acne washes, acne toners, acne leave-on treatments, and acne masks. We'd lay them out on a table and invariably ask: "Do you realize that you used all these different products but they all have the same active ingredient?" How would the average consumer know this? It isn't your fault if you don't.

Maybe the formula is different. Maybe the label is different. But the active ingredient inside is the same. Even more confusing is that some active ingredients appear in both over-the-counter *and* prescription medicines. So these patients were often wasting their money and their time. They were not getting results and were becoming very frustrated.

When you look at the list of active ingredients on acne products, you'll see that the most common is salicylic acid. Salicylic acid works on comedones and plugged pores. Salicylic acid is *not* effective on red inflammatory acne lesions. So if acne products claim to "clear and prevent breakouts," it depends on what they mean by breakouts. If they mean those little blocked pores, fine. But what about those painful red bumps? Salicylic acid alone won't work.

Benzoyl peroxide is a great medicine for acne. It removes the bacteria that cause the red bumps and, to a lesser extent, helps unplug pores. Sulfur functions to unplug pores, and may reduce bacteria while minimizing redness and swelling. Topical and oral antibiotics prescribed by your doctor also remove the *p. acnes* bacteria and quell inflammation. And glycolic acid works as an exfoliator. It doesn't unplug pores as well as salicylic acid, but it can be an effective acne remedy.

Given the diverse benefits of these medicines, we figured that the best way to get maximum results was to use them in combination, specifically combining benzoyl peroxide, salicylic or glycolic acid, and sulfur. Here's how it works:

1. **Unplug pores**　　　*salicylic acid* or *glycolic acid* (and, to a lesser extent, *benzoyl peroxide*)

   products:　　　cleanser, toner, leave-on lotion, or mask

2. **Remove bacteria**　　　*benzoyl peroxide*

   products:　　　cleanser, leave-on lotion, or mask

3. **Reduce swelling**　　　*sulfur*

   products:　　　leave-on lotion or mask

In other words, you'll wash your face with a medicated cleanser, then apply your medicated lotions, toner, or both, and leave them on your entire face. Sometimes you might need a mask, too. Not so complicated, is it? This routine will take you only a few minutes every day for a lifetime of clear skin.

Why does this approach work when so many others fail? The reasons are simple: If you just unplug pores, you may still have acne, and if you just remove bacteria, you may still have acne. The number one mistake people unwittingly make, as our patients so often showed us, was to use a salicylic acid cleanser, a salicylic acid toner, and a salicylic acid leave-on lotion. This medicine can't fight acne on its own. But if you unplug pores, remove bacteria, and reduce swelling using several *different* medicines, you can control acne. As long as you're getting the right combination of medicine on your skin, you'll be successful. Some products are even dual action, which means they have more than one function. Using them will make your acne-busting routine even easier.

In each of the following sections, we give you a range of products to choose from. If you don't like the scent or texture of one product, you can replace it with another one in that section. You will still always need to have a combination of benzoyl peroxide, salicylic acid or glycolic acid, and sulfur to be used on the entire face every day. But you don't always have to follow the order of unplug pores, remove bacteria, and reduce swelling. You can use any of the three products in whichever order you like, as long as you cleanse, tone, treat, and end up with a leave-on lotion on your face.

Our combination philosophy and providing freedom of choice are two of the reasons we have both our Proactiv Solution line and our Rodan & Fields line. Proactiv Solution is successful at treating mild or moderate acne in people of all ages with all skin types. Rodan & Fields CALM was created to treat acne blemishes and also the acne component of rosacea and is designed for teenagers with truly sensitive skin as well as adult women with drier skin and a bit of redness.

Having two lines of acne treatments is also part of our ongoing philosophy of continuous research. If some people don't respond well to a certain ingredient, we want to make sure there is another system that will work for them. And if our clients are able to make changes in their skin-care regimen to find the perfect combination, they're more likely to stick with it to achieve and maintain results.

before you start

How to Wash Your Face and Apply Products

When she was growing up, Katie's next-door neighbor Loretta was a lovely woman with glowing skin, a former runner-up for Miss California. She taught Katie her method of washing. First, Loretta always rinsed her face with steaming hot water to "open her pores." Then she scrubbed it with soap. Then she rinsed with cold water to "close her pores."

We've modified Loretta's method (since it's not possible to "open" or "close" pores) to make it more user-friendly. We've found that some patients never learned how to cleanse and apply products properly, so their acne treatments are not going to work properly either. Let's now debunk some of the myths about washing:

Hot water means better cleansing

False. Hot water does not remove bacteria. It increases blood flow and dilates blood vessels. It just makes an already red face more red.

Hot water will open your pores

False. You can't open pores with heat. Pores don't open and close like little mouths or windows!

Cold water will close your pores

False. Cold water will only make you cold!

Scrubbing will make acne go away

False. Teenagers tend to scrub and scrub and scrub, often till they're red. Overzealous cleaning can really hurt your skin. Washing more than twice a day is not better; it only strips the essential oils that healthy skin needs.

Rubbing alcohol will clean your face

False. Rubbing, or isopropyl, alcohol is an astringent that strips oil off the surface of your skin. It doesn't maintain prolonged removal of the *p. acnes* bacteria. Worse, it breaks down the skin's natural barrier, exposing it to rashes and infections. We never recommend astringents with rubbing alcohol, even for the oiliest faces. Drying out the complexion is not the answer to acne, so read those labels and stay away from products that list rubbing or isopropyl alcohol as the major ingredient.

The astringent that we recommend for most skin types is witch hazel, a far less irritating form of alcohol, which acts as a drying agent.

Exfoliation will make you break out

False. If your skin has been properly and gently exfoliated, medicated products and moisturizers will penetrate better without having to dig through that extra top layer of skin.

As we get older, the rate of skin-cell turnover slows down. And when it's not sloughing off as rapidly, you get a buildup of your stratum corneum, the dead overlapping skin cells that sit on the surface of skin like shingles on a roof. If this layer is thick, your skin will look dull and dry, and makeup will cake and streak. Exfoliation gives you back that glow and polish.

The exceptions to exfoliation are red skin with what appears to be "broken" blood vessels, and sensitive, eczema-prone skin. We do not recommend exfoliation in these cases.

Washing Basics

- Use lukewarm water;
- Use a very soft, cotton terry washcloth. Or try your fingertips or a facial Buf-Puf type of sponge in different grades;
- Pat your skin dry with a soft, cotton towel.

Don't Forget Your Hands

Make sure your hands are clean before you wash your face or apply any products.

With all the media-hyped fears about germs, antibacterial hand wipes have been overused. If you're away from home without access to soap and water, these towelettes serve a purpose. Overuse, on the other hand, contributes to bacterial resistance, which may render useless conventional antibiotics for common infections.

Application Basics for Medicated Products

For Cleansers

- Remove any eye makeup with a noncomedogenic cleanser or oil-free makeup remover pads;
- Dampen skin with lukewarm water;
- Use your fingertips to apply cleanser in a circular motion over your entire face;
- Avoid the sensitive area closest to your eyes;
- Massage for twenty seconds to one minute;
- Rinse with lukewarm water;
- Pat dry.

For Leave-on Products

- Make sure your cleansed skin is dry. If it's wet, you may experience unnecessary irritation;
- Use gauze pads or cotton balls for thin liquids, such as toners or astringents;
- For creams or lotions, use your fingertips;
- Apply the product over your entire face;
- Avoid the sensitive eye and mouth areas;
- Let it dry;
- In the morning, gently pat on sunscreen. You need about a teaspoon for your entire face;
- If you use moisturizer, apply it before the sunscreen.

What If My Skin Becomes Irritated?

Everyone's skin type is different, and so is its ability to tolerate topical medications. We have found that a 2.5 percent benzoyl peroxide solution is just as effective as a 5 percent or 10 percent solution, the standard percentage in over-the-counter products, so we recommend starting with a 2.5 percent product for most people. With benzoyl peroxide, more does not necessarily mean more bacteria removal—it often means more dryness and irritation. The exception is for those with extremely oily skin and moderate to severe acne, who can often tolerate a higher benzoyl peroxide dose without irritation.

No matter what your skin type, always start by using a medicated program once a day. After gradually building up your tolerance, over one to three weeks increase to twice daily. Some people are never able to use medicated products twice a day; their skin simply becomes too irritated. If you can only use them once a day, it's best to apply everything at night. If your skin gets red, dry, dehydrated, or irritated, stop using them every day; try every other day. It is okay to take a few days off to allow your skin to recover, using gentler, nonmedicated products, such as mild cleansers, in the meantime.

the rodan and fields approach: programs 1 through 6

What follows are unique and comprehensive programs for treating acne in different ages and different skin types. Each of these six programs has differ-

CLEANSERS TO USE WHEN NOT USING MEDICATED TREATMENTS

In some cases, medicated treatment may be inadvisable more than once a day. In other cases, your skin will need time to adjust before using treatments twice a day. What should you use to cleanse your skin without aggravating your acne in the meantime? Here are some tips for using other products:

- Foaming cleansers are good for oily skin, although lathering isn't necessary for a cleanser to work properly;
- For dry skin, creamy cleansers are good. Moisturizing bar soaps, such as Dove or Olay, can work as well, although many people prefer soap-free cleansers;
- Cetaphil Gentle Skin Cleanser is one of the most effective cleansers for sensitive skin, especially for those with rosacea;
- Other cleansers that are mild and noncomedogenic are:
  - Avance Algae Deep Gentle Cleanse
  - Aveeno Clear Complexion Foaming Cleanser
  - Biotherm Acnopur Purifying Cleanser
  - Biotherm Biopur Matifying Astringent Lotion Alcohol-Free
  - Cetaphil Daily Facial Cleanser for Normal to Oily Skin
  - Clearasil Daily Face Wash Sensitive Skin
  - Elemis Rehydrating Ginseng Toner
  - Ellen Lange Daily Maintenance Oil Control Cleanser
  - Eucerin Gentle Hydrating Cleanser
  - Eucerin Pore Purifying Foaming Wash
  - Jurlique Face Wash Cream
  - L'Oréal Ideal Balance Foaming Cream Cleanser
  - L'Oréal Ideal Balance Foaming Gel Cleanser
  - Physicians Formula Deep Pore Cleansing Gel
  - Rodan & Fields COMPOUNDS Gentle Wash
- Toners containing alcohol are much too drying for the skin. They strip superficial oil, which your body quickly replaces. A toner is not necessary for cleansing, but it can be an effective means to deliver moisture or medicine. Look for a toner or a serum that contains an alpha hydroxy or beta hydroxy acid, one with Vitamins C and E or other antioxidants, or one with hyaluronic acid, a humectant, which restores moisture in the skin. Avance Vitamin C Cerum, EmerginC Topical Vitamin C (cream or gel), Elemis Active Skin Complex, Ellen Lange Daily Maintenance Peel Plus Pads with alpha and beta hydroxy acids, and Rodan & Fields CALM 2 Prepare with salicylic acid are good examples.

ent product options. Remember, use these products on your *entire face*, not only on acne-prone areas, except where noted. The sensitive eye area should be avoided, of course, except where eye creams are indicated.

Every day you need to clean, tone, and treat your skin. The products you use need medicines to unplug pores, remove bacteria, and reduce swelling. The active ingredients in some of these products are applicable in several categories. For example, salicylic acid, which unplugs pores, is often an active ingredient in cleansers, toners, leave-on lotions, and moisturizers; and benzoyl peroxide, which removes bacteria and helps to unplug pores, is often an active ingredient in cleansers and leave-on lotions. This explains why Proactiv Solution Renewing Cleanser and Proactiv Solution Repairing Lotion, which contain benzoyl peroxide, both unplug pores and remove bacteria. However, we are listing cleansers only in Step 1—Unplug Pores and not Step 2—Remove Bacteria. The reason is simple: Leave-on lotions, such as Proactiv Solution Repairing Lotion, must be applied *after* cleansing and toning.

You will also notice that the order of the three steps is different for Proactiv Solution products from that for Rodan & Fields CALM products. That's because the formulation in each system is different, even though some ingredients are similar and the purpose remains the same. The order of use of ingredients is interchangeable as long as you cleanse, tone, and treat with salicylic acid or glycolic acid, benzoyl peroxide, and sulfur in some combination and end up with a leave-on lotion.

Note: "Apply sparingly" means you should use a dime-sized amount of product. It should be enough to have a thin coat applied over the entire surface of the skin where needed. It is always better to use less product rather than more!

Note: In the Extra Help sections, you may choose more than one product, such as a mask, a leave-on lotion, or a moisturizer, if needed.

program 1—teenage girl with persistent acne

Lacey is seventeen and desperate. "I don't want to go anywhere—especially prom and homecoming," she explains. "I don't like wearing makeup, but I have to put it on so people won't look at me." She smiles ruefully and continues, "I don't have problems dating because I've been with my boyfriend for a long time, but some girls say to him, 'Ugh, I don't know why you're with her. She has acne!' " He's such a great guy that he doesn't listen to them, but sometimes I feel like acne makes me very ugly. My boyfriend and my parents try to make me feel better and tell me that I'm a beautiful girl, but that only makes me cry. Some people don't understand about acne because they never had it—they don't know the pain and embarrassment it causes. I've tried so many products; you name it. My parents have spent so much money on dermatologists, department store products, and over-the-counter medicine, and nothing has worked. I need help!"

Despite her acne, Lacey's skin isn't especially oily, but it is raw and red from her overzealous washing and scrubbing. She can choose from three treatment options.

IT'S OKAY TO WEAR MAKEUP WHEN YOU HAVE ACNE

Many teenage girls and women are afraid to wear makeup because they worry it will make their acne worse. And in truth, the wrong makeup *can* make acne worse. Comedogenic foundation will definitely clog pores. We also see a lot of teens and women with little blackheads right on the edge of their lips, because they are constantly reapplying thick, waxy, comedogenic lip glosses.

Scientists have investigated what happens to makeup after it is applied. They discovered that it either migrates into pores or comes off on the hands. This does not mean, however, that all foundations are comedogenic. In fact, most are not. Comedogenicity occurs only in formulas that contain occlusive or irritating ingredients. And because makeup does tend to travel into the pore, if medicine is incorporated into a foundation formulation, it will help unplug or clear that pore. Therefore, a good, noncomedogenic foundation, medicated with such ingredients as benzoyl peroxide, salicylic acid, or sulfur, can help clear up acne. It can also provide protection from the sun's harmful rays.

If you use the right noncomedogenic makeup, it can go a very long way toward improving your appearance and self-confidence. For more information about how to use makeup effectively when you have acne, see chapter 17.

TREATMENT 1: PROACTIV SOLUTION
Start by using this treatment once a day for two weeks, then increase to twice a day. Until you are able to tolerate its use twice a day or if you remain at once

a day, use a mild cleanser, such as Cetaphil Gentle Skin Cleanser or Rodan & Fields COMPOUNDS Gentle Wash, when not using Proactiv Solution products.

1. Unplug Pores—glycolic acid, benzoyl peroxide

a) Renewing Cleanser	Wash off and pat dry.
b) Revitalizing Toner	Apply with gauze or cotton ball. Let dry.

2. Remove Bacteria—benzoyl peroxide

Repairing Lotion*	Apply with fingertips. Let dry. Use in the morning only.

3. Reduce Swelling—sulfur

Concealer Plus	Lightly dot on with applicator. Blend with concealer brush or fingertips. Use once or twice a day.
Refining Mask	Apply to clean, dry face or other affected area. Let dry ten minutes. Rinse with lukewarm water. Use once or twice a week for maintenance or every night for the five nights leading up to menstruation.

4. Extra Help—Proactiv Solution

Clarifying Night Cream*	Apply sparingly to dry skin. Use at night only.
Daily Oil Control (for slightly oily skin)	Apply to entire face or other affected area with fingertips after toner. Let dry. Use daily or as needed.
Green Tea Moisturizer	Apply sparingly to dry skin.
Matte Skin Finish (for very oily skin)	Apply sparingly to oily areas. Brush off residue when dry.
Sheer Finish Compact Foundation	Apply sparingly.
Sheer Finish Loose Powder	Apply sparingly over foundation.
Skin-Clearing Cream to Powder Foundation	Apply sparingly.

* If skin becomes dry when using Repairing Lotion twice a day, Repairing Lotion can be used in the morning, and Clarifying Night Cream can be used at night.

TREATMENT 2: RODAN & FIELDS CALM

Start by using this treatment once a day for two weeks, then increase to twice a day. Until you are able to tolerate its use twice a day or if you remain at once a day, use a mild cleanser, such as Cetaphil Gentle Skin Cleanser or Rodan & Fields COMPOUNDS Gentle Wash, when not using Rodan & Fields CALM products.

1. Reduce Swelling—sulfur

Rodan & Fields CALM 1   Wash off and pat dry.
  Wash (cleanser)

2. Unplug Pores—salicylic acid

Rodan & Fields CALM 2   Apply with gauze or cotton ball. Let dry.
  Prepare (toner)

3. Remove Bacteria—benzoyl peroxide

Rodan & Fields CALM 3   Apply with fingertips. Let dry.
  Treat (leave-on lotion)

4. Extra Help

Proactiv Solution Green Tea Moisturizer	Apply sparingly to dry skin.
Proactiv Solution Sheer Finish Compact Foundation	Apply sparingly.
Proactiv Solution Sheer Finish Loose Powder	Apply sparingly over foundation.
Proactiv Solution Skin-Clearing Cream to Powder Foundation	Apply sparingly.
Rodan & Fields CALM Soothe (mask)	Mix ingredients into a paste. Apply to face or other affected area. Let dry ten minutes. Peel off. Use once or twice a week or every night for the five nights leading up to menstruation.
Rodan & Fields COMPOUNDS Moisture	Apply to dry or irritated skin.

TREATMENT 3: OTHER PRODUCTS

Start by using this treatment once a day for two weeks, then increase to twice a day. Until you are able to tolerate its use twice a day or if you remain at once a day, use a mild cleanser, such as Cetaphil Gentle Skin Cleanser or Rodan & Fields COMPOUNDS Gentle Wash, when not using other products. Remember to pick only one product from each list, except in the Extra Help section, where you may choose more than one product, such as a moisturizer, if needed.

1. Unplug Pores—salicylic acid

Clean & Clear Blackhead   Wash off and pat dry.
  Clearing Scrub

Clinique Acne Solution
 Cleansing Foam
Iman Perfect Response
 Oil-Free Cleanser
L'Oréal Ideal Balance
 Foaming Cream Cleanser
L'Oréal Pure Zone Skin
 Balancing Cream
 Cleanser
Neutrogena Multi-
 vitamin Skin Therapy
Peter Thomas Roth Beta
 Hydroxy Acid 2% Acne
 Wash

2. Remove Bacteria—benzoyl peroxide

Clear By Design Gel 2.5%   Apply with fingertips. Let dry.
Neutrogena On-the-Spot
 Acne Treatment

3. Reduce Swelling—sulfur

Clearasil Adult Care   Apply sparingly with fingertips. Let dry.
 Acne Treatment Cream
Origins Out of Trouble   Apply with fingertips to face or other affected area.
 Mask   Let dry ten minutes. Rinse with lukewarm water. Use
                              once or twice a week, more if needed.

4. Extra Help

Clean & Clear Oil-Free   Apply sparingly to dry skin.
 Dual Action Moisturizer
Clearasil Total Control
 Daily Skin Perfecting
 Treatment
L'Oréal Pure Zone Oil-
 Free Moisturizer
Neutrogena SkinClearing
 Moisturizer

Don't Forget the Sunscreen

For all three treatments, applying sunscreen in the morning is the all-important final step. Apply after all treatment products have dried.

Clinique Sun Care Face SPF 15
Estée Lauder In the Sun Sunblock For Face SPF 15
Neutrogena Ultra Sheer Dry-Touch Sunblock SPF 30
Olay Complete UV Defense Moisture Lotion
Ombrelle Sunscreen Lotion SPF 30
Prescriptives All You Need Broad Spectrum Oil Absorbing Lotion SPF 15
Proactiv Solution Daily Protection Plus SPF 15
Proactiv Solution Oil Free Moisture SPF 15
Rodan & Fields COMPOUNDS Protect SPF 15

program 2—teenage boy with persistent acne

John is a nineteen-year-old college student with persistent acne since puberty. "My face is eaten up by pimples and zits, and I am so ashamed of it that I feel like going to school with a bag over my head," he says. "Plus I always have huge red bumps that make shaving a total pain. I feel that fighting my acne is like fighting a modern battle with guns left over from the Civil War—I never feel I have the weapons to fight my acne, it is always that bad. Every time I feel a bump coming up I say, 'Oh, great, here comes another one.' There is nothing I can do."

John can tolerate a fairly aggressive approach because he has very oily skin.

TREATMENT 1: PROACTIV SOLUTION

Start by using this treatment once a day for two weeks, then increase to twice a day. Until you are able to tolerate its use twice a day or if you remain at once a day, use a mild cleanser, such as Cetaphil Gentle Skin Cleanser or Rodan & Fields COMPOUNDS Gentle Wash when not using Proactiv Solution products.

1. Unplug Pores—salicyclic acid, glycolic acid
a) Deep Cleansing Wash   Wash off and pat dry.
b) Revitalizing Toner   Apply with gauze or cotton ball. Let dry.

2. Remove Bacteria—benzoyl peroxide
Repairing Lotion   Apply with fingertips. Let dry.

3. Reduce Swelling—sulfur
Concealer Plus   Lightly dot on with applicator. Blend with concealer brush or fingertips. Use once or twice a day.

Refining Mask	Apply to clean, dry face or other affected area. Let dry ten minutes. Rinse with lukewarm water. Use once or twice a week, more often if needed.

4. Extra Help—Proactiv Solution

ClearZone Body Pads*	Use in place of cleanser.
Daily Oil Control (for slightly oily skin)	Apply to entire face or other affected area with fingertips after toner. Let dry. Use daily or as needed.
Matte Skin Finish (for very oily skin)	Apply sparingly to oily areas. Brush off residue when dry.
Mild Exfoliating Peel	Apply thin layer. Let dry one to two minutes. Remove with fingertips. Rinse with lukewarm water. Use once a week.
Oil Blotter Sheets	Use as needed to pat away excess oil.
Rodan & Fields CLEAN Regimen for Blackhead Extraction	Follow instructions in kit.

* Body pads may be used on the face for a quick midday facial cleansing without a trip to the sink. They can also be used after playing sports.

TREATMENT 2: PROACTIV SOLUTION EXTRA STRENGTH

This treatment includes a 7 percent benzoyl peroxide cleanser and leave-on lotion, which is usually well tolerated by those with extremely oily skin and stubborn acne who have failed treatment with products containing 2.5 percent benzoyl peroxide. Start by using this treatment once a day for two weeks, then increase to twice a day. Until you are able to tolerate its use twice a day or if you remain at once a day, use a mild cleanser, such as Cetaphil Gentle Skin Cleanser or Rodan & Fields COMPOUNDS Gentle Wash when not using Proactiv Solution Extra Strength products.

Please note that you can also use the regular Proactiv Solution (Treatment 1, above) in the morning and Proactiv Solution Extra Strength at night if you find that the Extra Strength treatment is too drying for your skin when used twice a day.

1. Unplug Pores—salicylic acid

a) Extra Strength Cleanser	Wash off and pat dry.
b) Extra Strength Toner	Apply with gauze or cotton ball. Let dry.

2. Remove Bacteria—benzoyl peroxide

Extra Strength Lotion   Apply with fingertips. Let dry.

3. Reduce Swelling—sulfur

Extra Strength Mask   Apply to clean, dry face or other affected area. Let dry ten minutes. Rinse with lukewarm water. Use once or twice a week.

4. Fade Brown Spots—hydroquinone

Skin Lightening Lotion   Use at night only. Apply with fingertips to affected area.

Rodan & Fields RADIANT Regimen   Follow directions in kit.

5. Extra Help—Proactiv Solution

ClearZone Body Pads*   Use in place of cleanser.

Daily Oil Control (for slightly oily skin)   Apply to entire face or other affected area with fingertips after toner. Let dry. Use daily or as needed.

Matte Skin Finish (for very oily skin)   Apply sparingly to oily areas. Brush off residue when dry.

Oil Blotter Sheets   Use as needed to pat away excess oil.

Rodan & Fields CLEAN Regimen for Blackhead Extraction   Follow instructions in kit.

* Body pads may be used on the face for a quick midday facial cleansing without a trip to the sink. They can also be used after playing sports.

TREATMENT 3: OTHER PRODUCTS

Start by using this treatment once a day for two weeks, then increase to twice a day. Until you are able to tolerate its use twice a day or if you remain at once a day, use a mild cleanser, such as Cetaphil Gentle Skin Cleanser or Rodan & Fields COMPOUNDS Gentle Wash, when not using other products. Remember to pick only one product from each list, except in the Extra Help section, where you may choose more than one product, such as a cleansing pad or a leave-on lotion, if needed.

1. Unplug Pores—salicylic acid

Clean & Clear Blackhead Clearing Scrub   Wash off and pat dry.

Clearasil 3-in-1 Acne Cleanser

L'Oréal Ideal Balance
  Foaming Gel Cleanser
Neutrogena Oil-Free
  Acne Wash

2. Remove Bacteria—benzoyl peroxide

Clean & Clear Persa-   Apply with fingertips. Let dry.
  Gel 5
Fostex 5 Cream
Neutrogena On-the-
  Spot Therapy
Oxy 5 Sensitive Skin
  Vanishing Lotion
PanOxyl 5 Gel

3. Reduce Swelling—sulfur

Clearasil Adult Care   Apply sparingly with fingertips. Let dry.
  Acne Treatment Cream

4. Extra Help

Clearasil Pore Cleansing   Wipe on. Let dry.
  Pads*
Clinique Night   Apply with fingertips. Let dry.
  Treatment Gel
Neutrogena Clear Pore
  Shine Control Gel
Oxy Daily Cleansing Pads* Wipe on. Let dry.
Stri-Dex Sensitive Skin
  Triple Action Acne Pads*

* Body pads may be used on the face for a quick midday facial cleansing without a trip to the sink. They can also be used after playing sports.

Don't Forget the Sunscreen

For all three treatments, applying sunscreen in the morning is the all-important final step. Apply after all treatment products have dried.

  Clearasil Acne Treatment Cream SPF 15*
  Neutrogena Ultra Sheer Dry-Touch Sunblock SPF 45
  Olay Complete UV Defense Moisture Lotion
  Ombrelle Sunscreen Lotion SPF 30
  Proactiv Solution Daily Protection Plus SPF 15

Proactiv Solution Sheer Tint Moisture SPF 15*
Rodan & Fields COMPOUNDS Protect SPF 15

* These are excellent solutions for boys as they're cover-ups, not makeup, and the slight tint helps camouflage redness while they protect the skin from the sun.

program 3—twenty-eight-year-old woman with adult-onset acne and oily skin

Marie is twenty-eight and horrified by her adult-onset acne. "As a teenager I had beautiful, clear skin. But then it happened: I wake up one day and notice I have a breakout. I can't believe my eyes! I think it will go away, but it doesn't. I start breaking out more and more—it's horrifying. My husband is wondering what's happening, and my young son asks me why I have so many boo-boos on my face. I'm so depressed I quit my job, because I feel people are looking at my blemishes and not at me. I am so ashamed. I don't want my family members to see me, not even my own husband. I turn off the lights in our house, because they make the blemishes more noticeable. It's so bad and I am so depressed, I only want to go out when it's dark. I buy so many products, but they only make things worse, which makes me feel totally hopeless."

Marie needs the benefit of full-face medicine and makeup. She doesn't need to fear using the amount of concealing makeup she desperately needs to make her feel better and be able to leave the house without shame.

TREATMENT 1: PROACTIV SOLUTION

Start by using this treatment once a day for two weeks, then increase to twice a day. Until you are able to tolerate its use twice a day or if you remain at once a day, use a mild cleanser, such as Cetaphil Gentle Skin Cleanser or Rodan & Fields COMPOUNDS Gentle Wash, when not using Proactiv Solution products.

1. Unplug Pores—glycolic acid, benzoyl peroxide
a) Renewing Cleanser   Wash off and pat dry.
b) Revitalizing Toner   Apply with gauze or cotton ball. Let dry.

2. Remove Bacteria—benzoyl peroxide
Repairing Lotion   Apply with fingertips. Let dry. Use in the morning only.

3. Reduce Swelling—sulfur

Concealer Plus	Lightly dot on with applicator. Blend with concealer brush or fingertips. Use once or twice a day.
Refining Mask	Apply to clean, dry face or other affected area. Let dry ten minutes. Rinse with lukewarm water. Use once or twice a week for maintenance or every night for the five nights leading up to menstruation.

4. Extra Help—Proactiv Solution

Clarifying Night Cream	Apply sparingly to dry skin. Use only at night.
Daily Oil Control (for slightly oily skin)	Apply to entire face or other affected area with fingertips after toner. Let dry. Use daily or as needed.
Green Tea Moisturizer	Apply sparingly to dry skin.
Mild Exfoliating Peel	Apply thin layer. Let dry one to two minutes. Remove with fingertips. Rinse with lukewarm water. Use once a week.
Oil Blotter Sheets	Use as needed to pat away excess oil.
Sheer Finish Compact Foundation	Apply sparingly.
Sheer Finish Loose Powder	Apply sparingly over foundation.
Skin-Clearing Cream to Powder Foundation	Apply sparingly.

TREATMENT 2: RODAN & FIELDS CALM

Start by using this treatment once a day for two weeks, then increase to twice a day. Until you are able to tolerate its use twice a day or if you remain at once a day, use a mild cleanser, such as Cetaphil Gentle Skin Cleanser or Rodan & Fields COMPOUNDS Gentle Wash, when not using Rodan & Fields CALM products.

1. Reduce Swelling—sulfur

Rodan & Fields CALM 1 Wash (cleanser)	Wash off and pat dry.

2. Unplug Pores—salicylic acid

Rodan & Fields CALM 2 Prepare (toner)	Apply with gauze or cotton ball. Let dry.

3. Remove Bacteria—benzoyl peroxide

Rodan & Fields CALM 3 Treat (leave-on lotion)	Apply with fingertips. Let dry.

4. Extra Help

Proactiv Solution Green Tea Moisturizer	Apply sparingly to dry skin.
Proactiv Solution Sheer Finish Compact Foundation	Apply sparingly.
Proactiv Solution Sheer Finish Loose Powder	Apply sparingly over foundation.
Proactiv Solution Skin-Clearing Cream to Powder Foundation	Apply sparingly.
Rodan & Fields CALM Soothe (mask)	Mix ingredients into a paste. Apply to face or other affected area. Let dry ten minutes. Peel off. Use once or twice a week or every night for the five nights leading up to menstruation.
Rodan & Fields COMPOUNDS Moisture	Apply to dry skin.

TREATMENT 3: OTHER PRODUCTS

Start by using this treatment once a day for two weeks, then increase to twice a day. Until you are able to tolerate its use twice a day or if you remain at once a day, use a mild cleanser, such as Cetaphil Gentle Skin Cleanser or Rodan & Fields COMPOUNDS Gentle Wash, when not using other products. Remember to pick only one product from each list, except in the Extra Help section, where you may choose more than one product, such as a mask, toner, or a moisturizer, if needed.

1. Unplug Pores—salicylic acid

Clearasil Deep Pore Cream Cleanser	Wash off and pat dry.
Iman Perfect Response Oil-Free Cleanser	
L'Oréal Ideal Balance Foaming Cream Cleanser	
L'Oréal Pure Zone Skin Balancing Cream Cleanser	
Neutrogena Deep Cleaning Wash	

Neutrogena Multi-
vitamin Skin Therapy

Peter Thomas Roth Beta
Hydroxy Acid 2% Acne
Wash

2. Remove Bacteria—benzoyl peroxide

Clear By Design Gel 2.5%   Apply with fingertips. Let dry.

Neutrogena On-the-
Spot Acne Treatment

3. Reduce Swelling—sulfur

Clearasil Adult Care   Apply sparingly with fingertips. Let dry.
Acne Treatment Cream

Prescriptives Blemish
Specialist

4. Extra Help

Biotherm Acnopur   Apply with gauze or cotton ball. Let dry.
Exfoliating Toner

Clean & Clear Oil-Free   Apply sparingly to dry skin.
Dual Action Moisturizer

Neutrogena Clear Pore   Apply with fingertips. Let dry five to ten minutes.
Cleanser/Mask   Rinse with lukewarm water. Use once or twice a
                             week or every night for the five nights leading up to
                             menstruation.

Neutrogena Skin-   Apply sparingly to dry skin.
Clearing Moisturizer

Don't Forget the Sunscreen

For all three treatments, applying sunscreen in the morning is the all-
important final step. Apply after all treatment products have dried.

Clinique Sun Care Face SPF 15

Estée Lauder In the Sun Sunblock For Face SPF 15

Neutrogena Ultra Sheer Dry-Touch Sunblock SPF 30

Olay Complete UV Defense Moisture Lotion

Ombrelle Sunscreen Lotion SPF 30

Prescriptives All You Need Broad Spectrum Oil Absorbing Lotion SPF 15

Proactiv Solution Daily Protection Plus SPF 15

Proactiv Solution Oil Free Moisture SPF 15

Rodan & Fields COMPOUNDS Protect SPF 15

EMERGENCY SPOT KILL: QUICK FIXES FOR THE ZIT THAT GOT AWAY

Let's say the prom is coming up. Or you're getting married. Or you're about to make the biggest presentation of your life at work in front of hundreds of your colleagues. Naturally, you wake up with a huge stress pimple.

The fastest way to get rid of it is to hurry to your dermatologist for a cortisone injection. Cortisone is an anti-inflammatory medication—it shrinks swelling. The cortisone a dermatologist injects directly into the pimple is stronger and more effective than the over-the-counter hydrocortisone 1 percent cream you'd normally buy at the drugstore.

If you can't get to the dermatologist, don't worry! We've got a few little tricks for you to try. But remember, these suggestions are *only* for emergency pimples. Using spot treatment as your only acne treatment is contrary to our combination, full-face philosophy.

Note: Use only one of these treatments at a time.

- *Proactiv Solution Advanced Blemish Treatment* with a higher dose of benzoyl peroxide than Proactiv Solution Repairing Lotion. This can be irritating if used full face, but it concentrates the medicine where you need it.
- *Proactiv Solution Refining Mask.* Normally you'd use it on your entire face once or twice a week for ten to twenty minutes only, but for emergency treatment, put a healthy dollop of it on that pesky pimple before you go to bed. By the time you wake up, the sulfur and clay in the mask should have reduced the swelling. It's miraculous!
- *Salicylic acid spot-treat pads*—for the spot only. We like Clean & Clear Concealing Treatment Stick or Maximum Strength Persa-Gel 10. These pads help deliver the medicine right into the pimple.
- A drop of *Visine* and a small dab of over-the-counter *hydrocortisone* cream. The anti-inflammatory properties really do help take the red out!

Tip 1

For superspecial occasions, like your wedding, have an appointment ready with your dermatologist. It's easy enough to cancel if it becomes unnecessary, and it will be much more difficult to get in on short notice.

Tip 2

Use Proactiv Solution Refining Mask every day for five days *before* the special occasion as an extra preventive measure. It's gentle enough not to irritate your skin, and it helps reduce inflammation. But remember: While it's okay to leave a dab on overnight for emergency zits, never leave a full-face mask on for more than ten to twenty minutes.

What to Do If You Are Allergic to Benzoyl Peroxide

Some 1 to 3 percent of acne sufferers are allergic to or are irritated by benzoyl peroxide. They need another treatment program to combat acne. We created a line of products. Proactiv Solution Gentle Formula, which combine other acne-fighting ingredients. Along with salicylic acid, the four products contain alpha hydroxy acids and retinol. Be sure to use it on your entire face.

Proactiv Solution Gentle Formula

Start by using this treatment once a day for two weeks, then increase to twice a day. Until you are able to tolerate its use twice a day or if you remain at once a day, use a mild cleanser, such as Cetaphil Gentle Skin Cleanser or Rodan & Fields COMPOUNDS Gentle Wash, when not using Proactiv Solution Gentle Formula products.

1. Unplug Pores—salicylic acid

a) Gentle Formula Clarifying Cleanser	Wash off and pat dry.
b) Gentle Formula Clarifying Toner	Apply with gauze or cotton ball. Let dry.
c) Gentle Formula Clarifying Day Lotion A.M.	Apply sparingly with fingertips. Use only in the morning.
d) Gentle Formula Clarifying Night Cream P.M.	Apply sparingly with fingertips. Use only at night.

2. Remove Bacteria and Reduce Swelling—sulfur

Proactiv Solution Concealer Plus	Lightly dot on with applicator. Blend with concealer brush or fingertips. Use once or twice a day.
Proactiv Solution Refining Mask	Apply to clean, dry face or other affected area. Let dry ten minutes. Rinse with lukewarm water. Use once or twice a week, more often if needed.

3. Extra Help—Proactiv Solution

Green Tea Moisturizer	Apply sparingly to dry skin.
Sheer Finish Compact Foundation	Apply sparingly.
Sheer Finish Loose Powder	Apply sparingly over foundation.
Skin-Clearing Cream to Powder Foundation	Apply sparingly.

program 4—forty-five-year-old woman with adult-onset acne and dry skin

Melanie is forty-five and has had her life turned upside-down by adult-onset acne. "As I started going through perimenopause, all of a sudden my body went haywire from hormones—weight gain, losing my hair, and acne all over my face. It's been devastating," Melanie says. "I never had acne as a teenager, and this is truly disturbing my life. I'm around a lot of professional people every day, and having acne makes it really tough to go into work and face the people that I have to face. I've been on everything people take for acne—antibiotics, topical solutions, Retin-A, even Accutane. I've gone to three dermatologists in my area, but nothing's helped. I was advised not to take any hormone replacement pills, and I've been convinced that my acne will never go away and I'll wind up being the only little old lady in the nursing home with zits!"

Melanie has been trying to mask her acne with heavy makeup and concealer. She's also worried about aging and wrinkles. The following treatments work to heal Melanie's acne even while concealing it, without the drying effects that can exacerbate wrinkles.

TREATMENT 1: RODAN & FIELDS CALM

Start by using this treatment once a day for two weeks, then increase to twice a day. Until you are able to tolerate its use twice a day or if you remain at once a day, use a mild cleanser, such as Cetaphil Gentle Skin Cleanser or Rodan & Fields COMPOUNDS Gentle Wash, when not using Rodan & Fields CALM products.

1. Reduce Swelling—sulfur
Rodan & Fields CALM 1   Wash off and pat dry.
  Wash (cleanser)

2. Unplug Pores—salicylic acid
Rodan & Fields CALM 2   Apply with gauze or cotton ball. Let dry.
  Prepare (toner)

3. Remove Bacteria—benzoyl peroxide
Rodan & Fields CALM 3   Apply with fingertips. Let dry.
  Treat (leave-on lotion)

4. Extra Help

Proactiv Solution Green Tea Moisturizer	Apply sparingly to dry skin.
Proactiv Solution Replenishing Eye Cream	Apply with your pinkie finger, gently patting cream on the upper and lower eyelids, including the crow's-feet area.
Proactiv Solution Sheer Finish Compact Foundation	Apply sparingly.
Proactiv Solution Sheer Finish Loose Powder	Apply sparingly over foundation.
Proactiv Solution Skin-Clearing Cream to Powder Foundation	Apply sparingly.
Rodan & Fields CALM Soothe (mask)	Mix ingredients into a paste. Apply to face or other affected area. Let dry ten minutes. Peel off. Use once or twice a week or every night for the five nights leading up to menstruation.
Rodan & Fields COMPOUNDS Moisture	Apply to dry skin.
Rodan & Fields COMPOUNDS Moisture Eye	Apply with your pinkie finger, gently patting cream on the upper and lower eyelids, including the crow's-feet area.

TREATMENT 2: PROACTIV SOLUTION

Start by using this treatment once a day for two weeks, then increase to twice a day. Until you are able to tolerate its use twice a day or if you remain at once a day, use a mild cleanser, such as Cetaphil Gentle Skin Cleanser or Rodan & Fields COMPOUNDS Gentle Wash, when not using Proactiv Solution products.

1. Unplug Pores—glycolic acid, benzoyl peroxide

a) Renewing Cleanser	Wash off and pat dry.
b) Revitalizing Toner	Apply with gauze or cotton ball. Let dry.

2. Remove Bacteria—benzoyl peroxide

Repairing Lotion	Apply with fingertips. Let dry. Use in the morning only.

3. Reduce Swelling—sulfur

Concealer Plus	Lightly dot on with applicator. Blend with concealer brush or fingertips. Use once or twice a day.
Refining Mask	Apply to clean, dry face or other affected area. Let dry ten minutes. Rinse with lukewarm water. Use once or twice a week for maintenance or every night for the five nights leading up to menstruation.

4. Extra Help—Proactiv Solution

Clarifying Night Cream	Apply sparingly to dry skin. Use only at night.
Daily Oil Control (for slightly oily skin)	Apply to entire face or other affected area with fingertips after toner. Let dry. Use daily or as needed.
Green Tea Moisturizer	Apply sparingly to dry skin.
Mild Exfoliating Peel	Apply thin layer. Let dry one to two minutes. Remove with fingertips. Rinse with lukewarm water. Use once a week.
Oil Blotter Sheets	Use as needed to pat away excess oil.
Sheer Finish Compact Foundation	Apply sparingly.
Sheer Finish Loose Powder	Apply sparingly over foundation.
Skin-Clearing Cream to Powder Foundation	Apply sparingly.

TREATMENT 3: OTHER PRODUCTS

Start by using this treatment once a day for two weeks, then increase to twice a day. Until you are able to tolerate its use twice a day or if you remain at once a day, use a mild cleanser, such as Cetaphil Gentle Skin Cleanser or Rodan & Fields COMPOUNDS Gentle Wash, when not using other products. Remember to pick only one product from each list, except in the Extra Help section, where you may choose more than one product, such as a mask or an eye cream, if needed.

1. Unplug Pores—salicylic acid

Aveeno Acne Treatment Bar	Wash off and pat dry.
L'Oréal Pure Zone Skin Balancing Cream Cleanser	

Neutrogena Multi-
vitamin Acne
Treatment
Neutrogena Oil-Free
Acne Wash Cream
Cleanser
Clear By Design Gel 2.5%

2. Remove Bacteria—benzoyl peroxide

| Neutrogena On-the-Spot Acne Treatment | Apply with fingertips. Let dry. |

Neutrogena On-the-
Spot Acne Treatment   Apply with fingertips. Let dry.

3. Reduce Swelling—sulfur

Clearasil Adult Care   Apply sparingly with fingertips. Let dry.
Acne Treatment
Cream
Prescriptives Blemish
Specialist

4. Extra Help

Neutrogena Clear Pore   Apply with fingertips. Leave on five to ten minutes.
Cleanser/Mask   Rinse with lukewarm water. Use once or twice a
                             week or every night for the five nights leading up to
                             menstruation.
Neutrogena Healthy   Apply with your pinkie finger, gently patting cream
Skin Eye Cream   on the upper and lower eyelids, including the
                             crow's-feet area.

Don't Forget the Sunscreen

For both treatments, applying sunscreen in the morning is the all-important
final step. Apply after all treatment products have dried.

Clinique Sun Care Face SPF 15
Estée Lauder In the Sun Sunblock For Face SPF 15
Neutrogena Ultra Sheer Dry-Touch Sunblock SPF 30
Olay Complete UV Defense Moisture Lotion
Ombrelle Sunscreen Lotion SPF 30
Prescriptives All You Need Broad Spectrum Oil Absorbing Lotion SPF 15
Proactiv Solution Daily Protection Plus SPF 15
Proactiv Solution Oil Free Moisture SPF 15
Rodan & Fields COMPOUNDS Protect SPF 15

program 5—thirty-year-old man with persistent acne and oily skin

Wayne is thirty years old and worries that his acne will jeopardize his career. "I'm a news anchor and reporter, and being on TV five days a week and doing the weather in front of the perfectly blue weather wall, I am very self-conscious about the state of my skin," he explains. "The pimples are large and hard to cover up, even with the heavy makeup that is always used for television. I am really worried about keeping my job."

Wayne can tolerate a fairly aggressive approach and rest assured that acne won't cause him anguish about his career for much longer.

TREATMENT 1: PROACTIV SOLUTION

Start by using this treatment once a day for two weeks, then increase to twice a day. Until you are able to tolerate its use twice a day or if you remain at once a day, use a mild cleanser, such as Cetaphil Gentle Skin Cleanser or Rodan & Fields COMPOUNDS Gentle Wash, when not using Proactiv Solution products.

1. Unplug Pores—salicylic acid, glycolic acid

a) Deep Cleansing Wash	Wash off and pat dry.
b) Revitalizing Toner	Apply with gauze or cotton ball. Let dry.

2. Remove Bacteria—benzoyl peroxide

Repairing Lotion	Apply with fingertips. Let dry.

3. Reduce Swelling—sulfur

Concealer Plus	Lightly dot on with applicator. Blend with concealer brush or fingertips. Use once or twice a day.
Refining Mask	Apply to clean, dry face or other affected area. Let dry ten minutes. Rinse with lukewarm water. Use once or twice a week, more often if needed.

4. Extra Help—Proactiv Solution

ClearZone Body Pads*	Use in place of cleanser.
Daily Oil Control (for slightly oily skin)	Apply to entire face or other affected area with fingertips after toner. Let dry. Use daily or as needed.
Matte Skin Finish (for very oily skin)	Apply sparingly to oily areas. Brush off residue when dry.
Oil Blotter Sheets	Use as needed to pat away excess oil.

| Rodan & Fields CLEAN Regimen for Blackhead Extraction | Follow instructions in kit. |

* Body pads may be used on the face for a quick midday facial cleansing without a trip to the sink. They can also be used after playing sports.

TREATMENT 2: PROACTIV SOLUTION EXTRA STRENGTH

This treatment includes a 7 percent benzoyl peroxide cleanser and leave-on lotion, which is usually well tolerated by those with extremely oily skin and stubborn acne who have failed treatment with products containing 2.5 percent benzoyl peroxide. Start by using this treatment once a day for two weeks, then increase twice a day. Until you are able to tolerate use twice a day or if you remain at once a day, use a mild cleanser, such as Cetaphil Gentle Skin Cleanser or Rodan & Fields COMPOUNDS Gentle Wash, when not using Proactiv Solution Extra Strength products.

Please note that you can also use the regular Proactiv Solution (Treatment 1, above) in the morning and Proactiv Solution Extra Strength at night if you find that the Extra Strength treatment is too drying for your skin when used twice a day.

1. Unplug Pores—salicylic acid

| a) Extra Strength Cleanser | Wash off and pat dry. |
| b) Extra Strength Toner | Apply with gauze or cotton ball. Let dry. |

2. Remove Bacteria—benzoyl peroxide

| Extra Strength Lotion | Apply with fingertips. Let dry. |

3. Reduce Swelling—sulfur

| Extra Strength Mask | Apply to clean, dry face or other affected area. Let dry ten minutes. Rinse with lukewarm water. Use once or twice a week. |

4. Fade Brown Spots—hydroquinone

| Skin Lightening Lotion | Use at night only. Apply to affected area. |
| Rodan & Fields RADIANT Regimen | Follow directions in kit. |

5. Extra Help—Proactiv Solution

| ClearZone Body Pads* | Use in place of cleanser. |
| Daily Oil Control (for slightly oily skin) | Apply to entire face or other affected area with fingertips after toner. Let dry. Use daily or as needed. |

Matte Skin Finish (for very oily skin)	Apply sparingly to oily areas. Brush off residue when dry.
Oil Blotter Sheets	Use as needed to pat away excess oil.
Rodan & Fields CLEAN Regimen for Blackhead Extraction	Follow instructions in kit.

* Body pads may be used on the face for a quick midday facial cleansing without a trip to the sink. They can also be used after playing sports.

TREATMENT 3: OTHER PRODUCTS

Start by using this treatment once a day for two weeks, then increase to twice a day. Until you are able to tolerate its use twice a day or if you remain at once a day, use a mild cleanser, such as Cetaphil Gentle Skin Cleanser or Rodan & Fields COMPOUNDS Gentle Wash, when not using other products. Remember to pick only one product from each list, except in the Extra Help section, where you may choose more than one product, such as a cleansing pad or a leave-on lotion, if needed.

1. Unplug Pores—salicylic acid

Clearasil 3-in-1 Acne Cleanser	Wash off and pat dry.
L'Oréal Ideal Balance Foaming Gel Cleanser	
Neutrogena Oil-Free Acne Wash Cream	
Oxy Oil-Free Maximum Strength Once A Day Acne Wash	

2. Remove Bacteria—benzoyl peroxide

Clean & Clear Persa-Gel 5	Apply with fingertips. Let dry.
Fostex 5 Cream	
Neutrogena On-the-Spot Therapy	
Oxy 5 Sensitive Skin Vanishing Lotion	
PanOxyl 5 Gel	

3. Reduce Swelling—sulfur

Clearasil Adult Care Acne Treatment Cream	Apply sparingly with fingertips. Let dry.

What About Moisturizing When You Have Acne?

You *can* have both acne and dry skin, especially if you live in a dry climate, work or live in an office or home with dry air (as most of us do), or travel frequently in airplanes. Using the right noncomedogenic moisturizer and sunscreen will not make your face break out! Ingredients such as retinol, Vitamin C, and skin-nourishing and soothing botanicals can improve skin's texture and aid in diminishing the appearance of wrinkles without aggravating your acne.

Moisturizers for Acne-Prone Skin

Products with an asterisk contain acne-fighting medicines, such as salicylic acid.

*Aveeno Clear Complexion Daily Moisturizer
Belladonna Botanical Balancer
Belladonna Clarifying Cream
*Biotherm Acnopur Anti-Acne Moisturizing Treatment Gel
Cetaphil Daily Facial Moisturizer SPF 15
Cetaphil Moisturizing Lotion
Chanel Skin Conscience Total Health Moisture Lotion SPF 15
*Clearasil Acne Fighting Facial Moisturizer
*Clearasil Total Control Daily Skin Perfecting Treatment
Clearasil Total Control Intensive Hydrating Moisturizer SPF 10
Clinique Skin Texture Lotion Oil-Free Formula
Cosmence Mission Perfection Daily Purifying Moisture Treatment
Crème de la Mer Lotion
Elemis Absolute Day Cream
Ellen Lange MicroThera AM Moisturizing Lotion SPF 15
EmerginC Crude Control Hydrating, Protecting, and Balancing Emulsion
Estée Lauder Verité Calming Fluid
Eucerin Daily Control & Care Moisturizer
Eucerin Renewal Alpha Hydroxy Lotion SPF 15
Iman Perfect Response Oil-Free Hydrating Gel
Joey Calm and Correct Gentle Soothing Moisturizer
Joey Pure Pores Tinted Moisturizer SPF 15
Jurlique Viola Cream
Lorac Oil-Free Moisturizer
L'Oréal Pure Zone Oil-Free Moisturizer
Lubriderm Daily UV Lotion
*Neutrogena Multivitamin Acne Treatment
*Neutrogena SkinClearing Moisturizer Daily Face Cream

Olay Oil-Free Active Hydrating Beauty Fluid

Olay Complete Lotion UV Defense Moisture Lotion

Origins Matte Scientist Oil Controlling Lotion

Physicians Formula Oil-Free Moisturizer

Physicians Formula Self-Defense Color Corrective Moisturizing Lotion SPF 15

*Proactiv Solution Daily Protection Plus SPF 15

Proactive Solution Oil Free Moisture SPF 15

Rodan & Fields COMPOUNDS Moisture

See the moisturizing sections on page 227 in chapter 10 and on page 326 in chapter 16 for more information on how to properly hydrate your skin.

---

4. Extra Help

Clearasil Pore Cleansing Pads*	Wipe on. Let dry.
Clinique Night Treatment Gel	Apply with fingertips. Let dry.
Neutrogena Clear Pore Shine Control Gel	
Oxy Daily Cleansing Pads*	Wipe on. Let dry.
Stri-Dex Sensitive Skin Triple Action Acne Pads*	

* Body pads may be used on the face for a quick midday facial cleansing without a trip to the sink. They can also be used after playing sports.

Don't Forget the Sunscreen

For all three treatments, applying sunscreen in the morning is the all-important final step. Apply after all treatment products have dried.

Clearasil Acne Treatment Cream SPF 15*

Neutrogena Ultra Sheer Dry-Touch Sunblock SPF 45

Olay Complete UV Defense Moisture Lotion

Ombrelle Sunscreen Lotion SPF 30

Proactiv Solution Daily Protection Plus SPF 15

Proactiv Solution Sheer Tint Moisture SPF 15*
Rodan & Fields COMPOUNDS Protect SPF 15

* These are excellent solutions for men as they're cover-ups, not makeup, and the slight tint helps camouflage redness while they protect the skin from the sun.

program 6—a fifty-eight-year-old woman with dry skin

Susan is fifty-eight and is seeing the effects of menopause on her skin. "I went off the birth control pills I'd been on most of my life, and my face started to look just blah. I have some blemishes, my pores seem really big, and my skin is blotchy and dull," she says. "I'm also noticing a lot more age spots, and this is making me look older than I feel."

Susan will be helped with a morning regimen of Rodan & Fields RADIANT, which has been designed specifically to brighten skin tone and soften lines, and a nighttime regimen of Rodan & Fields CALM, to heal and control blemishes.

Note: As both daytime treatments include a sunscreen in Step 3, no additional sunscreen is needed.

TREATMENT 1: (A) RODAN & FIELDS RADIANT

Use only in the morning—start by using this treatment every second or third day for two weeks, then increase to once a day. Until you are able to tolerate its use every morning or if you remain at every second or third morning, use a mild cleanser, such as Cetaphil Gentle Cleansing Lotion or Rodan & Fields COMPOUNDS Gentle Wash, when not using Rodan & Fields RADIANT products.

1. Exfoliate—alpha hydroxy acid

Rodan & Fields   Wash off and pat dry.
RADIANT 1 Wash
(cleanser)

2. Fade Brown Spots—hydroquinone

a) Rodan & Fields   Apply with gauze or cotton ball. Let dry.
RADIANT 2 Prepare
(toner)

b) Rodan & Fields   Apply with fingertips. Let dry.
   RADIANT 3 Treat
   (leave-on lotion)

3. Protect Skin from Sun—UVA/UVB Filters

Rodan & Fields   Apply to face and neck.
   RADIANT 4 Protect
   (sunscreen)

4. Extra Help

Start by using once a week. If needed, work up to two or three times a week.

Rodan & Fields RADIANT   Apply to dry skin. Gently massage with fingertips
   Microdermabrasion   for one to two minutes. Rinse with lukewarm water.
   Paste   Pat dry.

Rodan & Fields   Apply to dry skin.
   COMPOUNDS
   Moisture

TREATMENT 1: (B) RODAN & FIELDS CALM

Use only at night—start by using this treatment every second or third night for two weeks, then increase to once a night. Until you are able to tolerate its use every night or if you remain at every second or third night, use a mild cleanser, such as Cetaphil Gentle Cleansing Lotion or Rodan & Fields COMPOUNDS Gentle Wash, when not using Rodan & Fields CALM products.

Continue to use Rodan & Fields CALM once or twice daily to control breakouts when not using Rodan & Fields RADIANT.

1. Reduce Swelling—sulfur

Rodan & Fields CALM 1   Wash off and pat dry.
   Wash (cleanser)

2. Unplug Pores—salicylic acid

Rodan & Fields CALM 2   Apply with gauze or cotton ball. Let dry.
   Prepare (toner)

3. Remove Bacteria—benzoyl peroxide

Rodan & Fields CALM 3   Apply with fingertips. Let dry.
   Treat (leave-on lotion)

4. Extra Help

Proactiv Solution Green Tea Moisturizer	Apply sparingly to dry skin.
Proactiv Solution Nourishing Eye Cream *or* Proactiv Solution Replenishing Eye Cream	Apply with your pinkie finger, gently patting cream on the upper and lower eyelids, including the crow's-feet area.
Proactiv Solution Sheer Finish Compact Foundation	Apply sparingly.
Proactiv Solution Sheer Finish Loose Powder	Apply sparingly over foundation.
Proactiv Solution Skin-Clearing Cream to Powder Foundation	Apply sparingly.
Rodan & Fields CALM Soothe (mask)	Mix ingredients into a paste. Apply to face or other affected area. Let dry ten minutes. Peel off. Use once or twice a week, more often if needed.
Rodan & Fields COMPOUNDS Moisture	Apply to dry skin.
Rodan & Fields COMPOUNDS Moisture Eye	Apply with your pinkie finger, gently patting cream on the upper and lower eyelids, including the crow's-feet area.

TREATMENT 2: (A) OTHER PRODUCTS

Use only in the morning—start by using this treatment every second or third day for two weeks, then increase to once a day. Until you are able to tolerate use every morning or if you remain at every second or third morning, use a mild cleanser, such as Cetaphil Gentle Skin Cleanser or Rodan & Fields COMPOUNDS Gentle Wash, when not using other products. Remember to pick only one product from each list.

1. Exfoliate—alpha hydroxy acid

MD Formulations Face and Body Wash	Wash off and pat dry.
SkinCeuticals Body Polish	

2. Fade Brown Spots—hydroquinone

Esoterica Skin Discol-   Apply with fingertips. Let dry.
  oration Fade Cream
MD Forte Skin Bleaching
  Gel
Porcelana Medicated
  Fade Cream

3. Protect Skin from Sun—UVA/UVB filters

Clinique Sun Care Face   Apply to face and neck.
  SPF 15
Estée Lauder In the Sun
  Sunblock For Face
  SPF 15
Neutrogena Ultra Sheer
  Dry-Touch Sunblock
  SPF 30
Olay Complete UV
  Defense Moisture
  Lotion
Ombrelle Sunscreen
  Lotion SPF 30
Prescriptives All You
  Need Broad Spectrum
  Oil Absorbing Lotion
  SPF 15

4. Extra Help

Start by using once a week. If needed, work up to two or three times a week.

Prescriptives Derma-   Apply to dry skin. Gently massage with fingertips for
  polish System   one to two minutes. Rinse with lukewarm water.
                            Pat dry.

TREATMENT 2: (B) OTHER PRODUCTS

Use only at night—start by using this treatment once every second or third night for two weeks, then increase to every night. Until you are able to tolerate its use every night or if you remain at every second or third night, use a mild cleanser, such as Cetaphil Gentle Skin Cleanser or Rodan & Fields COMPOUNDS Gentle Wash, when not using other products. Remember to pick only one product from each list, except in the Extra Help section, where you may choose more than one product, such as a mask or an eye cream, if needed.

Continue to use an acne treatment regimen once or twice daily to control breakouts when not using a treatment regimen to brighten skin tone and soften lines.

1. Unplug Pores—salicylic acid

Aveeno Acne Treatment Bar Wash off and pat dry.

Clear By Design Gel 2.5%

L'Oréal Pure Zone Skin Balancing Cream Cleanser

Neutrogena Multi-vitamin Acne Treatment

Neutrogena Oil-Free Acne Wash Cream

Proactiv Solution Deep Cleansing Wash

USING PRODUCTS FROM THE HEALTH FOOD STORE

We're all for using products that are as natural as possible, and there are some wonderful alternatives to conventional treatments available in health food stores, such as Zia's Acne Mask, which contains sulfur. As with any products, however, if the hype sounds too good to be true, it probably is. Look for the same active ingredients—benzoyl peroxide 2.5 percent, salicylic acid 2 percent, and sulfur—and be sure they're in medicinal-level strengths or they won't be as effective as other over-the-counter products. Many alternative companies load their products with botanicals, such as arnica (reduces swelling), calendula (soothing), and green tea (antioxidant), which can smell lovely and help your skin be less irritated, but they can't specifically target acne. Unfortunately, acne is too powerful for these compounds alone.

2. Remove Bacteria—benzoyl peroxide

Neutrogena On-the-Spot Acne Treatment
Proactiv Solution Repairing Lotion

Apply with fingertips. Let dry.

3. Reduce Swelling—sulfur

Clearasil Adult Care Acne Cream
Prescriptives Blemish Specialist

Apply sparingly with fingertips. Let dry.

Proactiv Solution Refining Masque

Apply to clean, dry face or other affected area. Let dry ten minutes. Rinse with lukewarm water. Use once or twice a week for maintenance or every night for the five nights heading up to menstruation.

4. Extra Help

Neutrogena Clear Pore Cleanser/Mask

Apply with fingertips. Leave on five to ten minutes. Rinse with lukewarm water. Use once a week.

Neutrogena Healthy Skin Eye Cream

Apply with your pinkie finger, gently patting cream on the upper and lower eyelids, including the crow's-feet area.

chapter six
babies and children—
the preteen years

most babies and children are resistant to acne because their hair follicles are still immature and are therefore unlikely to become clogged and sticky. Still, acne can happen to children; when it does, parents are upset that their otherwise perfect and healthy child has a problem complexion. Luckily, nearly all acne in babies goes away on its own and is not necessarily a prediction of acne later in life. However, acne in children, while responsive to treatment, is usually an indication that the child will have more severe acne in his or her teen years.

acne in babies

Neonatal Acne (Acne Neonatorum)

To the shock of their parents, even newborns can suddenly sprout tiny pimples on their faces. Neonatal acne appears as tiny pink, white, or red bumps, usually across the bridge of the nose and on the cheeks and scalp. This acne is triggered by the transference of maternal hormones when the baby is in utero, by hyperactive adrenal glands in the baby, or both. In each scenario, excessive androgens are to blame. Recent studies have also looked into the possibility that neonatal acne is caused or worsened by the yeast called malassezia, which is also responsible for seborrheic dermatitis (dandruff or cradle cap).

Neonatal acne is not serious, and it is surprisingly common. Around 20 percent of all newborns have at least a few pimples. Nearly all neonatal acne starts at two weeks of age and rarely lasts longer than three months. Your pediatrician will reassure you that it will go away on its own. No treatment is needed in mild cases.

If neonatal acne persists longer than two or three months, however, parents may become justifiably anxious that something is wrong with their baby's skin. In many cases, the acne is lingering because it is caused by comedogenic products, such as heavy moisturizing creams or oils, which may smell delicious but are in truth clogging your baby's pores. Unbeknownst to parents, the use of prescription creams that contain strong topical steroids on the baby's face may also cause acne.

After the use of comedogenic products is discontinued, neonatal acne should resolve on its own. If not, gentle treatment may be indicated. Salicylic acid (0.5 or 1 percent) in a cream or lotion base or 2.5 percent benzoyl peroxide lotion should be effective. Babies usually tolerate topical treatment quite well, but consult your pediatrician before using any medicated products.

Parents should be aware that sometimes what's thought to be neonatal acne is in truth contact dermatitis, caused by a reaction to a cleanser, lotion, or laundry detergent; or candida, which is a yeast infection. Candida looks like little red pustules and is quite common in the drool areas around the mouth, on the cheeks, and in the neck folds. Both contact dermatitis and candida clear up quickly (usually within one week) with medicated, low-strength topical over-the-counter products, such as 1 percent hydrocortisone for contact dermatitis and Lotrimen for candida. And, of course, with contact dermatitis, you'll want to discontinue use of the product that caused the reaction in the first place.

Infantile Acne *(Acne Infantum)*

Very rarely, neonatal acne can become severe in babies—usually boys, from increased levels of testosterone—and is called *acne infantum,* or infantile acne. Infantile acne is usually more serious than neonatal acne. It appears when a baby is between three and six months old, consists of inflammatory papules and pustules, and is confined mostly to the nose, cheeks, and chin.

The treatment for infantile acne is the same as for an adolescent with mild acne: Lower strength topical retinoids applied once daily or every other day combined with topical erythromycin or 2.5 percent benzoyl peroxide. Please note that oral tetracycline can permanently discolor developing teeth and affect bone growth and should be avoided.

Most cases of infantile acne resolve spontaneously before a baby turns one. Some will last a year or two, but it is extremely rare for infantile acne to persist into adolescence.

preadolescent acne in children ages one through seven

Between the ages of one and seven, acne in children is extremely rare. Acne developing during this period may signal an underlying disease and should be taken seriously. In this age group, acne might be a manifestation of insulin-resistant diabetes, polycystic ovarian syndrome in preadolescent girls, or a marker for an underlying adrenal gland tumor.

Any young child who suddenly develops acne should see a pediatrician for a glucose tolerance test and a test for other hormonal levels and perhaps be referred to an endocrinologist. If tests are normal or borderline for hormone levels, yearly follow-up visits are crucial to monitor any possible changes.

early-onset puberty and acne

"My daughter is ten, but she's had acne for a year," one desperate mother told us. "I am puzzled, confused, and worried because it is totally embarrassing for her in elementary school, and she is maturing so much faster than I ever did."

"My son Eric is only ten and a half and started breaking out seriously across his forehead and in between his eyes," another mother added. "It is really agonizing for him, and I think he is way too young. I don't want him to take any drugs. What can we do?"

Early-onset acne can cause pimples in kids as young as eight. It's usually not related to any underlying disease; instead, it may be the first sign of the onset of puberty. It's a tough break for children and their parents to have to struggle with acne at such a young age, especially as embarrassment can be devastating and teasing by peers can be unmerciful. "I'm twelve years old now, and when

I was ten my skin was so bad, I cried all the time," our patient Olivia told us. "Nobody else had bad skin except for me, and I felt like a freak in the freak show."

Many parents are worried and confused about safe and effective treatment for their child's delicate skin. Parents who go to the drugstore for over-the-counter products are confused about what to buy, since almost everything is targeted at teenagers. "I don't know what to do with a nine-year-old with pimples," one anxious mom told us. "All I know is she's going to have a horrible school life."

Luckily, a combination of over-the-counter medications can be as safe and effective for youngsters as it is for teenagers and adults. Children tend to respond very fast to the medicated products available for treatment of acne, and few children have acne severe enough to require oral antibiotics. If they do, tetracycline should be avoided until the permanent teeth are in, as it can discolor developing teeth. For those rare severe cases of early-onset pubertal acne, Accutane is not recommended until the age of thirteen. Just to be on the safe side, we also recommend that any child under the age of twelve with severe acne be seen by an endocrinologist to rule out any hormonal abnormalities.

Parents should treat early-onset pubertal acne with the seriousness it deserves, helping their children maintain a regular skin-care regimen. It can be difficult for any child who just wants to be like all the other kids to start taking care of his or her skin at such a young age, but treating acne early and as aggressively as necessary will prevent acne from getting worse later on, which, statistically, it is likely to do. "We found that our young girls who presented very early with a lot of comedones were more likely to go on to have severe acne," reports Dr. Ann Lucky, a pediatric dermatologist and the director of the dermatology clinic at the Children's Hospital Medical Center in Cincinnati.

The good news is that early-onset pubertal acne can be successfully treated and self-esteem restored. Let's look at how Olivia's story turned out: "As soon as I started using the Rodan and Fields Approach, it changed how I feel about myself," Olivia told us, bursting with pride. "I always thought people were looking at my zits and pimples, thinking,'Ooh!' when they would talk to me. And I'd be like, talk to my face, you know, not my zits. I have a lot more to say about me than they do. Now when I talk to people, I don't have to think about my zits and pimples at all."

patient history

Alexandra is only nine years old and has just finished the fourth grade. Her mother stopped us in the hall and whispered, "There's lots of small bumps on her forehead and nose. What's going on?" Alexandra's physical exam revealed small whiteheads, blackheads, and tiny domed pink bumps on the forehead, nose, and cheek area. There were no pustules.

Alexandra has early-onset mild acne, which is not unusual in kids of eight or nine. Studies by Dr. Lucky show that this is a common occurrence and it is very easy to treat at this stage. It is, unfortunately, also a key indicator of more severe acne to come in the teen years.

Alexandra's treatment plan includes washing with a gentle scrub soap containing salicylic acid (Proactiv Solution Deep Cleansing Wash, Neutrogena Clear Pore Soothing Gel Astringent, or Clearasil Total Control Deep Pore Cream Cleanser). Or washing with a 2.5 percent benzoyl peroxide scrub cleanser (Proactiv Solution Renewing Cleanser). Following the cleanser, Alexandra applies a leave-on treatment with either a topical lotion containing 2 percent salicylic acid or 2.5 percent benzoyl peroxide (Proactiv Solution Repairing Lotion, Proactiv Solution Clarifying Night Cream, Neutrogena Multivitamin Acne Treatment, or Neutrogena SkinClearing Moisturizer).

Alexandra's acne is not severe enough yet to need a sulfur treatment. She responded well to the salicylic acid alone (some cases require a boost with a 2.5 percent benzoyl peroxide lotion). Complete clearing should occur within one to three months, then her acne should be further managed with a salicylic acid cleanser and salicylic acid lotion to help prevent future breakouts.

program for early-onset acne

Remember, use these products on your *entire face*, not only on acne-prone areas, except where noted. Because benzoyl peroxide has not been tested in children under the age of twelve, we recommend you check with your child's pediatrician first before initiating treatment.

Note: "Apply sparingly" means you should use a dime-sized amount of product. It should be enough to have a thin coat applied over the entire surface of the skin where needed. It is always better to use less product rather than more!

TREATMENT 1: PROACTIV SOLUTION

Start by using this treatment every other day for two weeks, then increase to once a day. Most preteens will respond to once-a-day treatment. Until you are able to tolerate its use once a day, use a mild cleanser, such as Cetaphil Gentle Skin Cleanser or Rodan & Fields COMPOUNDS Gentle Wash, when not using Proactiv Solution products.

1. Unplug Pores—glycolic acid, benzoyl peroxide
a) Renewing Cleanser   Wash off and pat dry.
b) Revitalizing Toner   Apply with gauze or cotton ball. Let dry.

2. Remove Bacteria—benzoyl peroxide
Repairing Lotion   Apply with fingertips. Let dry. Use in the morning only.

3. Reduce Swelling—sulfur
Refining Mask   Apply to clean, dry face or other affected area. Let dry ten minutes. Rinse with lukewarm water. Use no more than once a week.

4. Extra Help
Clarifying Night Cream   Apply sparingly to dry skin. Use at night only.
Daily Oil Control   Apply to entire face or other affected area with
  (for slightly oily skin)   fingertips after toner. Let dry. Use only if needed.

TREATMENT 2: RODAN & FIELDS CALM

Start by using this treatment once a day for two weeks, then increase to twice a day. Until you are able to tolerate its use twice a day or if you remain at once a day, use a mild cleanser, such as Cetaphil Gentle Skin Cleanser or Rodan & Fields COMPOUNDS Gentle Wash, when not using Rodan & Fields CALM products.

1. Reduce Swelling—sulfur
Rodan & Fields CALM 1   Wash off and pat dry.
  Wash (cleanser)

2. Unplug Pores—salicylic acid
Rodan & Fields CALM 2   Apply with gauze or cotton ball. Let dry.
  Prepare (toner)

3. Remove Bacteria—benzoyl peroxide
Rodan & Fields CALM 3   Apply with fingertips. Let dry.
  Treat (leave-on lotion)

4. Extra Help

Proactiv Solution Green Tea Moisturizer	Apply sparingly to dry skin.
Proactiv Solution Clarifying Night Cream	Apply sparingly to dry skin. Use at night only.
Proactiv Solution Daily Oil Control (for slightly oily skin)	Apply to entire face or other affected area with fingertips after toner. Let dry. Use only if needed.

TREATMENT 3: OTHER PRODUCTS

Start by using this treatment every other day for two weeks, then increase to once a day. Most preteens will respond to once-a-day treatment. Until you are able to tolerate its use once a day, use a mild cleanser, such as Cetaphil Gentle Skin Cleanser or Rodan & Fields COMPOUNDS Gentle Wash, when not using other products. Remember to pick only one product from each list, except in the Extra Help section, where you may choose more than one product, such as a leave-on lotion or a moisturizer, if needed.

1. Unplug Pores—salicylic acid

Clean & Clear Blackhead Clearing Scrub	Wash off and pat dry.
Clinique Acne Solution Cleansing Foam	
Iman Perfect Response Oil-Free Cleanser	
L'Oréal Ideal Balance Foaming Cream Cleanser	
L'Oréal Pure Zone Skin Balancing Cream Cleanser	

2. Remove Bacteria—benzoyl peroxide

Clear By Design Gel 2.5	Apply with fingertips. Let dry.
Neutrogena On-the-Spot Acne Treatment	

3. Reduce Swelling—sulfur

Origins Out of Trouble Mask	Apply with fingertips to face or other affected area. Let dry ten minutes. Rinse with lukewarm water. Use once a week.

4. Extra Help

Clearasil Daily Skin   Apply sparingly.
  Perfecting Treatment
Neutrogena Multi-
  vitamin Acne
  Treatment
Neutrogena Skin-
  Clearing Moisturizer

Don't Forget the Sunscreen

For both treatments, applying sunscreen in the morning is the all-important final step. Apply after all treatment products have dried.

> Clinique Sun Care Face SPF 15
> Estée Lauder In the Sun Sunblock For Face SPF 15
> Neutrogena Ultra Sheer Dry-Touch Sunblock SPF 30
> Olay Complete UV Defense Moisture Lotion with SPF 15
> Ombrelle Sunscreen Lotion SPF 30
> Prescriptives All You Need Broad Spectrum Oil Absorbing Lotion SPF 15
> Proactiv Solution Daily Protection Plus SPF 15
> Proactiv Solution Oil Free Moisture SPF 15
> Rodan & Fields COMPOUNDS Protect SPF 15

No child with pimples is too young to begin a medicated skin-care program, but always check with your pediatrician first. An early start to acne may mean a more difficult case of acne as a teen. The application of medicated products even once a day helps heal and prevent the later onset of more severe acne. Instilling these good skin-care habits early and continuing the use of safe, low-strength medications will help prevent devastating breakouts in the years to come and will especially reap rewards in self-esteem as the child matures through the teenage and adult years.

chapter seven
teenage girls

"Where do I begin? Being a teenager is hard enough. And acne makes it better. Ha! I'd had an ideal olive complexion, but at sixteen I began noticing pimples. At first, I had no idea it was acne. My mother told me to get used to it, because every month my zits would return. So I had a cluster of redness with monthly pimples on my forehead, and it was a disaster, especially when I made my school's dance team and the main focus was on my face. I thought it was hopeless. All the girls teased me. But I was determined not to let it get to me."

—Mariana, age sixteen

"I've tried everything—over-the-counter, doctor's prescriptions, scrubbing, no scrubbing. My parents used to say that they'd never had acne and I'd say, 'Well, I do!' At one point my mother said, 'Eat lemons.' I ate lemons, and I rubbed lemons on my face, and it still didn't work. Because I have combination skin, my acne literally had a mind of its own every day. I don't think there was a square inch of my face that wasn't covered in pimples, pustules, blackheads, or whiteheads. It got to the point where I would pinch them because I didn't want to have the acne sitting on my skin. I used to feel that my skin was crawling. And pinching only made things worse. I got scabs. It was horrible. I didn't want anyone to touch my face. I was scared; I literally was scared."

—Sondra, age seventeen

"When I was fourteen my friends started breaking out and I was like, 'Oh that will never happen to me. I'll just wash my face a lot. How do people get pimples? That's so nasty.' But a year later I was washing my face, and the acne wouldn't go away, and I was a wreck. I remember one time in world history class I felt like everybody was staring at me because my face was just so horrible. I was begging in my head, 'Please, just turn off the lights so my acne won't be so intense and no one can see my face.'"

—Leigh, age fifteen

the teenage years are extraordinarily challenging—socially, psychologically, and physically," says Dr. John Koo, the director of the psychodermatology
clinic at the University of California at San Francisco Medical Center. "When a
teenager has a disfiguring skin condition like acne on top of all the normal
traumas of adolescence, it can affect grades in school, limit social activities,
cause low self-esteem, and result in long-term psychological consequences,
such as depression and social anxiety."

Although almost all teens have acne at some point during adolescence—
up to 85 percent—only a scant 7 percent ever see a dermatologist for their
acne. Instead, they suffer. And oh, how they suffer! It can be truly heartbreaking. One of Katie's daughters came up with an apt description of her experience with acne: "It is sort of like a car wreck on your face," she said. "You know
you shouldn't look at it, but you can't help yourself. It's just there. It's a mess. It
needs to be cleaned up."

The focus should not be whether acne exists in the teenage population,
but how *much* it exists and therefore how much it affects teens. We live in a
society that places a premium on a flawless complexion and a slender body,
and the pressure on young women to look their best and conform to this
ideal is intense. They are highly self-critical, scouring the magazines targeted
at their age group and comparing themselves with impossible ideals, not
knowing that the photos of models are usually airbrushed so their every im-
perfection is erased. Teenage girls are frequently, and justifiably, hypersensitive to criticism as a result. It becomes second nature to feel that everyone in
the entire world is staring at your face and talking about you behind your
back.

As teenage girls search for their identity, coping with acne can compound
their already intense anxiety about who they are, who they want to be, and
how they appear to the world. They wonder: "What's happening to my body?
Where do I fit in? Will I ever get a date? Why is school so hard? Why don't my
parents understand me? Why won't they just leave me alone?" (For more
about the psychological aspects of acne, see chapter 3.)

There is no typical teenage girl with acne. Some teenage girls are bothered more by the rank-smelling, skin-drying medications they may have used in the past than by a few blackheads, while others are traumatized by one pimple the night before a date with the boy they've been longing for months to go out with. Some are highly impatient—they want results now. And others, whose acne is mild, are in denial when it starts to worsen—"I don't want to think about it" is their typical comment.

No matter how little they admit to it, though, it is the rare teenage girl who is not desperately worried about her acne. "When you are in high school, it's just the hardest time in your life anyhow," sixteen-year-old Elizabeth told us. "Then to have acne and worry about friends and guys and about being popular—it's too much. Because my acne was so bad, I never had the self-confidence I should have had."

Acne can also be as devastating to parents as it is to teenage girls. "I saw my daughter go from a beautiful, bubbly, outgoing lady to a very self-conscious introverted young child who went into her shell and wouldn't come out," one mom lamented.

The good news is teenage girls can easily learn to be proactive about treating their acne. While doing so, however, they need a healthy dollop of empathy and reassurance. As we've mentioned before, we always tell our teen patients, "That girl sitting next to you in math class with the perfect skin, the one who always finds something rotten to say, well, guess what? In about ten years we'll be seeing her in our office, crying about her pimples." That usually gets a laugh. And anything that makes a teenage girl with acne laugh about her skin is a big plus.

getting through puberty—hormones can be hell!

In the memorable words of one of our teenage patients: "Puberty sucks!"

Physiologically, puberty is the most stressful time in the life of a human—but that's no consolation to a girl with acne. Your body's changing, your breasts are sprouting, your body hair is appearing all over the place, your shape is transforming, you're growing, stretch marks erupt, you're moody, and you finally understand what your mother was muttering about when she complained about PMS and reached for the painkillers at the same time every month. For a teenager who needs to feel some sort of control over her life, one of the hardest things to accept is that these hormonal changes in her body are completely *out* of her control.

Prepuberty can begin as early as age seven. Little girls develop breast buds and hair on their legs, and their hair and skin begin to get oily. Most girls start puberty closer to age eleven or twelve; African Americans tend to be a little younger. At the turn of the twentieth century, girls were getting their period closer to age fifteen; in every subsequent generation, puberty's onset has occurred at an earlier age, which is scary. Although this issue is being studied by medical researchers, no one knows for sure what has triggered this shift in hormonal development.

With puberty, along with all the other changes in their bodies, girls usually see a few blackheads then little pimples around their noses. Acne then spreads out to the central face areas. The reasons for acne are always the same, but how acne spreads is different in every girl's body, even with twins (see page 25). Some girls have pimples only on their foreheads, while others have an explosive onset of teeny red papules and pustules on their cheeks or the T-zone. Still others have acne worsen on their faces then make an unwanted appearance on their chests and backs as well. But no matter the severity, teenage acne is always treatable.

treating teenage acne

Nearly all of the teenage girls we see have scoured the shelves at drugstores and department stores. Many of these products only contain salicylic acid, and may be in alcohol-based formulas that are extremely drying and irritating. Teenage girls may also use these products only to spot-kill the pimples, so they're not getting the benefit of full-face therapy.

This creates a double whammy: Not only do girls already feel ugly when they have acne but what they're using to treat this acne makes them feel uglier. Having dry, red, chapped faces is just as bad as having pimples. But girls who don't know better—because they are misinformed about acne, as are most people—keep thinking that acne is caused by dirt or eating chocolate, so they continue desperately washing several times a day; applying concealers, creams, the wrong kind of makeup, whatever they can get their hands on; and whatever their friends said might work.

The Rodan and Fields Approach

The Rodan and Fields Approach is highly effective for most teens. Pick whichever products from our lists on pages 165–72 that you like (boys, see pages 185–90). Remember that you can alternate your topical routine. If something has a scent or texture you're not crazy about, feel free to try something else. The heart of our system is to use a combination of benzoyl peroxide, salicylic acid, and sulfur on your entire face. Some combination of products on the lists is bound to work for you.

It is crucial, however, to realize that your new routine is not one that can be started then stopped. A few months of treating it will not be enough. Your acne will quickly return. You're going to have to be following some form of medicated skin-care regimen for years—yes, years! Find the routine that works best for you, and stay with it. You brush your teeth, and you do your three acne treatment steps. Simple as that. If you are proactive, you can prevent acne before it happens. And then, no one need ever know that you used to break out—because you won't be breaking out any longer.

We tell our teen patients to apply their medicines and take their pill (if prescribed) at the same time every day—at night. It's much easier to set up an evening routine, because in the morning you're busy trying to get ready for school, which makes it harder to treat your skin. If, however, you are super-organized, using your medicated products twice daily will allow you to achieve faster results. Line up your cleanser and creams (and pill, if needed) by your toothbrush. Go ahead and make it a routine.

when to see a dermatologist

If you have been following the three-step approach in this book without fail and still have not seen improvement within eight to twelve weeks, we recommend that you see a dermatologist. It's important to treat moderate to severe acne as quickly as possible because of the potential for scarring.

We've found that some teenagers are so embarrassed and nervous when they first visit a dermatologist that they leave out important information about what's going on in their lives or what they're doing to their bodies. That's because, from their standpoint, they may believe it's not relevant or they're worried we might be judgmental. It is important that you feel you can talk to your dermatologist and even more important that your dermatologist talks to *you* about your acne.

For example, when teens come to see us, we have the parent in the room with them for the first visit. After we've established a relationship, most parents drop their kids off and sit in the waiting room. We want our patients to feel entirely comfortable with us, and that means being able to talk freely without worrying about what Mom or Dad might say or think. Some teens like to have a parent in the room to answer basic questions about practicalities, such as refills. Even when parents are present, though, we talk *to* the *teen*. The teen has our undivided attention. Only if treatment is complicated or we need to switch gears, such as trying a course of Accutane, do we ask parents to join the conversation, as they need to sign the consent form.

We hope you will be able to see your dermatologist as an ally with whom you can share all your concerns about your skin. And don't be too embarrassed to tell your parents you'd be more comfortable talking to a woman dermatologist (or, for boys, a male dermatologist) if you feel that would make it easier for you to share information. Anything and everything you tell us is completely confidential. Sometimes we need to ask tough questions about drinking, sex, or illegal supplements, because they can have extremely serious consequences for teens going on Accutane or other oral medications.

Most follow-up appointments are in six weeks. We'd expect to see some improvement by that time. In the meantime, however, you should always call your dermatologist if *anything's* going wrong. Nothing is too trivial to discuss. Your health and your skin are of vital interest to your doctor. You need to know that if something is not quite right or if you have a question, the time to ask is *now*. Don't wait until your next appointment to ask that question. If your question is urgent, ask to speak to the nurse right away then ask for the doctor to call back as well.

At this follow-up appointment, we'll find out how you're doing and if you feel that the medicines are working. Often teens are either intimidated by their doctors or so kind and considerate that they're worried that we, their dermatologists, might feel bad if their treatment isn't yet successful. Don't be! If you are not happy with the results you're seeing, say so! You can even use this simple statement, word for word: "I'm not impressed with how well I'm doing. I don't think I'm clearing as well as expected. I think we should try something else."

Be honest about your worries, your progress once treatment starts, and what's realistic for you to do regarding treatment, given your already packed schedule. We know how busy you are. We know how crucial it is to get every extra second of sleep. The last thing we want to do is load you down with a complicated regimen. We want it to be as easy as possible. For this reason, we might give you a slightly different treatment in the summer when you are more likely to have extra time and be less overwhelmed with school commitments.

Following, we'll discuss the pros and cons of treatments your dermatologist may recommend for you. Remember, your treatment and its application are ultimately up to you, so keep yourself informed and ask questions.

Accutane (Isotretinoin)

Accutane is the best drug we have to treat moderate-to-severe cases of acne. As teen boys tend to have the most severe and recalcitrant cases, we discuss Accutane in chapter 8 on page 177. For general information, see page 53 in chapter 2.

antibiotics—oral

Teens, as well as their parents, are often skeptical about taking antibiotics for acne because they worry about long-term side effects and increased bacterial resistance. The antibiotics used to treat acne, however, are not the antibiotics you take if you develop pneumonia or a staph infection. These tetracycline-derived antibiotics are mainly prescribed for acne and Lyme disease.

There are many treatment options without the need to ingest antibiotics, and if a teen doesn't want them, we won't prescribe them. We do believe, though, that if topical medications don't work, it's a good idea to at least *try* a course of antibiotics for several weeks, which will help clear your skin. Then, once they work, you can go off the antibiotics and back to a strictly topical regimen. Acne may be a long-term issue, but antibiotics are *not* forever. Leaving teens on antibiotics for longer than six to twelve months is a thing of the past. Nor do we believe that antibiotics should be prescribed for severe acne when Accutane is a highly successful alternative.

Always call your dermatologist if you have any questions or if you're experiencing side effects. Stomach upset is fairly common, although the newer antibiotics are meant to be taken with food and are much better tolerated. Acidophilus and probiotic supplements can help alleviate this side effect, too.

You should call your dermatologist immediately if you experience headaches, vision problems, or joint pain while taking antibiotics. Another common reaction to the tetracycline-derived antibiotics, such as minocycline, is hives, an allergic reaction that manifests as a red, bumpy, itchy rash. Please note that hives usually appear two to three *weeks* after you begin your course of pills.

oral contraceptives (birth control pills)

For teens who are fifteen or older who have a hormonally triggered worsening of their acne and an irregular period, we may suggest going on birth control pills. These pills, which prevent pregnancy by stopping ovulation, also level out hormones. So for a teen whose hormones have yet to be regulated, the steadily released dose of hormones from the pill will give her a clockwork menstrual cycle and may improve her acne, especially when combined with a topical treatment program.

The birth control pill is not a necessity for a teenage girl with acne, but it is a treatment option. It may be worth trying, and should easily fit into your lifestyle. Sexually active teens, for example, might welcome the opportunity to prevent pregnancy while helping treat their acne. Just remember that the pill cannot prevent sexually transmitted diseases.

If you start taking the pill, you should give it at least three months to work. We usually start with Alesse, Ortho Tri-Cyclen, Orthocept, or Yasmin. If a three-month course of one type of pill fails, it's worth trying a different brand. There are several that may help. Each brand of pill is subtly different, and a subtle change can often have a dramatic effect on the skin.

Some dermatologists do not prescribe birth control pills. You'll then need to see your gynecologist for the prescription, and, in fact, this is what we recommend. Your gynecologist will discuss which pill will be the right one for you, and your dermatologist will follow your progress once you begin taking it.

Many teens don't want to go on the pill because they're worried about possible weight gain. In truth, the hormone levels in the newest pills are more than one-fifth lower than the original pill and they shouldn't make you gain weight. The weight gain comes from an increased appetite. If you pay attention to portion size and avoid high-calorie foods, weight gain should not result. If you do have any side effects, discuss them with your gynecologist; she or he may be able to switch you to another brand.

Anyone who smokes, is a diabetic, or obese should never go on the pill. Those with a family history of breast cancer and blood clots should also discuss their options with a gynecologist.

For more information about hormones and a woman's monthly cycle, see the section on page 197 in chapter 9.

Topical Treatments—Antibiotics and Retinoids

Topical antibiotics, such as azeleic acid, clindamycin, erythromycin, and sodium sulfacetamide, remove bacteria. Retinoids, such as Differin, Retin-A, and Tazorac, work to unplug pores.

MONITORING YOUR MONTHLY CYCLE

Part of being a proactive patient is keeping track of your monthly cycle, especially if your acne flares around the time of your period.

Mark on a calendar:

- When you're expecting your period
- How long your periods last
- If you break out in the week before the arrival of your period. Be specific about how bad your acne gets on each successive day
- When you're beginning to feel bloated and moody

If you're not yet ovulating, your periods won't be as regular and your breakouts won't happen as consistently at the same time of the month. When you do start ovulating and your periods become regulated, you'll notice a trend of when your breakouts happen. This can be helpful for tweaking your treatment plan. For example, perhaps you are using your products only once a day. If you know that you're prone to a premenstrual flare-up, you can increase usage to twice a day the week before your period. By doing so you may well save yourself a whole new crop of pimples that otherwise would have lasted two to three weeks beyond your period.

We usually create a treatment plan that includes a cleanser with an antibiotic to be used in the morning, and an antibiotic cleanser/toner followed by a retinoid to be used at night. Some retinoids may be deactivated by sunlight, so they are best used at night. For example, you might wash with a salicylic acid cleanser, then apply an azelaic acid cream or gel in the morning and wash with a benzoyl peroxide cleanser and apply Differin at night.

Each program will be specifically tailored to your needs until success is achieved.

compliance

Compared with the teenage boys we treat, teenage girls make our jobs much easier! Because they are so image-conscious, girls are vastly more commu-

---

MICHELLE'S STORY

"I started getting acne when I was twelve, before any of my other girlfriends. It started with pimples on my forehead, then they moved everywhere. Plus, I had terrible, huge cysts on my chest and back. They hurt so much! It even hurt to sleep.

"I was teased every day because no one else had acne at twelve. I felt like I didn't belong, like I was being singled out. It wasn't fair when everyone else had perfect skin. My girlfriends were really supportive, and they kept telling me I should be glad I had zits now because they'd be gone by the time I got to high school. But I didn't believe them. The zits weren't going away. They were with me all the time; they were *part* of me. And they were getting worse.

"So when I heard about the Rodan and Fields Approach, I told my mom I had nothing to lose by trying it. I was desperate.

"About a week after I started using the Rodan and Fields products, my face was feeling better. I didn't think it was a lot of work at all to do the three steps. I did the cleansing in the shower so that took care of one step anyway. After two weeks I could notice the acne starting to clear up on my face. It wasn't so red and blotchy anymore. After two months there was no acne anywhere. I couldn't believe it!

"Now I'm sixteen, and I try to talk to other kids who have acne. They look at my beautiful clear skin and wonder why they should listen. They think I don't know what I'm talking about! But I do. I was there. I'm still doing the three-step approach every day, and my acne doesn't happen. I'm never going back there again."

nicative, more interested in what they need to do, and tend to follow through religiously. They talk to their friends about skin care, comparing what works and what doesn't. For example, if one of our teen patients goes on Accutane and it works, she is likely to tell her friends what it did for her. Sharing accurate information with your peers is a terrific way to help them and to dispel so many of the myths and misinformation that still abound about acne and its treatment.

There will still be teens who are so busy, stressed, and preoccupied with worries about the reality of their lives that they are forgetful about their treatment. But what all teenage girl acne patients need to do is follow a nightly routine to treat their acne, because being a proactive patient is the only way to control your acne. Constantly monitor your skin, and tell your dermatologist if there are any changes. Even if you get impatient at times, do your utmost to stick to the routine. You'll be glad you did.

tips for parents

We constantly hear from teenage girls that their parents don't understand them, especially when it comes to acne. Perhaps these parents didn't have bad acne and, because they don't understand all the ramifications, either downplay its seriousness or tell their daughters they'll "grow out of it." Or "It isn't so bad." Or "It's normal." Or "Stop complaining." Parents who believe all the myths and misinformation often nag their teens about what they eat and how they cleanse their faces, which makes everybody upset. If there's one thing guaranteed to push teens' wrong buttons, it's having their feelings invalidated and discounted by their parents.

On the other hand, there are so many touchy topics for already stressed teens that many equally stressed parents worry about lowering their kids' self-esteem by bringing up their complexion. The last thing they want to do is make an already self-conscious girl *more* self-conscious. Whenever they gently try to broach the subject, they're likely to hear, "Mom, what're you staring at? Quit looking at me like I just grew ten new pimples!"

There *is* a way for parents to help. After a teen has been to see us, we encourage parents to call us with any questions or information, especially right before the follow-up appointments. We want to know how their child is doing and whether there's improvement, side effects, or depression. Parents who are advocates for their children help us, especially with issues we may not be aware of, and parents help their children receive appropriate treatment.

Consider Counseling

Be aware of your daughter's moods. Aside from the usual ups and downs of adolescence, is she showing any signs of depression? (Refer to the checklist on page 98 in chapter 4.) If so, it's up to you to be an advocate for your child. Counseling with a therapist who specializes in adolescent issues can provide a safe haven for a girl to vent feelings she may otherwise have difficulty articulating. Therapy can help a teen learn how to express her thoughts and feelings about significant events that affect her life and remove barriers impeding her goals and dreams. It is a valuable, lifelong tool to learn that feelings are important and that recognizing and expressing them frees you to cope with tough times in constructive ways.

patient history—mild to moderate acne

Ashley is sixteen. She is a little overweight, doesn't like sports, and is sliding by in school. She has persistent red bumps (pustules) on her cheeks, particularly near her ears, and admits she can't help picking them constantly. She also has pink patches and a few pustules on her nose and back and often hides behind her hair. She has tried several drugstore lines in the past, all containing salicylic acid—cleansers, toners with alcohol, and lotions—none of which offered any relief. Her skin is dry from these previous therapies.

Ashley has mild to moderate acne, but she is only using one medicine—salicylic acid—which merely unplugs the pores. She also needs to remove the p. acnes bacteria and stop the swelling. We put her on the Proactiv Solution full-face treatment, which includes washing with a gentle scrub cleanser containing 2.5 percent benzoyl peroxide (Proactiv Solution Renewing Cleanser), followed by an alcohol-free toner with glycolic acid (Proactiv Solution Revitalizing Toner). Once the toner dries, Ashley applies a leave-on lotion with 2.5 percent benzoyl peroxide (Proactiv Solution Repairing Lotion).

Within six weeks, Ashley's face was completely clear of active acne lesions. The old blemishes were fading well, too. By her final follow-up visit, she had of her own volition lost five pounds, appeared more confident, and was performing better at school.

KEEP YOUR FINGERS OFF YOUR FACE— AND THAT MEANS TRY NOT TO PICK

It's almost impossible not to touch your face when pimples pop up. But it's never a good idea. If you've put medicine on your pimples, playing with those pimples will remove the medicine. And constant touching leads to constant picking and more swelling.

Most pickers have a magnifying mirror at home. As soon as you peer into it, you notice things you wish you hadn't. Before you know it, you've been picking your face for forty-five minutes, which is a bad idea. It can hurt. And it can most definitely lead to permanent scarring and new flare-ups of acne in the zone around the picked pimple.

Here's a handy tip: Put a timer in your bathroom, right next to the mirror. If you can't stop yourself from picking and you know you're going to do it—even if your mother said she'd ground you for life if you went after one more zit—set your timer for five minutes and allow yourself that amount of time at the mirror. The second the timer goes off, step back from the mirror and leave the room.

For more about picking, see page 36 in chapter 1 and page 83 in chapter 3.

patient history—severe acne

Laurie is fifteen and has very irregular periods. She is athletic and doing well at school. She has friends but is teased ruthlessly because her skin is so bad. She has tender nodules and cysts on her forehead, cheeks, and back. She is the oldest child, and none of her relatives remember having significant acne— but all of them have advice. The topical tretinoins, such as Retin-A and Differin, high-strength benzoyl peroxides, and combinations of benzoyl peroxide and clindamycin or erythromycin all failed to treat her acne effectively. In fact, all these medications made her face redder and drier, so she would only use them occasionally to spot-treat. She also has some difficulty swallowing antibiotic pills and is afraid of Accutane. Her parents are very concerned, so the options of topical care plus antibiotics, even Accutane, were reviewed.

We put Laurie on the Proactiv Solution full-face treatment, which includes washing with a scrub cleanser containing 2.5 percent benzoyl peroxide (Proactiv Solution Renewing Cleanser), followed by an alcohol-free toner with glycolic acid (Proactiv Solution Revitalizing Toner). After the toner dries, Laurie applies a leave-on lotion with 2.5 percent benzoyl peroxide (Proactiv Solution

Repairing Lotion). And, as needed, Laurie uses a mask containing sulfur (Pro-activ Solution Refining Mask).

This treatment program was used once daily for the first week, then increased to twice daily, with the mask applied for five to ten minutes every night until the redness subsided.

Full-face topical care was very helpful for Laurie, though not perfect, as several nodules continued to appear monthly. Blood tests to rule out excessive androgen hormones were negative. Because of her very irregular menstrual cycle and hormone-triggered acne, she was referred to a gynecologist to consider an antiandrogen birth control pill. She was placed on Yasmin, a new low-dose birth control pill. Within four months her skin was completely clear. She will stay on Yasmin and continue with the Proactiv Solution full-face treatment for approximately four months. We will then reevaluate her condition.

treatments for a teenage girl

Remember, use these products on your *entire face*, not only on acne-prone areas, except where noted.

Every day, you need to clean, tone, and treat your skin, and the products you use will contain medicines to unplug pores, remove bacteria, and reduce swelling. The active ingredients in some of these products are applicable in several categories. For example, salicylic acid, which unplugs pores, is often an active ingredient in cleansers, toners, leave-on lotions, and moisturizers, and benzoyl peroxide, which removes bacteria and helps to unplug pores, is often an active ingredient in cleansers and leave-on lotions. This explains why Proactiv Solution Renewing Cleanser and Proactiv Solution Repairing Lotion, which contain benzoyl peroxide, both unplug pores and remove bacteria. However, we are listing cleansers only in Step 1—Unplug Pores and not Step 2—Remove Bacteria. The reason is simple: Leave-on lotions, such as Proactiv Solution Repairing Lotion, must be applied *after* cleansing and toning.

You will also notice that the order of the three steps is different for Proactiv Solution products from that for Rodan & Fields CALM products. That's because the formulation in each system is different, although the ingredients are similar and the purpose remains the same. The order of use of ingredients is interchangeable as long as you cleanse, tone, and treat with salicylic acid or glycolic acid, benzoyl peroxide, and sulfur in some combination and end up with a leave-on lotion.

Note: "Apply sparingly" means you should use a dime-sized amount of product. It should be enough to have a thin coat applied over the entire surface of the skin, where needed. It is always better to use less product rather than more!

Note: In the Extra Help sections, you may choose more than one product, such as a mask or a moisturizer, if needed.

Normal Skin

TREATMENT 1: PROACTIV SOLUTION

Start by using this treatment once a day for two weeks, then increase to twice a day. Until you are able to tolerate its use twice a day or if you remain at once a day, use a mild cleanser, such as Cetaphil Gentle Skin Cleanser or Rodan & Fields COMPOUNDS Gentle Wash, when not using Proactiv Solution products.

1. Unplug Pores—glycolic acid, benzoyl peroxide

a) Renewing Cleanser	Wash off and pat dry.
b) Revitalizing Toner	Apply with gauze or cotton ball. Let dry.

2. Remove Bacteria—benzoyl peroxide

Repairing Lotion*	Apply with fingertips. Let dry. Use in the morning only.

3. Reduce Swelling—sulfur

Concealer Plus	Lightly dot on with applicator. Blend with concealer brush or fingertips. Use once or twice a day.
Refining Mask	Apply to clean, dry face or other affected area. Let dry ten minutes. Rinse with lukewarm water. Use once or twice a week for maintenance or every night for the five nights leading up to menstruation.

4. Extra Help—Proactiv Solution

Clarifying Night Cream*	Apply sparingly to dry skin. Use at night only.
Daily Oil Control (for slightly oily skin)	Apply to entire face or other affected area with fingertips after toner. Let dry. Use daily or as needed.
Green Tea Moisturizer	Apply sparingly to dry skin.
Matte Skin Finish (for very oily skin)	Apply sparingly to oily areas. Brush off residue when dry.

Sheer Finish Compact Foundation	Apply sparingly.
Sheer Finish Loose Powder	Apply sparingly over foundation.
Skin-Clearing Cream to Powder Foundation	Apply sparingly.

* If skin becomes dry when using Repairing Lotion twice a day, Repairing Lotion can be used in the morning, and Clarifying Night Cream can be used at night.

TREATMENT 2: OTHER PRODUCTS

Start by using this treatment once a day for two weeks, then increase to twice a day. Until you are able to tolerate its use twice a day or if you remain at once a day, use a mild cleanser, such as Cetaphil Gentle Skin Cleanser or Rodan & Fields COMPOUNDS Gentle Wash, when not using other products. Remember to pick only one product from each list, except in the Extra Help section, where you may choose more than one product, such as a leave-on lotion or a moisturizer, if needed.

1. Unplug Pores—salicylic acid

Clean & Clear Blackhead Clearing Scrub	Wash off and pat dry.
Clinique Acne Solution Cleansing Foam	
Iman Perfect Response Oil-Free Cleanser	
L'Oréal Ideal Balance Foaming Cream Cleanser	
L'Oréal Pure Zone Skin Balancing Cream Cleanser	
Neutrogena Multi-vitamin Skin Therapy	
Peter Thomas Roth Beta Hydroxy Acid 2% Acne Wash	

2. Remove Bacteria—benzoyl peroxide

| Clear By Design Gel 2.5% | Apply with fingertips. Let dry. |
| Neutrogena On-the-Spot Acne Treatment | |

3. Reduce Swelling—sulfur

Clearasil Adult Care
  Acne Treatment
  Cream

Apply with fingertips. Let dry.

Origins Out of Trouble
  Mask

Apply with fingertips to face or other affected area.
Let dry ten minutes. Rinse with lukewarm water. Use
once or twice a week, more if needed.

4. Extra Help

Clean & Clear Oil-Free
  Dual Action
  Moisturizer
Clearasil Daily Skin
  Perfecting Treatment
L'Oréal Pure Zone Oil-
  Free Moisturizer
Neutrogena Skin
  Clearing Moisturizer

Apply to dry skin.

Dry or Sensitive Skin

TREATMENT 1: RODAN & FIELDS CALM

Use only at night. Start by using this treatment every second or third night for
two weeks, then increase to every night. Until you are able to tolerate its use
every night or if you remain at every second or third night, use a mild cleanser,
such as Cetaphil Gentle Skin Cleanser or Rodan & Fields COMPOUNDS Gentle
Wash, when not using Rodan & Fields CALM products.

1. Reduce Swelling—sulfur

Rodan & Fields CALM 1
  Wash (cleanser)

Wash off and pat dry.

2. Unplug Pores—salicylic acid

Rodan & Fields CALM 2
  Prepare (toner)

Apply with gauze or cotton ball. Let dry.

3. Remove Bacteria—benzoyl peroxide

Rodan & Fields CALM 3
  Treat (leave-on lotion)

Apply with fingertips. Let dry.

4. Extra Help

Proactiv Solution Green
  Tea Moisturizer

Apply sparingly to dry skin.

Proactiv Solution Sheer Finish Compact Foundation	Apply sparingly.
Proactiv Solution Sheer Finish Loose Powder	Apply sparingly over foundation.
Proactiv Solution Skin-Clearing Cream to Powder Foundation	Apply sparingly.
Rodan & Fields CALM Soothe (mask)	Mix ingredients into a paste. Apply to face or other affected area. Let dry ten minutes. Peel off. Use once or twice a week, or more often if needed.
Rodan & Fields COMPOUNDS Moisture	Apply to dry skin.

TREATMENT 2: PROACTIV SOLUTION GENTLE FORMULA

Start by using this treatment once a day for two weeks, then increase to twice a day. Until you are able to tolerate its use twice a day or if you remain at once a day, use a mild cleanser, such as Cetaphil Gentle Skin Cleanser or Rodan & Fields COMPOUNDS Gentle Wash, when not using Proactiv Solution Gentle Formula products.

1. Unplug Pores—salicylic acid

a) Gentle Formula Clarifying Cleanser	Wash off and pat dry.
b) Gentle Formula Clarifying Toner	Apply with gauze or cotton ball. Let dry.
c) Gentle Formula Clarifying Day Lotion A.M.	Apply sparingly with fingertips. Use only in the morning.
d) Gentle Formula Clarifying Night Cream P.M.	Apply sparingly with fingertips. Use only at night.

2. Remove Bacteria and Reduce Swelling—sulfur

Proactiv Solution Concealer Plus	Lightly dot on with applicator. Blend with concealer brush or fingertips. Use once or twice a day.
Proactiv Solution Refining Mask	Apply to clean, dry face or other affected area. Let dry ten minutes. Rinse with lukewarm water. Use once or twice a week, more often if needed.

3. Extra Help—Proactiv Solution

Green Tea Moisturizer	Apply sparingly to dry skin.
Sheer Finish Compact Foundation	Apply sparingly.

Sheer Finish Loose Powder	Apply sparingly over foundation.
Skin-Clearing Cream to Powder Foundation	Apply sparingly.

Oily Skin

TREATMENT 1: PROACTIV SOLUTION

Start by using this treatment once a day for two weeks, then increase to twice a day. Until you are able to tolerate its use twice a day or if you remain at once a day, use a mild cleanser, such as Cetaphil Gentle Skin Cleanser or Rodan & Fields COMPOUNDS Gentle Wash, when not using Proactiv Solution products.

1. Unplug Pores—salicylic acid, glycolic acid

a) Deep Cleansing Wash	Wash off and pat dry.
b) Revitalizing Toner	Apply with gauze or cotton ball. Let dry.

2. Remove Bacteria—benzoyl peroxide

Repairing Lotion	Apply with fingertips. Let dry.

3. Reduce Swelling—sulfur

Concealer Plus	Lightly dot on with applicator. Blend with concealer brush or fingertips. Use once or twice a day.
Refining Mask	Apply to clean, dry face or other affected area. Let dry ten minutes. Rinse with lukewarm water. Use once or twice a week for maintenance or every night for the five nights leading up to menstruation.

4. Extra Help—Proactiv Solution

Daily Oil Control (for slightly oily skin)	Apply to entire face or other affected area with fingertips after toner. Let dry. Use daily or as needed.
Matte Skin Finish (for very oily skin)	Apply sparingly to oily areas. Brush off residue when dry.
Oil Blotter Sheets	Use as needed to pat away excess oil.
Sheer Finish Loose Powder	Apply sparingly over foundation.
Skin-Clearing Cream to Powder Foundation	Apply sparingly.

TREATMENT 2: OTHER PRODUCTS

Start by using this treatment once a day for two weeks, then increase to twice a day. Until you are able to tolerate its use twice a day or if you remain at once a day, use a mild cleanser, such as Cetaphil Gentle Skin Cleanser or Rodan & Fields COMPOUNDS Gentle Wash, when not using other products. Remember to pick only one product from each list, except in the Extra Help section, where you may choose more than one product, such as blotting sheets or a moisturizer, if needed.

1. Unplug Pores—salicylic acid

Clean & Clear Oil-Free Continuous Control Acne Wash — Wash off and pat dry.

Clearasil 3-in-1 Acne Defense Cleanser

Clinique Acne Solution Cleansing Foam

Iman Perfect Response Oil-Free Cleanser

L'Oréal Ideal Balance Foaming Cream Cleanser

L'Oréal Pure Zone Skin Balancing Cream Cleanser

Neutrogena Multi-vitamin Skin Therapy

Oxy Skin Wash

2. Remove Bacteria—benzoyl peroxide

Clear By Design Gel 2.5% — Apply with fingertips. Let dry.

Clean & Clear Oil-Fighting Astringent — Apply with gauze or cotton ball. Let dry.

3. Reduce Swelling—sulfur

Clearasil Tinted Acne Treatment — Apply with concealer brush or fingertips. Use once or twice daily.

Origins Out of Trouble Mask — Apply with fingertips to face or other affected areas. Let dry ten minutes. Rinse with lukewarm water. Use once a week for maintenance or every night for the five nights leading up to menstruation.

4. Extra Help

Clearasil Daily Skin Perfecting Treatment — Apply sparingly to dry skin.

Lancôme Matte Finish Shine-Control Blotting Sheets — Use as needed to pat away excess oil.

Don't Forget the Sunscreen

Whether your skin is normal, dry, sensitive, or oily, applying sunscreen in the morning is the all-important final step. Apply after all treatment products have dried.

Clinique Sun Care Face SPF 15
Estée Lauder in the Sun Sunblock For Face SPF 15
Neutrogena Ultra Sheer Dry-Touch Sunblock SPF 30
Olay Complete UV Defense Moisture Lotion with SPF 15
Ombrelle Sunscreen Lotion SPF 30
Prescriptives All You Need Broad Spectrum Oil Absorbing Lotion SPF 15
Proactiv Solution Daily Protection Plus SPF 15
Proactiv Solution Oil Free Moisture SPF 15
Rodan & Fields COMPOUNDS Protect SPF 15

once your acne goes away, you *will* have acne amnesia

Kathy recently removed a deep cyst from the face of a young girl who had been teased unmercifully and unrelentingly in school about it. Two weeks after the procedure, all that remained was a tiny pink dot, barely a freckle, and no one has said a word about it. They literally forgot the cyst had even existed.

It may be impossible to believe when you're suffering from acne, but once it's gone, it's forgotten. The torture goes away. The embarrassment disappears. No acne, no teasing. *You'll* even have acne amnesia. And it's one of the most wonderful feelings in the world! Teens who look back at photographs taken of themselves are shocked by how bad their skin once was. Acne amnesia protects them.

One teen whose skin is now radiant and clear summed it up perfectly: "Having clear skin has changed the way people look at me, the way they think of me," she said. "I really think this is going to be a new life for me."

We encourage every teenage girl to start her acne treatment program right away. There's no reason to prolong the agony. We want you to have acne amnesia—immediately! Compared with when we were teenage girls, there are an abundance of effective, readily available medicated treatments that heal and prevent acne without punishing your complexion in the process.

One ecstatic mom told us, "My daughter had been in hiding due to her acne. After a couple of weeks with the Rodan and Fields Approach, I saw a difference. The redness went away, and she felt beautiful. She's doing more things, and she's not feeling so embarrassed and using makeup to cover it all up. It's great! She can just go out and be herself in front of people she doesn't know. I'm getting to see a side of my daughter I haven't seen in years."

CARRY AROUND AN EMERGENCY FACE KIT

We love the idea of creating a small emergency face kit that you can throw in your backpack or purse to have handy whenever you might need it the most. Load it up with the following:

- **Concealer.** Proactiv Solution Concealer Plus is medicated with sulfur and comes in a tube with a wand applicator. It's available in different shades for all skin colors. Clearasil Tinted Acne Treatment is a concealer containing sulfur and resorcinol. Both have a pleasant scent and can be used to cover blemishes. You don't need to use concealer more than once or twice a day.
- **A Small Makeup Brush.** Use this to apply the concealer. It's easier to be precise with a brush than with a finger and more hygienic. If you don't like using a brush, Q-tips are a good alternative.
- **Salicylic Acid Pads.** These are great to use after you've worked out. Simply keep a few in a Ziploc bag, and give your face a wipe-off to remove sweat and dirt. We like Noxzema's 2 in 1 Extra-Strength Salicylic Acid Acne Medicine Pads, or Proactiv Solution Clear Zone Body Pads.
- **Salicylic Acid Dot Pads.** Clean and Clear Maximum Strength Overnight Acne Patches, pHisoDerm Clear Confidence Swab sticks, or Ponds Clear Solutions Overnight Blemish Reducers are designed to be dabbed on a pimple. The downside is the cost. The plus side is they are easily transportable and sterile.
- **Antibiotic Towelettes.** If you've seen a dermatologist, he or she can give you a prescription for clindamycin or erythromycin towelettes, which can be used any time during the day.
- **Small Mirror.** You're not always near a bathroom mirror when having a face emergency. Keep a portable one handy!

For emergency treatment for the zit that, naturally, pops up right before a crucial event, see the sidebar on page 127 in chapter 5.

chapter eight
teenage boys

"I was tired of putting my hand over my face when I was walking down the hall in school or acting like my face itched just to hide it. It was really painful, and I couldn't stand it. Plus, my face was usually so oily that five minutes after I cleaned it, if I wiped my hands on it, they looked as greasy as if I'd stuck them in a jar of Vaseline."

—Steven, age fifteen

"I looked like I had a third eye on my chin. I was ready to rip my skin off."

—Jeremy, age seventeen

"I don't think anyone could feel more like a geek than when they're walking around with all that stuff on their face. My acne got so bad that when I smiled, the pimples felt like they would pop."

—Matt, age sixteen

Who would want to go out with me?" Toby, a shy sixteen-year-old, mumbled as he sat in our office, staring at his shoes. "I mean, come on, look at me! I'm a mutant!"

Toby's not a mutant, although he feels like one. He just has acne.

Nearly every teenage boy in the world has acne—and it tends to be more severe for them than it does for girls. We do our utmost to reassure boys that for them, unlike for girls and women, whose hormones can wreak havoc for a lifetime, their acne will most likely go away when puberty is over and they hit their twenties. For a fifteen-year-old, though, that's an eternity! In the mean-time, teenage boys are a challenge to treat. Their pain is immense, but they tend to suffer in silence, and they're not used to putting anything on their faces other than shaving cream!

Acne as a visible disease exacerbates every teenage boy's insecurities about his developing sense of self. Because there is a stigma attached to skin care, boys can be taunted unmercifully for performing a skin-care ritual. And wearing concealer or any type of makeup is inconceivable, so few boys risk using a product to cover up their pimples when they're with their peers. Unlike girls, who can learn to artfully disguise their acne, boys have nowhere to hide. And unlike girls, who eagerly share tips and information with each other about products and treatments, boys tend not to discuss their acne, even with their closest friends. They don't know where to turn for advice. For them, acne is personal. It's private. Which means teenage boys often live in their own personal, private hell of embarrassment and shame. We often worry that their suffering is even worse than girls'.

Parents are often at a loss when it comes to helping their teenage sons with acne. "My fourteen-year-old son used to say things to me like 'Mom if you buy me cool jeans and cool shoes and stuff, the kids won't make fun of my face,' " one heartsick mother told us.

The good news is kids *will* stop making fun once that acne is gone, and this fourteen-year-old won't need designer jeans and shoes to feel cool. With a little cooperation, successful treatment of acne in teenage boys is assured.

getting through puberty—hormones can be hell!

Physiologically, puberty is one of the most stressful times in the life of a human, but that's no consolation to a boy with acne. Your voice is changing dramatically, your shape is transforming (but probably not fast enough!), your body hair is thickening, you're growing, your moods are all over the place. Let's not even begin to discuss what's going on down there in the region you *really* don't want to talk about!

Girls tend to hit adolescence earlier than boys, which is one of the reasons girls are often taller than boys until the midteen years. Most boys start seeing acne around the age of twelve or thirteen. It tends to come on quickly, first appearing in the middle of the face. Initially boys tend to have blackheads and whiteheads, then pustules and pimples. Cysts and nodules appear last. Unfortunately, teenage acne can worsen dramatically, sometimes seemingly overnight. It is also quite common for boys to have acne appear on their chests and backs as well, especially if they play sports.

FOOTBALL SEASON IS ACNE SEASON

As soon as practice starts, our offices are full of boys. Acne is aggravated by the friction and rubbing of football helmets, chin straps, and shoulder pads. Plus, the guys who get a good workout are sweaty and often overheated. That's a recipe for an acne flare-up.

Any boy who is physically active needs to be able to clean his skin properly after practice. We suggest you throw a bottle of Proactiv Solution Extra Strength Cleanser in your backpack or keep one in your locker at school, so you can use it as soon as you jump in the shower. If you don't want anyone to know what acne products you're using, go to the drugstore, where you'll find small travel-sized plastic bottles. Simply fill up the unmarked bottle with whatever product you like, and take it with you wherever you go without worrying about being teased.

Body pads with salicylic acid, such as Proactiv Solution Clear Zone Body Pads, Clearasil Pore Cleansing Pads, Oxy Daily Cleansing Pads, or Stri-Dex Sensitive Skin Triple Action Acne Pads, are also easily transportable. Keep a few in a plastic Ziploc bag. That way, if you can't get to a shower, you can still easily wipe off the sweat and grime. Don't worry, the medicine won't stain your clothes. And here's a strategy: If you don't want to be seen with your body pads, hide in the toilet stall for a quick swipe—no one but you will be the wiser.

For more information about acne on the body, see chapter 14. For more information about exercise, acne, and sports equipment, see page 333–34.

treating teenage acne

Please read the sections The Rodan and Fields Approach and When to See a Dermatologist on pages 156–58 in chapter 7 about treatment, because much of what you may need to do for your acne will be the same as it is for girls. (Well, you can skip the stuff about birth control pills!)

Unlike girls, though, many of the boys who come to our office are not in the mood to talk. They sit, slumped in a chair, unable to make eye contact. If their mom is with them, it's often more embarrassing if she answers the questions.

After the first appointment, we gently suggest that parents of boys read a magazine in the waiting room. Acne is *your* problem, not your mother's. And if you don't want to talk about it, that's okay too. We can do the talking for you. We know what a drag acne is—we both had it. We draw pictures of what causes acne and why. And then we stress that we *are* going to beat this thing—together. However, we need you to be involved, because we can't help you if you don't want to help yourself.

We need to know what supplements you're taking, if any, and any products you may already have tried. For example, anabolic steroids used by body builders can cause explosive cystic acne. If you can't remember the names of what you've used, don't worry—just throw them in a brown bag and bring it to your next appointment.

It's also very important to communicate to your dermatologist what treatments are realistic for you. This can make your life a lot easier in the long run. For example, your dermatologist can figure out how to include two-in-one types of products so you have one less step to do. He or she will also try to find a way to help you remember to take your medicines consistently. For example, it often helps to leave your oral prescription on the kitchen table so you're reminded to take your pill with a meal.

We believe in the KISS rule—Keep It So Simple. With KISS, you can easily follow your routine every day and put an end to your acne.

accutane (isotretinoin)

Accutane is a serious drug, which we discuss in depth starting on page 53 in chapter 2. Please read that section first. Accutane is also one of the most effective treatments available for moderate to severe acne.

We often see teens who have been prescribed Accutane by their general practitioners whose acne hasn't gotten better. *We don't believe that any physicians other than dermatologists should prescribe Accutane.* It demands constant monitoring, for one thing, and only dermatologists who work with this drug on a daily basis understand how best to prescribe it effectively. With Accutane, you might take one or two five- to six-month courses of pills in your lifetime to get rid of the pimples. You want to take Accutane under the strict supervision of your dermatologist to ensure that you will achieve dramatic improvement and minimize potential side effects.

One of the main reasons teens who have previously tried Accutane did not see improvement is, paradoxically, *under*treatment. Generally, many of these teens were treated at too low a dose for too short a time. The standard prescription of one mg/kg may not be enough for some teens. Others may not be absorbing it properly and may therefore require a higher dose. It is imperative to prescribe Accutane in a precise dosage that is calibrated with your body weight and, if needed, adjusted by the dermatologist depending on your clinical response. It should be taken for a minimum of twenty to twenty-four weeks, which is five to six months. When accurately prescribed and properly absorbed by the body, Accutane can work wonders on stubborn cases of acne. Take it at the same time every day. We suggest dinnertime. Leave the pill on the table near a glass of water so you don't forget it. Medications like Accutane work best when taken at the same time every day *with food*.

Many teens are afraid of the monthly blood tests that accompany taking Accutane. We've seen captains of football teams as well as diminutive shy girls nearly keel over at the thought! But you really don't have to worry about the pain of the needle prick. A cream available over the counter, called ELA-Max, is a topical anesthetic that quickly numbs the skin. If you apply it over the vein twenty to thirty minutes before getting your blood drawn, you won't feel the needle stick. Be sure to tell the phlebotomist (the person who draws your blood) that you're nervous, so she or he will do her or his best to be reassuring. Lie down and try to relax. Wearing headphones and listening to music can help. Turn your head away and close your eyes so you don't have to see anything—and when your skin is numb it'll be over before you know it. Don't be shy or embarrassed about speaking up if you're upset by blood! Nearly everyone dreads needles.

When taking Accutane, blood tests are required monthly because there are several extremely important health risks when it is taken improperly. Teens must be aware of the following issues before taking Accutane:

Drinking Alcohol Must Be Avoided

Accutane is hard on your liver, and alcohol is hard on your liver. The double whammy of consuming both is going to create problems, and you won't be able to fudge the truth because the effects will show up in your monthly blood tests. We know that drinking goes on, but while we're prescribing Accutane and you're under our care, you must not drink. No exceptions.

You Must Not Take Any Body-Building Supplements

Creatine, a commonly used supplement for body building, can also affect your liver. You must not take it while on Accutane. Also, anabolic steroids not only make acne worse but can be dangerous and may affect your liver. In general, we recommend not taking steroids unless prescribed for specific medical conditions by a physician and certainly not while taking Accutane.

Accutane Will Make You Sun-Sensitive

You can still enjoy outdoor activities, such as skiing or swimming, but only if protected with sunscreen. Always keep sunscreen handy, apply it religiously, and reapply it after any outdoor activity. Use a lip balm with SPF, too, as your lips will be very dry and will become easily chapped while you're taking Accutane.

Accutane and Depression

One of the very rare side effects of Accutane is serious depression. Spontaneous suicide not related to Accutane use is one of the leading causes of death in teenagers, especially boys. Acne is depressing, as you know. Clearing your acne can lift depression, which is why we encourage all teens to treat their acne proactively.

Girls Must Be on Birth Control Pills or Abstinent

Accutane causes birth defects by affecting a developing fetus. It has no adverse effects on male reproductive function.

compliance

Before we choose a therapy program for a sixteen-year-old with a tough case of acne, we always ask him a simple question: "What are the odds that you'll use this?"

Most teenage girls are eager participants in the fight against acne. Most teenage boys, however, are not. It's not for lack of *wanting* to comply with instructions. Daily rituals are not yet the norm for them.

The last thing we want to do is make a teen feel guilty or worse about himself by suggesting he use a complicated routine that he can't possibly follow. Many guys already feel that they've disappointed their parents, who are spending money on medications and doctor visits. A guy who admits he'll have a problem following instructions is a better candidate for oral medications, which take only a second to swallow, than more time-consuming topical regimens. When a treatment program is customized for a teen, it helps him feel that he is being listened to and his needs are being addressed.

Some boys, of course, are more than happy to try whatever it takes. One of our patients is a wonderful guy who likes to style his hair in spikes, gelled to

ONE FAMILY'S WAY TO ENCOURAGE COMPLIANCE

Deborah and Richard are the parents of active children, ranging in age from eight to thirteen. They live in Houston and have always had a proactive attitude toward skin care. Richard is a tennis professional, which means he's out in the sun every day, and he understands the vital importance of sunscreen. So when their eldest son, Chris, started developing acne at age twelve, they were determined to use his treatment as a teaching tool for their entire family.

"Children see Mom putting on her creams and makeup, but they don't usually see Dad take care of his skin," Deborah explains. "But because Richard needs to use sunscreen every day, he makes sure he puts it on in front of the kids, right after breakfast, before he leaves for the day. When he comes home from work—he's already had a shower in the locker room at his tennis club—he makes a point of putting on moisturizer, one for his face and a different lotion for his arms and legs. He lets the little kids rub it in, and they fight over the chance to do it!

"When Chris started getting pimples then blackheads near his nose and in his ears, which really bothered him, his dad showed him how to use Proactiv Solution in front of all the kids. Now, all the kids watch Chris wash his face with the cleanser, then apply the toner and lotion. He uses the mask twice a week, and the kids watch him do that, too. Sometimes Richard and I both put on masks at the same time. All the kids want to use masks now!

"Chris's skin quickly cleared up, and he never has to be reminded to keep taking care of his skin. He's got all his self-confidence back, and our little ones understand the importance of a regular skin-care regimen. By the time they hit puberty, we'll be ready!"

perfection. He wears three silver rings, he's in a band, he plays soccer, and he's on the school yearbook committee. And he'll wash his face twice a day in a three-step program for however long he needs to in order to keep his acne in check. For the rest of our teenage boy patients, we assure them that we will try to make their program as simple as possible. What often helps motivate them is to take Polaroid pictures at each appointment. This way they can see the benefits as their treatments progress and be encouraged.

Remember, your treatment can't work if you participate only now and then. We can't make you do anything you don't really want to do, but we still hope that all boys stick to the program, because it can take up to two months to work. Don't give up. It *will* work if you give it a chance.

Finally, for parents looking for a way to motivate their teens to comply with their treatment, one mom has a great solution: "When my boys start grumbling or avoiding their regular routine, I pull out a photo of me at age sixteen—the one where I look hideous, covered with pimples and juicy red cysts—and tape it to their bathroom mirror," she explains. "That usually works like a charm!"

all about shaving

Boys have the lifelong hassle of everyday shaving. Whenever there are pimples, cysts, or irritation on the tender skin of the face and neck, shaving can become a painful and bloody experience. It hurts physically, and it hurts emotionally for any boy to look at the nicks and scrapes on his face and realize he's going to have to wake up and go through the same torturous process the next day and the next. And for most, growing a mustache or beard is hardly a viable option.

Here are some useful tips to make shaving less an ordeal:

- Change your razor blade more frequently. Once a month is not enough. The duller the blade, the more drag there is on the skin. You'll need to change it as often as every day when you have acne or irritation, as a used blade has microscopic tears in it and can cut skin. Once your skin has improved, you can change the blade every other day.
- Experiment with double-blade or triple-blade sensitive-skin razors and electric shavers to find the one that causes the least amount of irritation.
- Shave from the chin down your neck. Shaving from the neck up, though it gives a closer shave, causes more skin irritation.
- Have your skin as soft and warm as possible before shaving. Shaving during or after a nice hot shower is a good idea.
- Exfoliating before shaving to help lift up curly hairs is a great idea to achieve a close shave and minimize shaving bumps. Try an exfoliating cleanser, such as Proactiv Solution Deep Cleansing Wash or a Buf-Puf type of cleansing pad, before you shave.
- Use your acne medicines, such as Rodan & Fields CALM 1 Wash, instead of shaving cream. A medicated cleansing product for shaving helps deliver medicine down into the pores, because the act of shaving creates exfoliation.

Your dermatologist can also prescribe Benzashave, which is a medicated shaving cream containing benzoyl peroxide.

- For bleeding after you shave, apply two seconds of pressure with a clean cotton gauze pad. Tissues and toilet paper, as you know, stick to skin. And styptic pencils sting.
- Many aftershave lotions smell great, but they can cause irritation, especially if they're alcohol-based and heavily fragranced. If you like a scent, try applying some to your wrist or at the pulse points in your neck (away from any breakouts).
- If you can avoid shaving on a particular day, by all means do so.

tips for parents

Parents of teenage daughters hear, "I need help. You know, I can't stand this acne one more minute. I look horrible. Fix this now! Get me to the dermatologist tomorrow!"

Boys are seldom that blunt. One of our friends likes to joke that when talking to their parents, teenage boys have a vocabulary of three words—and two of them are grunts!

No matter how uncommunicative or sullen your teen, you must be sensitive to his needs. That he is not talking about his acne doesn't mean he's not suffering. If you wait for him to bring up his worries, you might wait for a very long time. One mom we spoke to told us she kept wondering when her son was going to bring up that he desperately wanted to see a dermatologist. She didn't want to make him more self-conscious than she knew he was already, so she said nothing. Finally, after months and months had gone by and his acne was raging out of control, she couldn't stand it any longer, and she gently broached the topic when they were discussing his college applications. "Yeah," he said casually. "Make me an appointment." She was waiting for *him* to say something, while he was waiting for *her* to say something. In the meantime, her son was suffering needlessly.

Of course, had this mom brought up the idea of treatment at the wrong time—let's say they'd just had a fight or he had a bad day at school—she would've been ignored. It's up to parents to read their kids' moods, finding a receptive, nonthreatening time to bring up sensitive topics. A good time to talk is when you're alone in the car, with no other family members present. Bringing up acne in front of teens' friends or their little brothers is often a recipe for disaster. (For more guidance on talking to your teen about acne, see page 90 in chapter 4.)

Moreover, parents should never tease teens about acne. Don't belittle your son's pain and self-esteem by making comments such as "Take it like a man"; "Scars look manly"; "Who cares, because you're a guy your appearance isn't as important as it is for girls"; "All your friends have it—misery loves company— so stop complaining."

More than anything, you need to be an ally for a son suffering with acne. If you had acne as a teen, encourage your son to start an acne regime as soon as his pimples appear. Doing so will help avoid permanent scarring. Talk to him in a nonjudgmental way about compliance, since the sooner his acne improves, the sooner his self-esteem will skyrocket. Check the levels of medicine in his tubes and bottles so you know whether the products are being used appropriately. Be sure he understands what to do. One observant mother discovered that her son had unwittingly been doing his three steps wrong. He'd use the Proactiv Solution Renewing Cleanser, then wash it off. He'd use the Revitalizing Toner, then wash it off. He'd use the Repairing Lotion, then wash it off. So he actually washed all the medicines down the drain. As soon as he stopped washing off his toner and lotion, his acne improved dramatically and his bathroom time was cut in half.

When you take the time to connect with your son about his acne, the results can be formidable. "My son is now eighteen, and my heart ached for him during high school when he would hide and try to fix his acne on his own," one single dad told us. "He finally asked me to order Proactiv Solution and help him figure out the regimen. Two months later he asked me to order it again. His face cleared up, and his confidence jumped. Now, we are truly getting along for the first time in our lives. He's socializing better, he's dressing better, he looks better, his face is cleared up for the first time. We're both completely thrilled."

Consider Counseling

Be aware of your son's moods. Aside from the usual ups and downs of adolescence, is he showing any signs of depression? (Refer to the checklist on page

98 in chapter 4.) If so, it's up to you to be an advocate for your child. Counseling by a therapist who specializes in adolescents can provide a safe haven for a boy to vent feelings he may otherwise have difficulty articulating. Therapy can help a teen learn how to express his thoughts and feelings about significant events that impact his life and remove barriers impeding his goals and dreams. It is a valuable, lifelong tool to learn that feelings are important and that recognizing and expressing them frees you to cope with tough times in constructive ways.

patient history—mild-to-moderate acne

Roy was fourteen. Everything was going well—he was athletic, smart, and had lots of girlfriends. Then he started breaking out.

Roy has blackheads and whiteheads on his forehead under his baseball cap, a few red bumps on his nose, and small pimples where he shaves his neck. His sister, who is sixteen, already sees a dermatologist because her skin is far worse, so he figured it wouldn't be long before acne ruined his life. He gladly ran to the dermatologist when his mother suggested he, too, see one.

Roy's diagnosis is mild-to-moderate acne. We put him on the Proactiv Solution full-face treatment, which includes washing with a scrub cleanser containing 2.5 percent benzoyl peroxide (Proactiv Solution Renewing Cleanser), followed by an alcohol-free toner with glycolic acid (Proactiv Solution Revitalizing Toner). After the toner dries, Roy applies a leave-on lotion with 2.5 percent benzoyl peroxide (Proactiv Solution Repairing Lotion). And as needed Roy uses a mask with 8 percent sulfur (Proactive Solution Refining Mask) or a sulfur concealer (Clearasil Acne Treatment Cream).

Roy's skin cleared easily in one month. He will maintain his complexion with this treatment because acne is not curable, only treatable through regular, consistent care. He can also use Proactiv Solution Deep Cleansing Wash—a 2 percent salicylic acid cleanser with fine scrubbing granules as an alternative to the Proactiv Solution Renewing Cleanser.

patient history—severe acne

Adam is seventeen. Both his parents have mild scarring on their faces as reminders of their teen years. Lucky Adam got a double genetic dose! He also goes to a competitive private high school and is studying hard to get into a top college. His stress level is high, and his self-esteem is crushed.

Adam has painful red nodules on his cheeks and forehead. He also has some comedones, several pustules, and evidence of depressed scars. His acne is severe. He is a very quiet and intense young man; he replies when questioned but does not offer information freely. He has trouble looking our staff in the eye.

Because of his family history of nodular cystic acne, we are very concerned about scarring. Adam and his parents discussed options with us, including full-face topical therapy using several medications, topical therapy plus oral antibiotics, and Accutane. Adam admits that because of his hectic schedule, he has neither the time nor the desire to apply one to two medicines over his full face twice a day. His parents are desperately concerned about scarring, so the best, most aggressive course of action was chosen: Accutane, the most powerful drug available for nodular cystic acne. The major side effects were reviewed at great length, and the appropriate blood tests were ordered. Adam's parents were required to call the office immediately if they noticed any signs of depression, though we explained that this was a rare side effect.

After one month on Accutane, Adam has no new acne. The original blemishes are shrinking nicely, and his self-esteem is rising. He will complete a five-month course of Accutane. Following its completion he will continue on topical maintenance therapy, which includes the Proactiv Solution full-face treatment.

With severe acne, it is imperative not to wait but to begin a course of Accutane if there are signs of scarring and when compliance might be an issue. It is important to note that even with Accutane, acne isn't curable, but it is treatable and preventable. After the use of Accutane, acne may have been minimized, but it will still require topical care.

treatments for teenage boys

Remember, use these products on your *entire face*, not only on acne-prone areas, except where noted.

Every day you need to clean, tone, and treat your skin, and the products you use contain medicines to unplug pores, remove bacteria, and reduce swelling. The active ingredients in some of these products are applicable in several

YES, YOU TOO CAN USE A MASK

We do want to stress that it's okay for guys to use any of the products that girls use. In fact, we encourage it. It's up to you to be proactive. Ask your mom or sister, a trusted cousin, or even a friend for help and advice.

Sulfur-based masks are a tremendous help for excess oil absorption and in reducing inflammation. And no one has to know you've got one on. You can lock yourself in the bathroom, apply it, leave it on for ten minutes, then rinse it off with lukewarm water.

We recommend Proactiv Solution Refining Mask, with sulfur, and Neutrogena Oil-Absorbing Acne Mask, which has benzoyl peroxide.

Also, it's okay for guys to get facials, have their blackheads removed by a professional, or remove blackheads themselves with our extractor. Dare to be different!

categories. For example, salicylic acid, which unplugs pores, is often an active ingredient in cleansers, toners, leave-on lotions, and moisturizers; and benzoyl peroxide, which removes bacteria and helps to unplug pores, is often an active ingredient in cleansers and leave-on lotions. This explains why Proactiv Solution Renewing Cleanser and Proactiv Solution Repairing Lotion, which contain benzoyl peroxide, both unplug pores and remove bacteria. However, we are listing cleansers only in Step 1—Unplug Pores and not Step 2—Remove Bacteria. The reason is simple: Leave-on lotions, such as Proactiv Solution Repairing Lotion, must be applied *after* cleansing and toning.

Note: "Apply sparingly" means you should use a dime-sized amount of product. It should be enough to have a thin coat applied over the entire surface of the skin, where needed. It is always better to use less product rather than more!

Note: In the Extra Help sections, you may choose more than one product, such as a peel, a leave-on lotion, or a cleansing pad, if needed.

Oily Skin

TREATMENT 1: PROACTIV SOLUTION
Start to use this treatment once a day for two weeks, then increase to twice a day. Until you are able to tolerate its use twice a day or if you remain at once a day, use a mild cleanser, such as Cetaphil Gentle Skin Cleanser or Rodan & Fields COMPOUNDS Gentle Wash, when not using Proactiv Solution products.

1. Unplug Pores—salicylic acid, glycolic acid

a) Deep Cleansing Wash   Wash off and pat dry.

b) Revitalizing Toner   Apply with gauze or cotton ball. Let dry.

2. Remove Bacteria—benzoyl peroxide

Repairing Lotion   Apply with fingertips. Let dry.

3. Reduce Swelling—sulfur

Concealer Plus   Lightly dot on with applicator. Blend with concealer brush or fingertips. Use once or twice a day.

Refining Mask   Apply to clean, dry face or other affected area. Let dry ten minutes. Rinse with lukewarm water. Use once or twice a week, more often if needed.

4. Extra Help—Proactiv Solution

ClearZone Body Pads*   Use in place of cleanser.

Daily Oil Control
  (for slightly oily skin)   Apply to entire face or other affected area with fingertips after toner. Let dry. Use daily or as needed.

Matte Skin Finish
  (for very oily skin)   Apply sparingly to oily areas. Brush off residue when dry.

Mild Exfoliating Peel   Apply thin layer. Let dry one to two minutes. Remove with fingertips. Rinse with lukewarm water. Use once a week.

Oil Blotter Sheets   Use as needed to pat away excess oil.

Rodan & Fields CLEAN
  Blackhead Extractor   Follow instructions in kit.

* Body pads may be used on the face for a quick midday facial cleansing without a trip to the sink. Can also be used after playing sports.

TREATMENT 2: RODAN & FIELDS CALM

Start by using this treatment once a day for two weeks, then increase to twice a day. Until you are able to tolerate its use twice a day or if you remain at once a day, use a mild cleanser, such as Cetaphil Gentle Skin Cleanser or Rodan & Fields COMPOUNDS Gentle Wash, when not using Rodan & Fields CALM products.

1. Reduce Swelling—sulfur

Rodan & Fields CALM 1   Wash off and pat dry.
  Wash (cleanser)

2. Unplug Pores—salicylic acid

Rodan & Fields CALM 2   Apply with gauze or cotton ball. Let dry.
  Prepare (toner)

3. Remove Bacteria—benzoyl peroxide

Rodan & Fields CALM 3 Treat (leave-on lotion)	Apply with fingertips. Let dry.

4. Extra Help

Rodan & Fields CALM Soothe (mask)	Mix ingredients into a paste. Apply to face or other affected area. Let dry ten minutes. Peel off. Use once or twice a week.
Rodan & Fields COMPOUNDS Moisture	Apply to dry skin.

TREATMENT 3: OTHER PRODUCTS

Start to use this treatment once a day for two weeks, then increase to twice a day. Until you are able to tolerate its use twice a day or if you remain at once a day, use a mild cleanser, such as Cetaphil Gentle Skin Cleanser or Rodan & Fields COMPOUNDS Gentle Wash, when not using other products. Remember to pick only one product from each list, except in the Extra Help section, where you may choose more than one product, such as a cleansing pad or a leave-on lotion, if needed.

1. Unplug Pores—salicylic acid

Clean & Clear Blackhead Clearing Scrub	Wash off and pat dry.
Clearasil 3-in-1 Acne Cleanser	
L'Oréal Ideal Balance Foaming Gel Cleanser	
Neutrogena Oil-Free Acne Wash	

2. Remove Bacteria—benzoyl peroxide

Clean & Clear Persa-Gel 5	Apply with fingertips. Let dry.
Fostex 5 Cream	
Neutrogena On-the-Spot Therapy	
Oxy 5 Sensitive Skin Vanishing Lotion	
PanOxyl 5 Gel	

3. Reduce Swelling—sulfur

Clearasil Adult Care Acne Treatment Cream	Apply sparingly with fingertips. Let dry.

4. Extra Help

Clearasil Pore Cleansing Pads*	Wipe on. Let dry.
Clinique Night Treatment Gel	Apply with fingertips. Let dry.
Neutrogena Clear Pore Shine Control Gel	
Oxy Daily Cleansing Pads*	Wipe on. Let dry.
Stri-Dex Sensitive Skin Triple Action Acne Pads*	

* Body pads may be used on the face for a quick midday facial cleansing without a trip to the sink. They can also be used after playing sports.

Very Oily Skin

TREATMENT 1: PROACTIV SOLUTION EXTRA STRENGTH

This treatment includes a 7 percent benzoyl peroxide cleanser and leave-on lotion, which is usually well tolerated by those with extremely oily skin and stubborn acne who have failed treatment with products containing 2.5 percent benzoyl peroxide. Start to use this treatment once a day for two weeks, then increase to twice a day. Until you are able to tolerate its use twice a day or if you remain at once a day, use a mild cleanser, such as Cetaphil Gentle Skin Cleanser or Rodan & Fields COMPOUNDS Gentle Wash, when not using Proactiv Solution Extra Strength products.

Note that you can also use the regular Proactiv Solution (Treatment 1, above) in the morning and Proactiv Solution Extra Strength at night if you find that the Extra Strength treatment is too drying for your skin when used twice a day.

1. Unplug Pores—salicylic acid, glycolic acid

a) Extra Strength Cleanser	Wash off and pat dry.
b) Extra Strength Toner	Apply with gauze or cotton ball. Let dry.

2. Remove Bacteria—benzoyl peroxide

Extra Strength Lotion   Apply with fingertips. Let dry.

3. Reduce Swelling—sulfur

Extra Strength Mask   Apply to clean, dry face or other affected area. Let dry
ten minutes. Rinse with lukewarm water. Use once or
twice a week.

4. Fade Brown Spots

Skin Lightening Lotion   Use at night only. Apply to affected area.
Rodan & Fields RADIANT   Follow instructions in kit.
  Regimen

5. Extra Help—Proactiv Solution

ClearZone Body Pads*   Use in place of cleanser.
Daily Oil Control   Apply to entire face or other affected area with
  (for slightly oily skin)   fingertips after toner. Let dry. Use daily or as needed.
Matte Skin Finish   Apply sparingly to oily areas. Brush off residue
  (for very oily skin)   when dry.
Oil Blotter Sheets   Use as needed to pat away excess oil.
Rodan & Fields CLEAN   Follow instructions in kit.
  Regimen for Blackhead
  Extraction

* Body pads may be used on the face for a quick midday facial cleansing without a trip to
the sink. They can also be used after playing sports.

Don't Forget the Sunscreen

For all three treatments, applying sunscreen in the morning is the all-
important final step. Apply once all treatment products have dried.

Clearasil Acne Treatment Cream SPF 15*
Neutrogena Ultra Sheer Dry-Touch Sunblock SPF 45
Olay Complete UV Defense Moisture Lotion with SPF 15
Ombrelle Sunscreen Lotion SPF 30
Proactiv Solution Daily Protection Plus SPF 15
Proactive Solution Sheer Tint Moisture SPF 15*
Rodan & Fields COMPOUNDS Protect SPF 15

* These are excellent solutions for boys as they're cover-ups, not makeup, and the slight
tint helps camouflage redness while they protect the skin from the sun.

YES, YOU CAN CONCEAL YOUR ACNE— ITS REALLY JUST TINTED SUNSCREEN

Teenage girls with acne have already spent days and weeks of their lives in the bathroom covering up their pimples. Boys don't use makeup, so they can't camouflage the worst of the redness and pimples and are usually unfairly stigmatized if they try. We hope this inescapable reality will be an incentive to get your acne treated so you won't have anything to hide.

In the meantime, here's a great tip: Use a tinted sunscreen moisturizer. It's *not* makeup. Sunscreen is a necessity for every man, woman, and child, and when it's got a slight bit of color in it, it can downplay red skin and pimples while providing necessary protection from harmful solar radiation. We like Clearasil Tinted Acne Cream SPF 15 and Proactiv Solution Sheer Tint Moisture with SPF 15. Consider them bronzers, not makeup!

Some topical prescription medications, such as Sulfacet, are also available in tinted formulations. Ask your dermatologist about them.

once your acne goes away, you *will* have acne amnesia

Treat the acne and it goes away—and with it all of the unbearable memories.

"The Rodan and Fields Approach was such a help," seventeen-year-old Jackson told us. "I mean it wasn't just something to put on my face—it was almost like a psychiatrist for me. It made me confident again. It gave me back everything I had before the blemishes. When my face was so messed up, it didn't feel like I would ever get rid of the acne. I'd use something, and the zits would come back, and then I'd try something expensive, and that didn't work, either, and the zits came back, and I thought I was going to go crazy. I'm not depressed and unhappy anymore. I look people in the eye now instead of looking at the ground."

"There was a profound change in my son's self-esteem and his social esteem at school," Jackson's delighted mom told us when his acne disappeared. "Now I have a whole different child—he's confident, he's making straight A's, he's popular, and every morning he tells me he looks good. Because he does!"

• • •

Remember, for boys, learning to care about acne-prone skin can be challenging, from mastering the ritual of a multistep cleansing and treatment program to finding "masculine" ways to camouflage breakouts. Once achieved, however, the rewards may seem miraculous. Self-esteem and social confidence soar once pimples vanish.

chapter nine
adult women

"After I had my first miscarriage, my skin went downhill. I never had acne as a teenager, and then all of a sudden I started developing these horrible cysts all over my face that would last nearly an entire month. My life was destroyed; I couldn't go without makeup. I didn't even want to face people because I was so afraid they'd see nothing but these huge lumps on my face."

—Miranda, age twenty-nine

"I'm a flight attendant and in the public eye all the time, and I was always broken out. It was terrible. I've used every excuse from being premenopausal, to being pregnant, to stress, to jet lag. Even my three-year-old son said, 'Mom, you need Band-Aids on those boo-boos.' My husband is so wonderful, he never said a word—but I was just nuts about my pimples."

—Jane, age thirty-six

"People used to call me 'Ivory girl,' but when I hit twenty-eight I don't know what happened. I woke up one day with a lump on the side of my nose. I went to the dermatologist, and he told me I was beginning adult acne. From that one spot, the acne began to cover my entire face. It was awful! Suddenly I turned into the creature from the black lagoon. There were pimples on top of pimples. I literally hid from society for three years."

—Belinda, age thirty-three

many women think they've left their teenage acne dilemma behind only to be devastated when it suddenly reappears fifteen years later. Others who have never had acne before are shocked when pimples and cysts sprout on their chins. When acne appears on a woman's face, it can not only alter her appearance but have an intense effect on everything in her life. To deal with what is erroneously perceived as a teenage problem can be extremely embarrassing for a grown woman—especially when she begins to see visible signs of aging on her skin in addition to the pimples.

Those who managed to escape acne as teens find themselves entering an unfortunate new world of stares and humiliation. Job performance suffers, especially in those who need to work with the public. Social withdrawal is also common. We've seen outgoing, vivacious women become housebound and withdrawn because they're too ashamed and embarrassed by the condition of their skin. Single women stop dating. Married women wonder if their husbands find them unattractive. Stress and worry compound, and the frustration becomes intense. Furthermore, because nearly all over-the-counter acne products are geared toward teenagers, women often have no idea what to buy or how to treat their skin. If they do buy teenage-oriented products, they often find them harsh and irritating. For those who have children entering puberty, it can be particularly mortifying to have the same skin condition as their kids. Will they ever outgrow acne? What *will* make it go away?

Although dermatologists are seeing a tremendous upsurge in acne in adult women who come for treatment, this acne has actually existed for decades. It simply wasn't discussed or treated before, because women often had no idea where to turn for advice. And it certainly wasn't called acne. It was a breakout. It was a monthly rash. It was a stress bump. Since women often didn't realize that these breakouts were indeed acne, they didn't think their problem was serious enough to take to a doctor. Unfortunately, when this happens, acne can persist for years. "Acne for some patients may be close to a life-long process," said Dr. Diane M. Thiboutot, an associate professor of medicine/dermatology at Pennsylvania State University College of Medicine.

When we started our practices and saw adult women day after day with the same problem, we realized something serious was going on. We had one of those wonderful Eureka! moments validating our experience when we went to a medical conference over a decade ago. One area of the conference was called the Poster Section. Posters are descriptions of early-stage research that has been done or is ongoing that may not be part of a large, scientifically controlled study and has not yet been published in any of the medical journals. We love these posters, because the research on view is cutting-edge, fascinating, and informative.

We stood there, skimming some of the abstracts, furiously scribbling notes, when we came upon a survey done by a dermatologist we greatly respected. In this survey, taken in a shopping center, the dermatologist claimed that 70 percent of the adult women they sampled had acne. Most of the breakouts occurred on the chin, followed by the nose, forehead, and cheeks. Their skin was usually normal to dry—not oily, as with teens. Sometimes there were microcomedones present. Most felt their acne did not worsen with food but that it did worsen with the use of over-the-counter acne medications, which were highly irritating. It also worsened with cosmetic use, menstrual irregularities, stress, tension, and sun exposure. Few had seen a dermatologist for treatment or asked their regular doctors for advice.

This informal survey reinforced what we had already seen in our adult women patients. Huge numbers of women all over America have acne. The responses to the survey questions were the same responses we heard to the very same questions we asked in our offices. This made us more determined than ever to create a skin-care program that would help adults get rid of their acne for good as much as it would help teenagers. Acne is a complicated skin condition. Studies show it lasts twenty years on average in adult women. There's no quick fix to *cure* it, as you know, and for some it may be a lifelong process—but it can be *treated* just as easily as teenage acne.

is all acne the same?

Adult acne in women is caused by the same process as teenage girl acne: too much oil formation leading to clogged pores, an overgrowth of bacteria, and inflammation. The devastation is equally painful. We see acne in females as part of a spectrum that some go in and out of throughout their lifetimes. Some are genetically programmed to suffer with acne for decades; others only now and then, depending on other cofactors, such as environment and cosmetics. Some will spontaneously manifest with explosive nodular acne; others will have a few monthly bumps that they see as annoyances more than anything else.

However, there are some significant differences between adult and teen female acne. "Teenagers tend to have much more severe, inflammatory acne, with many comedones. In adult females, however, the acne tends to be a low-grade persistent mild or moderate type, so the treatment effect is not as dra-

matic," says Dr. Thiboutot. We've also found that teen acne is often concentrated in the T-zone, while women are more likely to have deeper nodules in
the chin area that seemingly arrive out of nowhere and feel like tender rocks.
They take longer to form, and they're harder to eliminate than the smaller
comedones.

Dermatologists are not yet sure why the appearance of acne differs so
greatly in adults from that of teenage females, although much research is ongoing. Some believe stress in working women trying to juggle both difficult
jobs and the demands of family and children is a critical cofactor. We know
that stress definitely exacerbates acne and that working women, for whom
unblemished complexions are vital to livelihood and self-esteem, are more
likely to seek out treatment.

As always, genetics is a major factor. Acne's causes may be hormonal, but
a woman's *response* is genetically determined. This explains why some
women have big pimples and no scars while others suffer from small pimples
that leave angry red spots for months and sometimes dell or ice-pick scars to
boot.

We wish we could tell you that you'll grow out of adult acne. You won't.
Some months may be better than others. You may even go for six months
without seeing a blemish and stop your medicated skin-care regime, then,
one day, out of the blue, pimples suddenly make a most unwelcome reappear-
ance. As women age from puberty to the fertile years, to perimenopause, to
postmenopause, the only constant is that their hormones continuously
change. As a result their acne fluctuates. When acne arrives on top of wrinkles, it seems extraordinarily unfair. But you can no more change the genetic
destiny that programs your body for acne than you can change the color of
your eyes or the size of your feet. The plus side of what we jokingly refer to as
hormone hell is the ability to conceive and bear children. The minus side is the
zits that come along with the diapers.

Triggers for Adult-Onset Acne
(in descending order of importance)

- Hormonal changes;
- Pregnancy;
- Stress;

- Comedogenic cosmetics, particularly heavy occlusive sunscreen (see chapter 17);
- Overeating food such as sushi, seaweed, and fish, or taking supplements that are heavy in iodides;
- Strenuous exercise with inadequate cleansing afterward. This usually flares acne on the chest, back, and buttocks (see chapter 15).

the hormonal double whammy

Why do adult women break out?

The answer is simple: hormones. The physiology of the female, whose hormones fluctuate each month and throughout her lifetime, creates the potential for adult acne. This explains why adult women have so much more chronic and unremitting acne than adult men. It also explains why women often have flare-ups of their acne at specific times in their monthly cycles, when hormones are most active. The first questions we always ask adult women acne sufferers are:

- How often do you get your period? Every twenty-eight days, etc.?
- Is your cycle regular?
- At which point do you break out in your cycle? Midcycle? The week before your period? The day before?
- How long do these breakouts last?
- Are you on birth control pills?
- Have you had weight gain or loss?
- Do you have facial hair?

Monthly hormonal fluctuation is one factor in the hormonal double whammy. The other is the dreaded aging whammy.

The Aging Whammy

"As women age, hormonal levels begin to fluctuate," explains Dr. Risa Kagan, a board-certified obstetrician and gynecologist with a private practice in Berkeley, California, who is also an associate clinical professor at the University of California, San Francisco, and a specialist in women's health care issues, particularly hormonal disorders, menopause, and osteoporosis. "When the femi-

A HAIRY POINT

When those pesky hairs begin to appear on the chin or cheeks, sometimes even on the neck, women naturally want to get rid of them in a hurry. Tweezing and plucking hairs, however, often triggers acne or makes preexisting acne worse by inflaming the area.

Permanent hair removal will stop these hairs from sprouting. Any future pimples will, therefore, be prevented. If you can afford laser hair removal or electrolysis, we suggest you try it. (Lasers work better on the combination of fair skin and dark hair, so be judicious with their use if you are a woman of color.) If not, the prescription cream Vaniqa, used twice a day, retards hair regrowth, but it needs to be used constantly to be effective. Please note that temporary hair-removal methods, such as waxing and depilatories, tend to be extremely irritating to the skin and can trigger acne-like reactions.

For many women, as new hairs appear on their chins, scalp hair may be thinning. This can be extremely embarrassing, and some women go to great lengths to hide any noticeably bare spots on the scalp. Studies have shown that Rogaine works better for women than it does for men, even though it is targeted at balding males. We suggest you try Rogaine twice a day. In the morning use Rogaine for Women (2 percent strength); in the evening use Rogaine for Men (5 percent strength). The greater concentration tends to weigh hair down, so it's easier to use at night when you don't have to worry about styling it.

---

nizing hormones [those from the estrogen family, produced by your ovaries] decrease, this allows for a relative increase in the masculinizing hormones [those from the androgenic family, such as testosterone, dihydrotestosterone, and cortisol, produced by your ovaries and adrenal glands], already present in the body. Decreased estrogen and progesterone levels, which affect a woman's fertility, are a normal part of the aging process. With less of these hormones, though, the masculinizing hormones become more prominent, which explains why your chin suddenly seems to sprout hairs when you least want to see them. These hairs grow on the facial target tissue most susceptible to androgens."

With acne, though hormone levels may be appropriate for your age, the sensitivity of each woman's hair follicles to the shift in androgens is genetically determined. It's intrinsic and unchangeable. So for women who have a genetically determined sensitivity to androgens, once the feminizing hormone levels begin to drop, acne can develop and quickly worsen.

A Closer Look at the Monthly Whammy

There are always fluctuations in every woman's hormonal levels throughout the month. These are perfectly normal and allow you to ovulate and menstruate. Men, whose hormonal levels increase during puberty and remain fairly constant throughout most of their lives, don't have these bouncing hormonal levels.

"During the first half of your monthly cycle [the follicular phase], the pituitary gland is stimulated to secrete follicle-stimulating hormone [FSH] and luteinizing hormone [LH], which cause the follicles, the tiny sacs in each ovary which contain the oocytes [the immature egg cells], to enlarge," Dr. Kagan says. "Estrogen and progesterone are then released to prepare the uterine lining for implantation of a fertilized egg.

"At midcycle, there's a surge of LH, which stimulates ovulation, the release of the egg from the ovary. At this time, in the second half of the cycle [the luteal phase], the ovaries produce high levels of progesterone. Together, estrogen and progesterone provide the delicate balance needed by the body to create a lush environment for a fertilized egg to be able to implant in the uterus: If fertilization does not occur, estrogen and progesterone levels begin to decline, and your period will begin."

For women prone to acne, the progesterone rise during the luteal phase of the monthly cycle may work in tandem with the androgens in the body to overstimulate the sebaceous glands. The acne tends to appear in the same area each month, often around the same time. Scientists aren't yet able to pinpoint how exactly this happens, but when they do, we may be able to develop more treatments for acne in adult women. In the meantime, birth control pills can work by suppressing this cycle.

If your acne suddenly becomes worse and your normal menstrual cycles suddenly begin to change in length or duration, we recommend that you see your gynecologist right away for a complete hormonal workup, which involves simple blood tests. Your monthly cycle is a reflection of the state of your hormones. There may be a metabolic disorder affecting the thyroid, an iron deficiency, or simply a normal fluctuation.

Because of the hormonal double whammy, we can't stop all the hormones

POLYCYSTIC OVARIAN SYNDROME

Polycystic ovarian syndrome (PCOS) is a serious condition caused when many follicles develop on the ovaries but none become fully mature and therefore ovulation can't occur. Most women who have this condition have years of irregular menstrual cycles, often fewer than six a year. PCOS causes elevated levels of luteinizing hormone (which stimulates the ovaries), testosterone, and insulin, and the symptoms can be devastating: acne, weight gain, hair loss in a balding pattern on the head, increased hirsutism (facial hair), and deepening of the voice. If untreated, it can lead to infertility. When hormone balance is restored, these symptoms abate.

Any woman with these symptoms should see a gynecologist for treatment.

in your body from wreaking havoc on your skin. The acne that appeared on your face this morning didn't happen last night. It's a process that can take up to two weeks to manifest. The only solution is to treat your entire face on a regular basis to stop breakouts before they happen.

when should you see a dermatologist?

If you have been following our program religiously and have still not seen any improvement in eight to twelve weeks, we recommend that you see a dermatologist. It's important to treat stubborn adult acne as quickly as possible because of the potential for scarring.

Adult acne should be taken seriously, whether you have two tiny pimples or twenty large cysts reappearing every month. Acne is a disease, and dermatologists can help you. Ironically, many women who see us say, "Oh, today my skin's the best it's looked. I had three pimples yesterday." Your dermatologist should ask how your skin looks on a typical day. It's more difficult to prescribe an effective treatment based upon what is seen in only one visit.

Communicating your history of acne is vital. Also bring in either a detailed list or a bag full of the skin-care products, makeup, and sunscreen you use. Don't forget herbal and vitamin supplements.

treatment for acne in adult women

The Rodan and Fields Approach is as effective for adults as it is for teens. You can alternate your topical routine, too, so if something has a scent or texture you're not crazy about, feel free to try something else as long as you complete the three steps combining benzoyl peroxide, salicylic acid, and sulfur on your entire face.

Adults rarely have problems with compliance, because they are highly motivated to see improvement and responsible enough to understand the ramifications of sporadic treatment. For both adults and teens, it is crucial to remain on the new treatment program for at least four to six months. A few months of trying it may not be enough; your acne might quickly return.

If, however, eight to twelve weeks have passed and you see no improvement, make an appointment with a dermatologist, where the following treatments (listed in descending order of the most commonly prescribed) may be recommended in addition to, or in place of, the Rodan and Fields Approach: hormone therapy, spironolactone, oral antibiotics, topical antibiotics and retinoids, and Accutane.

Hormone Therapy (Oral Contraceptives or Birth Control Pills)

Birth control pills are often prescribed for acne because they suppress and level out the uneven surges of estrogen and progesterone, thereby stabilizing the hormonal stimulation that causes acne breakouts. They are often prescribed for women who have a history of menstrual irregularities, premenstrual flare-ups of acne, increased oil production, mild to moderate facial hair, and inflammatory nodular acne, particularly on the chin and jaw. For these women, birth control pills are a terrific option that we recommend trying, depending on your family history and your plans for pregnancy. However, birth control pills don't work instantly—at least three months are usually needed before any changes in acne are visible.

Approximately 50 percent of our adult women acne patients improve on the birth control pill. For some, it has no effect on acne whatsoever; in a few rare cases, it worsens it. Birth control pills have the best effect on women who have irregular cycles and whose acne is worsened specifically by hormonal triggers.

The pill works by stopping ovulation; thickening the cervical mucus, which makes it more difficult for the sperm to reach the egg; and thinning the uterine lining to make it less receptive to a fertilized egg. It does not prevent the transmission of sexual diseases, and it does not affect future fertility. In the past, the pill had much higher levels of the hormones estrogen and progesterone and therefore frequently caused weight gain, breast tenderness, and moodiness. The newest pills have much lower levels, so these side effects are minimal.

The pill can reduce the risk of ovarian and endometrial cancer and also fibroids, which are noncancerous growths within the uterus. It also helps prevent women with polycystic ovaries from developing more cysts. Because it levels out hormones, the pill helps relieve the uncomfortable symptoms of PMS.

We usually start patients with Yasmin or Ortho Tri-Cyclen. If results are not seen within three months, we recommend trying another brand. Each brand of birth control pill is subtly different, and a subtle change can have dramatic results on skin. Please note that you must see your gynecologist for a birth control pill prescription. You can use this opportunity to have both the yearly Pap smear test for cervical cancer, a must for all women, and a regular checkup.

Some women, especially those with a history of breast cancer or who plan to have a family, do not wish to take the pill. We understand this and respect any woman's wishes. There are alternative treatments available, and we will work together as a team to explore them all.

Birth control pills should never be taken if you smoke, or if you have a history of thrombosis (blood clots) or strokes, a heart abnormality, high blood pressure, severe migraines, breast cancer, liver or gall bladder disease, obesity, or diabetes. Women with acne who are advised not to take estrogen—such as those over age thirty-five who are smokers, breast-feeding mothers, and those with a family history of breast cancer—may sometimes be prescribed a progesterone-only pill, which is less effective for acne than a pill with both estrogen and progesterone but can provide a significant improvement in your acne nonetheless.

Spironolactone

Spironolactone is a mild diuretic, which means it makes you urinate excess water. It is often prescribed to treat high blood pressure. As it also has an antiandrogen effect, for women who tend to have more of the masculinizing hormones and symptoms, such as acne, facial hair, and thinning scalp hair, spironolactone can be very effective. (Because of these feminizing side effects, spironolactone is avoided when treating men.)

Because spironolactone is what's called a potassium-sparing diuretic, you need to have your potassium levels checked several weeks after you begin taking it and periodically while you are on it. You should also avoid taking potassium supplements. Spironolactone may make your breasts slightly tender, and it occasionally causes midmonthly spotting. It is safe to be on spironolactone for a year or more.

Spironolactone is generally prescribed in tandem with birth control pills, usually with an estrogen-dominant birth control pill, such as Lo Estrin, Ortho Tri-Cyclen, or Yasmin, because the pill regulates the feminizing hormones, and spironolactone blocks the masculinizing hormones. As a result, the combination of the two drugs is synergistic for the treatment of acne.

Oral Antibiotics

Oral antibiotics work by removing the *p. acnes* bacteria and decreasing inflammation. Acne may be a long-term issue, but antibiotics are *not* forever. As for teens, antibiotics are rarely prescribed for longer than six months. Nor do we believe that antibiotics should be prescribed for severe acne when Accutane is a highly successful alternative. Please refer to page 49 in chapter 2 for more information about oral antibiotics.

Always call your dermatologist if you have any questions or if you're experiencing side effects while taking oral antibiotics. Stomach upsets are fairly common, although the newer antibiotics are meant to be taken with food and are tolerated better. Acidophilus and probiotic supplements can help alleviate this side effect, too.

You should call your dermatologist immediately if you experience headaches, vision problems, or joint pain while taking antibiotics. Another common reaction to the tetracycline-derived antibiotics, such as minocycline, is hives, an allergic reaction that manifests as a red, bumpy, itchy rash. Please note that hives usually appear two to three *weeks* after you begin your course of pills.

Topical Antibiotics and Retinoids

Topical antibiotics, such as azeleic acid, clindamycin, erythromycin, and sodium sulfacetamide, remove bacteria. Retinoids, such as Differin, Retin-A, and Tazorac, work to unplug pores. We usually create a treatment plan that includes using benzoyl peroxide or topical antibiotics in the morning and a retinoid at night. For more information on topical antibiotics and retinoids, see pages 51 and 56 in chapter 2.

Accutane

Accutane is a serious drug that works best on cases of moderate to severe acne. In most women, results are seen in two months. It is imperative to pre-

DIANA'S STORY

"I'm now thirty-five and a former model who never had any sort of skin care problems. I used anything and everything and enjoyed trying all sorts of different products. About six months ago I started flaring up with the most horrendous acne, and nothing worked to get rid of it. I was going through gallons of concealer, and as I now have a job which puts me in the public eye, it was very embarrassing. Even my hairdresser commented, asking me what was going on with my skin. The acne was bumpy, on my cheeks and chin, and there was simply no hiding it. The heartbreak for me was knowing that I was getting married soon, and I would just cry and cry and cry to think of what my face would look like with me in my lovely gown standing beside my lovely new husband. He was so sweet and did not point out how bad my skin was looking, but it was obvious that he did notice. No amount of makeup on the *outside* can help clear your skin and cure it from the *inside*.

"Once I started using Proactiv Solution, my face cleared up almost right away. You have given me back my motivation and self-esteem, which I never thought I could have again. And you saved me from a costly chemical peel, as well as the drama of taking Accutane. I'm looking forward to a happy wedding, a happy career, and the knowledge that I can leave the house again without putting on big sunglasses, a baseball cap, and a whole ton of concealer."

scribe Accutane at a dose determined by your body weight for a minimum of five to six months. Once Accutane clears your acne, a topical regimen can be followed for maintenance of acne-free skin.

Unfortunately, a small number of women who have had more than two courses of Accutane, sometimes up to six, still fail to respond. Their hormone levels may be normal, but, we think, for some unknown reason, that the oil gland is supersensitive to the androgens that stimulate acne. When this happens, we try spironolactone or antibiotics plus a topical regimen.

Accutane causes birth defects, so it absolutely must *not* be taken during pregnancy. For more on this topic, see page 208. For more general information on Accutane, refer to page 53 in chapter 2 and page 177 in chapter 8.

acne and pregnancy

"I'm a wound-care nurse so I know a lot about skin. I always had pretty good skin as a teen and in my twenties, but after I became pregnant with my second child, my skin started breaking out. I thought after he was born, it would get better—it didn't. Then I thought after I weaned my baby when he was ten months old, my hormones would go back to normal and my skin would too—it didn't. I need help!"

—Anna, age thirty-three

"I had beautiful skin until I started having children. Then the texture of my skin changed—I had tiny little knots underneath my skin, with discoloration around them, plus red blotches everywhere on my face. This turned into cystic acne, where the large knots underneath my skin would linger for months before going away, and in the meantime I'd get new ones. The doctors kept telling me, 'It's hormonal, you know, so it'll go away,' which didn't make me feel any better, and it certainly didn't make me look any better. So I was going through nine months of pregnancy with bad skin and another nine months of nursing with bad skin."

—Samantha, age thirty-six

"All bets are off!" That's what we always tell our pregnant patients. You don't know the day you're going to deliver, how you're going to deliver, how much weight you'll gain, how bad your morning sickness will be, how you'll feel, or how your skin will look, so strap yourself in for a nine-month-long roller coaster ride.

For women who have heard so much about the glow of pregnancy, the sudden appearance of acne triggered by pregnancy's hormonal changes can put a large damper on their enthusiasm and diminish their joy. Many women also notice that their faces have become much redder during pregnancy (the medical term is *plethoric*). This is due to an increased blood volume, which nearly doubles during pregnancy, and, unfortunately, there is no medical solution to reduce pregnancy-induced facial redness. Your best bet is to tone it down with makeup.

Some women's bodies adjust easily; such women love being pregnant and sail through the nine months with relative ease. Others aren't quite so lucky. They spend three months enduring perpetual queasiness, then wake up with pimples. And sometimes these pimples persist for years after the pregnancies. It isn't fair.

Fortunately, having acne during one pregnancy doesn't mean you'll always have acne or that subsequent pregnancies will also trigger skin problems. It's simply impossible to predict. When you're pregnant you can wake up, look down at your blossoming belly, and exclaim, "Oh, my goodness, what the heck happened last night?!" Then you waddle into the bathroom, peer at your face, and say again, "Oh, my goodness, what the heck *did* happen last night?!"

Drugs and Pregnancy

Acne treatment is more challenging during pregnancy, but it is possible. The biggest dilemma pregnant women with acne face is that few drugs available are safe to use. There are alternatives. Many pregnant women falsely assume that their acne can't be treated at all, so they avoid going to the dermatologist. Don't wait! You might scar in the meantime by postponing treatment. In addition, the last thing you need to be doing while waiting for your baby to be born is worrying about pimples and cysts.

The FDA classification of drugs capable of causing congenital abnormalities, or birth defects, is teratogen. The risk factor is labeled as follows:

A   Controlled studies show no risk
B   No evidence of risk in humans

C   Risk cannot be ruled out because it hasn't been studied in humans

D   Positive human evidence of fetal risk

X   Contraindicated in pregnancy

The relative risk from topical medications is significantly low. FDA-approved drugs, for which no tests have been conducted on pregnant or nursing females (Category C), but are generally considered safe for use during pregnancy are:

Topical

erythromycin

benzoyl peroxide

salicylic acid

an alternative is <u>oral</u> erythromycin

Topical retinoids, such as Tazorac, however, are cousins to Accutane, the most potent teratogenic drug of all, and because of their classification in Category X, we will not prescribe them for any woman contemplating pregnancy. Topical sulfur is safe in the first two trimesters but should be withheld in the third, as in extremely rare cases it can contribute to a condition of the fetus called kernicterus, which may lead to birth defects, such as cerebral palsy, hearing loss, and mental retardation. Oral sulfurs are more dangerous, and we don't recommend their use during pregnancy. However, if acne is severe, oral erythromycin and low-dose prednisone may be used for short periods of time to prevent scarring. The patient should be closely monitored by both her dermatologist and obstetrician before using any medications. (A pregnant woman should always check with her obstetrician or gynecologist before using *any* medications.)

We always fully discuss potential treatments with our pregnant patients or patients who are contemplating pregnancy, then devise a suitable regimen. You should do the same with your dermatologist. To aid this process, once you're pregnant, you should write down the active ingredients in your medicated skin-care products and take that list to your obstetrician or gynecologist to ask his or her advice. Always discuss every drug that you ingest or put on your skin with your obstetrician or gynecologist, including herbal supplements and especially Vitamin A, to be on the safe side. Then you can determine your acne treatment with your dermatologist.

Although benzoyl peroxide has been safely sold over the counter for over forty years and has never been linked to any reported birth defects, we tell our patients that even though the FDA has cleared it, they should still check with their obstetrician or gynecologist for final approval. Topical salicylic acid in a 2 percent or less solution and topical erythromycin are also viable options. Oral erythromycin is usually prescribed during pregnancy only for a rare condition called acne conglobata, which is severe, explosive, nodular acne that has a high potential for scarring if left untreated. Dermatologists can also safely inject cysts with very low-strength steroids to shrink them.

We *do* recommend that pregnant women have facials (with noncomedogenic products, of course) as much-needed, relaxing stress-busters and as an acne treatment. You can also safely have comedone extractions performed and also microdermabrasion or glycolic peels.

Accutane and Pregnancy

According to the FDA, "Accutane is one of the most potent human teratogens and should not be used during pregnancy. This agent has been associated with a pattern of malformations involving craniofacial, cardiac, thymic, and central nervous system structures."

Any woman taking Accutane must also use birth control pills plus a barrier method of contraception (such as a diaphragm or condom) and be tested for pregnancy once a month.

If you have been on Accutane and wish to become pregnant, Accutane is technically completely out of your system twenty-four days after the last pill has been taken. However, just to be on the safe side, we suggest waiting a minimum of three months.

Be aware that if you take vitamin supplements, especially those with high doses of Vitamin A, you should show the bottles to your obstetrician or gynecologist. Accutane is derived from Vitamin A, so if you take excessive supplemental doses, you might be exposing yourself to a similar risk.

Note that Accutane causes birth defects only if ingested by a pregnant woman. It has absolutely no effect on your reproductive system if you are not pregnant. It has no effect on your chromosomes, either, nor does it affect sperm. Men can safely take Accutane at any point without worrying about potential effects on the baby.

MELASMA

Feminizing hormones and sun exposure, cosmetics, certain drugs, and a genetic predisposition can trigger an outbreak of melasma, which appears as a proliferation of brown spots on the face, neck, and ears. It resembles postinflammatory hyperpigmentation and is often called the mask of pregnancy, since it's most commonly seen in pregnant women. Melasma is also frequently seen in menopausal women on hormone replacement therapy (HRT).

Melasma can be as devastating to women as acne. It often fades on its own after pregnancy has ended, but women taking hormones, such as birth control pills or HRT, should discuss with their gynecologists discontinuing their use to effectively end melasma.

We often use a combination of hydroquinone with a topical retinoid to treat the spots caused by melasma. In fact, the Rodan & Fields RADIANT regimen was created to lighten melasma: the alpha hydroxy (AHA) cleanser aids with exfoliation, the hydroquinone toner and lotion lift the abnormal color, and the UVA/UVB zinc-based sunscreen helps stop the return of pigment.

Breast-feeding

With a few exceptions, all bets are still off while you continue to breast-feed.

We recommend that most women, to be on the safe side, stick to the same acne treatment they used during pregnancy. If there is no pressing need for a course of antibiotics, wait until your little one is weaned. Breast-feeding has so many benefits for both mother and child that we urge you to continue with it for however long you had planned to as long as your acne is not causing permanent scars. If it is, see your dermatologist. You can discuss with your doctor all the options available to you.

All Bets Are On, Again

Most women who have acne flare-ups during pregnancy or breast-feeding see them subside once hormone levels settle down. June's story is a good example: "Getting pregnant at forty just rained havoc on my face," June told us. "I just got so sick of the hormones screaming in my face and everything going wild. I felt ugly and awful, with huge boils everywhere, plus, I was no spring chicken and blew up like a beached whale!

"I started the Rodan and Fields Approach when I was nursing, and it's been great. I haven't had a boil buildup in a long time. I only wish I'd tried it sooner, as it would have made me a much less miserable pregnant lady!"

acne and stress

"I rarely had acne before, but at thirty-three the stress of starting school again to get a second doctoral degree really took a toll," Georgia said. "My face just went crazy. As a result, I only went out to attend classes. I studied at home and didn't socialize the entire first semester. I'm also a singer and was on stage a lot, and it was really, really difficult to sing in front of the faculty and my peers, because no matter how much makeup I caked on, all the acne just kind of soaked through."

As you can see from Georgia's story, stress influences adult acne. It affects the release of hormones from the adrenal glands, in addition to the androgens, which have a direct effect on the sebaceous (oil-producing) glands. More hormones can mean more acne, and more acne can mean more stress.

For information on how to manage stress and eliminate your stress-induced acne, see page 98 in chapter 4.

patient history—an adult woman: age thirty-one

Jamie had mild acne as a teen, which until her thirty-first birthday she had long forgotten. Then she began getting monthly nodules on her chin and jawline, with the occasional nodule on her neck. She averages two to five nodules a month, and as each lasts for a month, her face is never clear. Just as one nodule is about to resolve, a new one appears, often in the same location. The previous cysts often leave brown marks.

Jamie has a classic case of mild to moderate adult acne. Adult acne tends to be deeper and more long-lasting and has a very high probability of scarring. The location of eruption tends to be exclusively at the chin, jawline, and neck. Her adult acne also correlates well with her menstrual cycle, stress, and hectic lifestyle, which is also extremely typical.

Jamie's previous treatment consisted of products from an elegant skin-care line purchased at her local department store. Most of them contained salicylic acid, with occasional nonmedicated exfoliant cleansers. No other medicines were tried. Jamie stated that she would like to avoid pills at this point in her life.

We put Jamie on the Rodan & Fields CALM treatment, which includes washing with a cleanser containing sulfur (CALM 1 Wash), followed by an alcohol-free toner with salicylic acid (CALM 2 Prepare). After the toner dries, Jamie applies a leave-on lotion with 2.5 percent benzoyl peroxide (CALM 3 Treat). And daily on the five days preceding her menstrual cycle, Jamie applies a mask with sulfur (CALM Soothe).

It took approximately two months for Jamie's skin to clear. Her glowing complexion is easy to maintain with the same CALM regimen.

patient history—an adult woman: pregnant

Erin had the best skin in high school and college. She never saw a bump until she was twenty-eight, three months into her first pregnancy. Then the long-anticipated glow of pregnancy turned to fire. She had multiple red papules and nodules on her face with central facial pink patches in the middle of her face. She was not happy, but she was worried about taking any potentially harmful drugs. We explained to Erin that her moderate acne was due to the surge of estrogens her body was experiencing. It's quite common for pregnant women to go through many different stages of acne while the fetus is growing. We stressed that it's extremely important to treat acne conditions during pregnancy because scarring is a real possibility during this time.

Erin's initial therapy included topical use of salicylic acid, benzoyl peroxide, and prescription erythromycin. Her obstetrician felt these medicines were safe for use during pregnancy.

For optimum benefit, we put Erin on the Proactiv Solution full-face treatment; she washes with a gentle scrub cleanser containing salicylic acid (Proactiv Solution Deep Cleansing Wash), followed by a toner with glycolic acid (Proactiv Solution Revitalizing Toner). After the toner dries, Erin applies a leave-on lotion with 2.5 percent benzoyl peroxide (Proactiv Solution Repairing Lotion). And, as needed, a prescription topical erythromycin (ATS Solution) is applied.

Erin began her acne treatment in the third month of pregnancy. She was seen monthly throughout the course of her pregnancy and was easily maintained with topical care and occasional injections. While in the office, Erin sometimes underwent low-dose cortisone injections to the large painful nodules, which resolved within twenty-four hours.

treatments for adult women

Remember, use these products on your *entire face*, not only on acne-prone areas, except where noted.

Every day, you need to clean, tone, and treat your skin, and the products you use contain medicines to unplug pores, remove bacteria, and reduce swelling. The active ingredients in some of these products are applicable in several categories. For example, salicylic acid, which unplugs pores, is often an active ingredient in cleansers, toners, leave-on lotions, and moisturizers, and benzoyl peroxide, which removes bacteria and helps to unplug pores, is often an active ingredient in cleansers and leave-on lotions. This explains why Proactiv Solution Renewing Cleanser and Proactiv Solution Repairing Lotion, which contain benzoyl peroxide, both unplug pores and remove bacteria. However, we are listing cleansers only in Step 1—Unplug Pores and not Step 2—Remove Bacteria. The reason is simple: Leave-on lotions, such as Proactiv Solution Repairing Lotion, must be applied *after* cleansing and toning.

You will also notice that the order of the three steps is different for Proactiv Solution products from that for Rodan & Fields CALM products. That's because the formulation in each system is different, although the ingredients are similar and the purpose remains the same. The order of use of ingredients is interchangeable as long as you cleanse, tone, and treat with salicylic acid or glycolic acid, benzoyl peroxide, and sulfur in some combination and end up with a leave-on lotion.

Note: "Apply sparingly" means you should use a dime-sized amount of product. It should be enough to have a thin coat applied over the entire surface of the skin, where needed.

Note: In the Extra Help sections, you may choose more than one product, such as a mask, a leave-on lotion, or a moisturizer, if needed.

TREATMENT 1: PROACTIV SOLUTION

Start to use this treatment once a day for two weeks, then increase to twice a day. Until you are able to tolerate its use twice a day or if you remain at once a day, use a mild cleanser, such as Cetaphil Gentle Skin Cleanser or Rodan & Fields COMPOUNDS Gentle Wash, when not using Proactiv Solution products.

1. Unplug Pores—glycolic acid, benzoyl peroxide
a) Renewing Cleanser	Wash off and pat dry.
b) Revitalizing Toner	Apply with gauze or cotton ball. Let dry.

2. Remove Bacteria—benzoyl peroxide
Repairing Lotion	Apply with fingertips. Let dry. Use in the morning only.

3. Reduce Swelling—sulfur
Concealer Plus	Lightly dot on with applicator. Blend with concealer brush or fingertips. Use once or twice a day.
Refining Mask	Apply to clean, dry face or other affected area. Let dry ten minutes. Rinse with lukewarm water. Use once or twice a week for maintenance or every night for the five nights leading up to menstruation.

4. Extra Help—Proactiv Solution
Clarifying Night Cream	Apply sparingly to dry skin. Use only at night.
Daily Oil Control (for slightly oily skin)	Apply to entire face or other affected area with fingertips after toner. Let dry. Use daily or as needed.
Green Tea Moisturizer	Apply sparingly to dry skin.
Mild Exfoliating Peel	Apply thin layer. Let dry one to two minutes. Remove with fingertips. Rinse with lukewarm water. Use once a week.
Sheer Finish Compact Foundation	Apply sparingly.
Sheer Finish Loose Powder	Apply sparingly over foundation.
Skin-Clearing Cream to Powder Foundation	Apply sparingly.

TREATMENT 2: RODAN & FIELDS CALM

Start to use this treatment once a day for two weeks, then increase to twice a day. Until you are able to tolerate its use twice a day or if you remain at once a day, use a mild cleanser, such as Cetaphil Gentle Skin Cleanser or Rodan &

Fields COMPOUNDS Gentle Wash, when not using Rodan & Fields CALM products.

1. Reduce Swelling—sulfur

Rodan & Fields CALM 1
  Wash (cleanser)

Wash off and pat dry.

2. Unplug Pores—salicylic acid

Rodan & Fields CALM 2
  Prepare (toner)

Apply with gauze or cotton ball. Let dry.

3. Remove Bacteria—benzoyl peroxide

Rodan & Fields CALM 3
  Treat (leave-on lotion)

Apply with fingertips. Let dry.

4. Extra Help

Proactiv Solution Green
  Tea Moisturizer

Apply sparingly to dry skin.

Proactiv Solution Sheer
  Finish Compact
  Foundation

Apply sparingly.

Proactiv Solution Sheer
  Finish Loose Powder

Apply sparingly over foundation.

Proactiv Solution Skin-
  Clearing Cream to
  Powder Foundation

Apply sparingly.

Rodan & Fields CALM
  Soothe (mask)

Mix ingredients into a paste. Apply to face or other affected area. Let dry ten minutes. Peel off. Use once or twice a week or every night for the five nights leading up to menstruation.

Rodan & Fields
  COMPOUNDS
  Moisture

Apply to dry skin.

TREATMENT 3: OTHER PRODUCTS

Start to use this treatment once a day for two weeks, then increase to twice a day. Until you are able to tolerate its use twice a day or if you remain at once a day, use a mild cleanser, such as Cetaphil Gentle Skin Cleanser or Rodan & Fields COMPOUNDS Gentle Wash, when not using other products. Remember to pick only one product from each list, except in the Extra Help section, where you may choose more than one product, such as a mask, a toner, or a moisturizer, if needed.

1. Unplug Pores—salicylic acid

Clearasil Deep Pore
  Cream Cleanser

Iman Perfect Response
  Oil-Free Cleanser

L'Oréal Ideal Balance
  Foaming Cream
  Cleanser

L'Oréal Pure Zone Skin
  Balancing Cream
  Cleanser

Neutrogena Deep
  Cleaning Wash

Neutrogena Multi-
  vitamin Skin Therapy

Peter Thomas Roth Beta
  Hydroxy Acid 2% Acne
  Wash

Wash off and pat dry.

2. Remove Bacteria—benzoyl peroxide

Clear By Design Gel 2.5%

Neutrogena On-the-
  Spot Acne Treatment

Apply with fingertips. Let dry.

3. Reduce Swelling—sulfur

Clearasil Adult Care
  Acne Treatment Cream

Prescriptives Blemish
  Specialist

Apply sparingly with fingertips. Let dry.

4. Extra Help

Biotherm Acnopur
  Exfoliating Toner

Apply with gauze or cotton ball. Let dry.

Clean & Clear Oil-Free
  Dual Action Moisturizer

Apply sparingly to dry skin.

Neutrogena Clear Pore
  Cleanser Mask

Apply with fingertips. Let dry five to ten minutes. Rinse with lukewarm water. Use once or twice a week or every night for the five nights leading up to menstruation.

Neutrogena Skin-Clearing Moisturizer	Apply sparingly to dry skin.

Don't Forget the Sunscreen

For all three treatments, applying sunscreen in the morning is the all-important final step. Apply once all treatment products have dried.

Clinique Sun Care Face SPF 15
Estée Lauder In the Sun Sunblock For Face SPF 15
Neutrogena Ultra Sheer Dry-Touch Sunblock SPF 30
Olay Complete UV Defense Moisture Lotion
Ombrelle Sunscreen Lotion SPF 30
Prescriptives All You Need Broad Spectrum Oil Absorbing Lotion SPF 15
Proactiv Solution Daily Protection Plus SPF 15
Proactiv Solution Oil Free Moisture SPF 15
Rodan & Fields COMPOUNDS Protect SPF 15

once your acne goes away, you *will* have acne amnesia

"Thanks to you, I am not ugly anymore," twenty-nine-year-old Brandi told us. "My self-confidence is back, and I'm happy when my husband takes me out. My only regret is that I didn't take any before-and-after photos—I never wanted to have my picture taken before, and I'm sure you can understand why!"

We urge women, who are so often the caretakers in their families, to be proactive about their lives, too. Your health is as important as your children's and your partner's. Take time for yourself. There is no reason to live with acne and its emotionally devastating effects. With proper treatment, you too can have acne amnesia as Brandi does.

"Had I found your program, I would not have suffered through the remarks, through the depression, through the hurt and excruciating mental anguish for twenty years," Brandi explains. "I would not have changed as a person. I would not have quit participating in the sports I love. I would not have withdrawn from my friends and family. I would not have gone twenty years without having my pictures taken (including my high school prom, senior class picture, and wedding photos). I would not have spent thousands of dollars trying every product on the market and seeing dermatologists who could not find the right treatment for me.

"Now," she goes on, "I am returning to my old self again. I go out all the time; I am traveling. I don't mind having my picture taken—in fact, I insist on it! I am participating in sports again. I am not running to the mirror to count how many cysts have appeared since the day before. I have learned to find different friends, the ones who don't care about the outside. Now I feel like I can face the public every day with clear skin and a nice smile, and it's given me the confidence I need to do my job right.

"Most important, I have finally become pleased with my appearance again. I look forward to the future. You gave me back my life."

chapter ten

perimenopause, menopause, and your aging skin

"I never had acne before, and then at age forty-five, all of a sudden I started breaking out all over my face, neck, chest, and back. It was devastating because I couldn't understand why I had it. I tried changing my diet, reducing sugar and fat intake, spent hundreds of dollars on different products, and nothing worked. Not only that, but the time and agony of dealing with acne on both a daily basis and minute by minute was completely draining. I was so self-conscious when I spoke to anyone out in public. All I could think of was how bad my skin looked and how I wished I could just hide."

—Isabella, age forty-six

"Once I started to go through menopause, I went off the birth control pills I'd been on most of my life, and my face just blossomed. I would get breakouts where the cyst felt like it went right down to the bone, and it hurt to even smile. On some days I would miss work because I couldn't stand how my face looked. I was mortified."

—Clorinda, age fifty

"After I had a full hysterectomy, my acne flared up and became worse. I went on different hormones, and every time I had a hormone change my acne would flare up. After I got comfortable with the hormone level, though, I still couldn't shake the acne. I am very regimented with my skin-care routine, and I didn't pick my pimples. I even tried tanning, but all that did was give me crispy acne! Nothing worked."

—Deanna, age fifty-three

they are the forgotten women. Our youth-oriented society, which ignores anyone old enough to remember hearing the Beatles on the radio forty years ago, presents a particularly difficult dilemma to older women suffering from acne. These women are as devastated as teenagers when their skin breaks out, but they are completely discounted as consumers who need a skin-care regimen that works on acne and on the visible signs of aging. Menopause marks a hugely important turning point—an inevitable rite of passage—for all women, and its emotional effects can be difficult enough to face. To compound this, a face marked with pimples can be overwhelming and depressing.

Older women with acne are often bewildered and deeply mortified by problem skin. It affects them whenever they have to face the public. This can be an especially difficult problem for working women, who in the current competitive marketplace need to appear as youthful and polished as possible: "When I hit my forties, I guess my hormone balance went out of whack. As I became more successful professionally, I also broke out more," forty-eight-year-old Willa told us. "It was very difficult for me to be a speaker in front of my association and to introduce myself to professional people when my chin and forehead were broken out. I felt like I didn't look as professional as my position warranted."

There has been very little information published about acne in older women. With no resources to refer to, older women turn their pain inward and can become increasingly depressed. Shame from their appearance, along with concerns about aging, are often belittled as "trite" or "self-indulgent" by family members and peers. And acne has its own, unique stigma, because most people don't expect an older person to have boils on his or her face: "I went to a family gathering, and I felt so embarrassed because people stared at the big red bumps on my face, then turned their backs on me and just walked away," one sixty-three-year-old patient told us as she fought back tears. "I think that was the most terrible moment of my life. The embarrassment was unbearable. I can't ever forget how my relatives—people I've known all my life—just walked away from me."

It is a small comfort to these forgotten women when we tell them how common their acne is. Older women often see dermatologists for yearly skin-cancer check-ups, or for rosacea (a condition that manifests itself with red bumps and flushing, without blackheads, often has a natural progression, becoming worse with age. We'll discuss rosacea at length in chapter 13). Rosacea and acne often go hand in hand. Older women care just as much about their pimples as their teenage children or grandchildren do. "You know I'm going to die when I stop caring," one impeccably groomed patient in her seventies joked.

Many older women have been battling acne for decades. It may have started in their thirties, so when we see them, it's the tail end of what has become a chronic condition. It is possible, however, to have sudden-onset acne spring itself upon unsuspecting older women. This can happen to women who have had drastic hormone removal, such as with a hysterectomy, or if hormone replacement therapy is abruptly discontinued.

Acne in older women tends to manifest itself in the same way and in the same areas as it does in younger women, with painful, large, red nodules in the chin, jawline, and neck area. In women past their thirties we rarely see it on the chest, back, or buttocks. However, sometimes older women, especially smokers, have tiny comedones around the outside of the eye. These bumps have been triggered by photo-aging due to excessive sun exposure and are *not true acne*. This is a condition called Favre-Racouchot syndrome and is treated with a topical retinoid such as Tazorac along with acne surgery extractions. (For more information, see page 311 in chapter 15.)

Age aside, all women deserve a future free of blemishes and worries. No woman is ever too old to be helped by treatment. Read on to discover the causes of your acne and the treatments that will work for you.

the hormonal connection

Menopause is not a sudden process, and it is certainly not a disease. It is a gradual reduction of the output of the feminizing hormones (particularly estrogen) once the egg supply in the ovaries dwindles, and it often takes a decade or longer. Symptoms usually begin around a woman's midforties (often earlier) and usually consist of hot flashes, vaginal dryness, and irregular menstrual cycles. This period of time is called perimenopause. On average, it lasts several years.

Menopause is defined as the cessation of menses for a year. The average age for menopause is fifty-one. Menopausal and postmenopausal women still produce hormones, although in much smaller quantities. Because the feminizing hormones are in decline, the masculinizing hormones can become dominant, which accounts for increased facial hair, thinning scalp and pubic hair, weight gain—and acne.

POSSIBLE SYMPTOMS OF PERIMENOPAUSE

acne
back pain
bloating
breast changes
dry skin
fatigue
food intolerance
hair changes
headaches
insomnia
irritability
joint pain
memory loss and fuzzy thinking
mood changes
urinary dysfunction
vaginal dryness
vision changes
weight loss or gain

when should you see a dermatologist?

If you have been following our program religiously and still have not seen any improvement in eight to twelve weeks, we recommend that you see a dermatologist. It's important to treat stubborn adult acne as quickly as possible because of the potential for scarring.

Acne in older women should be taken seriously, whether it's two tiny pimples or twenty large cysts reappearing every month. Acne is a disease, and dermatologists can help you. Communicating your history of acne is vital. Bring in either a detailed list or a bag full of the skin-care products, makeup, and sunscreen you use. Don't forget herbal and vitamin supplements.

treatment for acne in older women

The Rodan and Fields Approach is as effective for older women as it is for younger. In fact, we designed our Rodan & Fields CALM and RADIANT regimens specifically for the needs of our adult female patients.

Older women rarely have problems with compliance, because they are highly motivated to see improvement and are responsible enough to understand the ramifications of sporadic treatment. As with all acne patients, it is crucial to remain on a new treatment program for at least four to six months. A few months of trying it may not be enough, and your acne might quickly return.

If, however, eight to twelve weeks have passed and you see no improvement, make an appointment with a dermatologist, who may recommend the following treatments (listed in descending order of the most commonly prescribed) in addition to, or in place of, the Rodan and Fields Approach: hormone replacement therapy (HRT), hormone therapy (oral contraceptives and spironolactone), and other treatments (oral antibiotics, topical antibiotics, retinoids, and Accutane).

Hormone Replacement Therapy (HRT)

Because estrogen levels decline during perimenopause, hot flashes and other symptoms can become unbearable and acne can flare. When women asked their gynecologists about treatment options, the standard protocol until very recently was hormone replacement therapy (HRT), which is successful at reducing perimenopausal symptoms. In addition, it was thought to reduce the risk of osteoporosis, fractures, cardiovascular disease, Alzheimer's, and colon cancer.

Many women have been on HRT for years if not decades. Yet the medical belief that HRT had significant health benefits was stunningly questioned by several recent studies. This data shocked physicians as well as millions of menopausal women, who now have additional health worries.

One study, "Effect of Hormone Replacement Therapy on Breast Cancer Risk: Estrogen versus Estrogen Plus Progestin," by Ronald K. Ross, Annlia Paganini-Hill, Peggy C. Wan, and Malcolm C. Pike of the University of Southern California/Norris Comprehensive Cancer Center in Los Angeles, in the February 16,

2000, issue of the *Journal of the National Cancer Institute*, reported that women who were current users or who had used HRT in the last two years before their cancer diagnosis had a slightly higher risk of breast cancer than women who had not used hormone replacement therapy. This risk was higher in women on estrogen/progestin therapy than in women who used estrogen therapy alone and was positively correlated to duration of use.

Even more astonishing were the reported results of a long-term study by the Women's Health Institute, sponsored by the National Institute of Health. The study was meant to last eight years and tracked the relationship between HRT and possible benefits for heart disease, bone fractures with risks of blood clots, and breast and endometrial cancers.

In July 2002 the trial was stopped after only five years and two months. The unanticipated data showed that instead of protecting women against heart disease, it slightly increased the risk. It also increased the risk of breast cancer, stroke, and blood clots. This study showed a lower risk for hip fractures and colon cancer, but these benefits were outweighed by the possibility of more serious disease. Indeed, the risk for heart disease and breast cancer appeared to be cumulative, which meant that the longer a woman stayed on HRT, the greater her risk.

More than ever, a perimenopausal woman must discuss her symptoms and their manageability with her gynecologist, weigh the pros and cons, and make an informed decision about whether HRT is a viable option. Rest assured, there are many women who decide that the benefits of a short course of HRT far outweigh the small possibility of increased risk of other diseases. "Hormone therapy is no longer recommended for prevention of illnesses such as colon cancer, osteoporosis, or heart disease," Dr. Risa Kagan, a board-certified obstetrician and gynecologist, says. "Gynecologists recommend the lowest dose possible for the shortest period of time for menopausal symptoms. This is extremely individual for every woman; the time frame may be as short as a few months or as long as several years."

According to the American College of Obstetricians and Gynecologists, "the effects of these menopausal symptoms on the quality of a woman's life can be considerable, and the severity and duration of symptoms can vary widely from woman to woman. Some women experience few or very short-lived symptoms, while others experience severe symptoms over many years.

Yet too often, women are made to feel guilty about how they respond to menopausal symptoms, which are often trivialized by such comments that women should simply be able to 'put up with it.' "

We find this comment to be most telling, as there is a significant similarity between the belittling of a woman suffering from menopausal symptoms and a woman suffering from acne. Sympathy is often in short supply, and misunderstanding and condescension abound.

If your acne is triggered or made worse by your menopausal symptoms, it is similar to acne triggered during pregnancy. Acne often appears because of unavoidable hormonal changes. Pregnancy will end, and perimenopause will also end—but it may take years.

We always work in tandem with our patients' gynecologists when HRT is an option for acne treatment. We usually try HRT for a period of three months. A medicated topical acne regimen plus HRT usually does the trick.

HRT is usually prescribed in an estrogen/progesterone (called progestin) form for women who still have their uterus. Estrogen on its own can cause an increased risk for endometrial cancer, but for women who've had hysterec-

BEWARE OF THE SUPPLEMENTS FOR MENOPAUSAL SYMPTOMS

If you scan the shelves at drugstores and health food stores, you'll see that they are groaning with products allegedly designed to help relieve the symptoms women experience during perimenopause. Many of these contain phytoestrogens, which are estrogenlike substances derived from a plant source, usually soy or flaxseed oil. Herbals such as black cohosh, wild yam, dong quai, and valerian root are also touted.

So far, there is no solid, scientific evidence that any phytoestrogens provide real relief from hot flashes and other symptoms. Because the herbal supplement industry is not regulated by the FDA, there could be any number of active or inert ingredients in these pills that may cause acne or other problems. Additionally, there may be risks associated with ingesting concentrated forms of soy over a long period of time.

We think it's always best to discuss treatment options with a physician, rather than self-medicating, because there are too many variables that can affect your overall health. As always, whenever you see a dermatologist or a gynecologist, bring whatever supplements you have been taking so their contents can be assessed.

tomies, that risk has been removed, so estrogen alone is permissible. HRT is supplied orally, through a patch on the skin, as a cream or gel, or with an intrauterine device (IUD) or vaginal ring (which is localized therapy for vaginal dryness and urinary tract problems).

A note about coming off a course of HRT: We advise women who have been on HRT and wish to stop to slowly taper off their use rather than go cold turkey. An abrupt withdrawal will have a dramatic effect on hormone levels and can often trigger acne outbreaks, even in women who have had no pimples for decades. It's almost always best to slowly wean yourself from the pills. You can work out a timetable with your gynecologist to do so.

Hormone Therapy
(Oral Contraceptives and Spironolactone)

There have been many studies about the long-term safety of birth control pills for healthy women to use until menopause. The risks of HT do not apply to the use of birth control pills. Regardless of the length of oral contraceptive use or the user's age, birth control pills have not been found to increase breast cancer risk.

Birth control pills are an option for acne treatment in perimenopausal women. "Unless contraindicated, they have been found to be quite safe for use until menopause," says Dr. Kagan. They are usually combined with the diuretic spironolactone, which increases their effectiveness.

For more information, see page 203 in chapter 9.

Other Treatments

Other acne treatments include oral antibiotics, topical antibiotics and retinoids, and Accutane. For women who do not wish to go on any form of HT or who are advised against it by their gynecologists, we often start with a topical regimen. Refer to page 204 in chapter 9 for more information.

acne and stress

Many women have found that their stress levels have *not* decreased as their lives progress and children move out of the house. An elderly parent may be ailing, children may be struggling with their own lives, or savings may be de-

Joyce's Story

"I'm fifty-nine, and when I started getting pimples five years ago, I felt like a teenager again. My skin got so bad that I didn't want to go out in public, and my makeup didn't do a very good job at concealing all the redness. I saw several dermatologists, but what they gave me didn't do the trick. In fact, the last one I saw gave me a bag of samples to try, which didn't make me feel any better. He told me I had rosacea, but I didn't. I had plain old acne. I felt I had nowhere to go for advice. I was starting to feel desperate. I needed a miracle!

"By the time I discovered Proactiv Solution, I was willing to try anything. Within two weeks, I started to see results. And I haven't had a problem since. Because so many of my friends comment on my skin, I'm happy to talk with them about what I use. I don't want anyone to have to go through what I did at my age."

pleted by downturns in the economy—these can all cause sleepless nights. In addition, divorce, death, and other losses in the family can be overwhelming. Acne can then be the last straw.

Women of a certain age, who may have grown up during the Depression or had parents who did, often feel that they are not entitled to pamper themselves and that stress-busting techniques, such as massages, facials, and other treatments, are an indulgence. Yet a small amount of time doing something lovely just for yourself can often have far-reaching and therapeutic benefits. There is no reason to feel ashamed about thinking you deserve to have something luscious. And that includes clear, glowing skin.

For more information on managing stress, see page 98 in chapter 4.

your aging skin

If we could find a wrinkle cure in a bottle, we'd be gazillionaires! Unfortunately, there is no such thing—despite all the hype in those breathless ads for wrinkle lotions and potions. According to the American Academy of Dermatology, over-the-counter wrinkle creams and lotions may soothe dry skin, but they do little or nothing to reverse wrinkles. The only skin-care products studied for safety and efficacy, and approved by the FDA to treat aging skin, are tretinoin creams, such as Avage or Renova.

As we age, skin-cell turnover slows down. When we're young, the turnover rate for the renewal of the epidermis's outer layer is once every twenty-eight days. As we move into our twenties and thirties, the renewal rate slows down by about 10 percent each decade. By the time we hit our fifties and sixties, skin can look dull, sallow, and blotchy. Pores can become packed with dead cells and appear larger. In addition, damage to the fibers in the skin (called elastin and collagen) by the sun's ultraviolet light and cigarette smoke decreases elasticity in the skin. The end result is unwanted wrinkles.

How your skin ages is in part genetically determined. There are, however, many products and treatments you *can* use to improve the health and quality of your skin: sunscreen, moisturizer, exfoliation, microdermabrasion, chemical peels, lasers, Botox, and surgery. We will discuss each of these proactive options below.

Sunscreen

First and foremost, never, ever leave the house without sunscreen on! Refer to the section on page 320 in chapter 16 for more information about the proper use of sunscreen.

Moisturizing Mature Skin

An unfortunate fallacy among women is that moisturizers are not good for acne-prone skin and that applying creams to the face will make acne worse. We often see fifty-five-year-old women who have flaky patches on their cheeks because they're afraid to use moisturizers. However, moisturizers are necessary for the skin, especially if you live in a dry environment.

The safe recommendation is to pick a moisturizer clearly labeled noncomedogenic. It needn't be 100 percent oil free, as long as your skin doesn't react to it. We tell our patients and friends shopping for moisturizers to buy only what they can afford. Realize that no moisturizer, whether it costs $10 or $100, can deeply penetrate the skin to stimulate the production of the thick layer of collagen you had as a twenty-year-old. Moisturizers primarily coat the dead outer layer of skin (stratum corneum), plumping up the moisture content and making the skin more pliable. Moisturizers are cosmetics, not over-the-

MOISTURIZERS AND EYE CREAMS FOR AGING, ACNE-PRONE SKIN

Moisturizers

Aveeno Clear Complexion Daily Moisturizer
Cetaphil Moisturizing Lotion
Chanel Skin Conscience Total Health Moisture Lotion SPF 15
Clearasil Acne Fighting Facial Moisturizer
Clearasil Total Control Daily Skin Perfecting Treatment
Crème de la Mer Cream or Lotion
Elemis Absolute Day Cream
Ellen Lange MicroThera AM Moisturizing Lotion SPF 15
EmerginC Crude Control Hydrating, Protecting, and Balancing Emulsion
Estée Lauder Verité Calming Fluid
Eucerin Renewal Alpha Hydroxy Lotion SPF 15
Jurlique Viola Cream
L'Oréal Pure Zone Oil-Free Moisturizer
Lubriderm SPF 15 Lotion
Neutrogena SkinClearing Daily Face Cream
Olay Complete UV Defense Moisture Lotion
Proactiv Solution Oil Free Moisture SPF 15
Rodan & Fields COMPOUNDS Moisture

Eye Creams

Crème de la Mer The Eye Balm
Neutrogena Healthy Skin Eye Cream
Proactiv Solution Nourishing Eye Cream
Proactiv Solution Replenishing Eye Cream
Rodan & Fields COMPOUNDS Moisture Eye

counter drugs. As cosmetics, according to the FDA, moisturizers do not change the structure and function of the skin. Therefore, if you like the scent and texture of a cream, your skin responds to it, and it makes you feel good, go for it. Expect subtle changes, like a softer complexion, and you may be pleasantly surprised. Expect a face-lift from applying salmon oil and your hopes may be deflated. And, as much as we wish it could, sun damage cannot be undone by over-the-counter moisturizers.

The cosmetics industry does its best to convince us that there's hope in a jar. We know better. There is no miracle cream to erase folds and wrinkles. There will always be, however, another Cream of the Week launched to much fanfare and consumers willing to try it. This isn't entirely a bad idea. The continual search for new and improved products keeps the cosmetic industry looking for beneficial (and lucrative) breakthroughs, as happened when alpha hydroxy acids (AHAs) were introduced. The AHA moisturizers can be helpful, but they can't instantly make anyone look ten years younger.

This simple test will help you reach past the hype to what truly works for you: If you like two different products, use one on half your face and one on the other half. Test eye creams the same way. Expect to see results in a few days or weeks.

For more information on moisturizing, see page 323 in chapter 16.

Exfoliation

Exfoliation strips off the unnecessary dead cells sitting on the surface of your skin that make your complexion look dull. We've always believed it is an important part of acne treatment because it helps medications penetrate better, thus increasing their effectiveness. Many people think exfoliating means scrubbing their faces with harsh products containing ground apricot pits or walnut shells, which can tear the skin, producing irritation and redness. The tiny, round, synthetic beads we use in our Proactiv Solution Renewing Cleanser and Deep Cleansing Wash and Rodan & Fields RADIANT 1 Wash are extremely gentle and promote safe daily exfoliation.

Exfoliants include:

Alpha hydroxy acids (AHAs)

These may help reduce wrinkles, spots, and other signs of aging in sun-damaged skin. AHAs cause greater sensitivity to the sun, so you must protect yourself with sunscreen and hats and avoid sun exposure altogether whenever possible.

Retin-A or Renova

Retin-A helps acne and signs of aging (brown spots, pore size, fine wrinkles), but it can be irritating. As with AHAs, you must protect yourself from the sun.

Retinol

For those who are too sensitive to AHAs or prescription retinoids, over-the-counter retinol is significantly milder, which means it is not as effective but is still worth adding to your treatment.

Not everybody can exfoliate. If you have rosacea, atopic dermatitis (eczema), or highly sensitive skin, you should not actively exfoliate. Use a light touch with your fingertips instead. Or try a soft cotton washcloth or a very soft buff-puff type of cleansing pad. Also, try using gauze pads when you apply toner rather than a cotton ball. These techniques provide gentle exfoliation.

Microdermabrasion

Microdermabrasion is a procedure performed with a vacuum suction machine that spews out extremely fine crystals of sodium bicarbonate or aluminum bicarbonate onto the skin, which are then quickly vacuumed up by the same machine. These crystals pull off the dead layer of cells, called the stratum corneum. Depending on how much pressure, how much vacuum, and the volume of crystal flow, exfoliation can continue down into the deeper levels of the skin. Microdermabrasion helps stimulate and restore collagen and the elastic fibers in your skin's dermis with a subtle rejuvenating benefit. It's also very helpful for acne scars.

We suggest that microdermabrasion be performed every one to two weeks for five to six sessions to achieve maximum results. After that, a monthly tune-up is suggested. Microdermabrasion can be performed by a dermatologist, nurse, or licensed esthetician.

Because microdermabrasion has a potent exfoliating effect, it helps both acne and wrinkles. It unplugs pores, allowing medicines better penetration, while reducing some mild acne scars and hyperpigmentation.

Chemical Peels

Dermatologists and estheticians also perform exfoliating peels, which help dissolve the sebum plug to unclog pores. These peels also aid in exfoliation and cell renewal. Dermatologists perform high-strength peels with glycolic acid (30 to 70 percent) or salicylic acid (20 to 30 percent). Most states limit estheticians to lower levels, less than 20 to 30 percent for glycolic acid. Over-the-counter at-home peels are 2 percent or less for salicylic acid and less than 10 percent for glycolic acid. If you want to use one of the over-the-counter peels, check the label to see that the active ingredients include glycolic acid or salicylic acid. Follow directions exactly. To avoid irritation, chemical peels should not be used more often than once a week, and stay away from the eyelids and mouth.

Lasers

Nonablative lasers and light sources, such as Pulsed Dye, Neodyndium YAG, and Intense Pulsed Light, spare the top layer of skin and heat the dermis, contracting the skin to stimulate the production of new collagen. This causes a very subtle improvement in wrinkles and scars, and is especially useful for shallow acne scars. The process is only mildly painful and has a short healing time but needs to be repeated every month for four months to be effective.

The FDA has approved the CO_2 and Er:YAG (erbium) lasers to treat wrinkles. These are high-tech devices that remove skin one layer at a time, and are performed under anesthesia in an outpatient surgical setting. It requires two to three weeks to heal. In addition, posttreatment redness can last three months followed by permanent loss of pigmentation in 30 percent of cases.

Botox

Botox injections are performed by a dermatologist, occuloplastic surgeon (an ophthalmologist with additional training in cosmetic surgery), or plastic surgeon. They consist of the botulinium toxin (it's not toxic!) and are generally injected into the forehead and crow's feet area. Botox injections work by temporarily paralyzing the muscles that contract to cause wrinkles. They are, however, not a permanent fix—they usually last for three to four months. Botox has no effect whatsoever on acne or acne scars.

Surgery

Some acne scars can be improved by dermatologic surgeons through such methods as excision or dermabrasion. Acne scars can be filled with collagen or other filler materials for temporary improvement.

WHEN ACNE SCARS TURN INTO WRINKLES

To add insult to injury, we've often seen women with acne scars that turn into wrinkles! This is quite common in the chin area or cheeks, where the skin becomes bound down by the scar adhesions. This creates a tethering effect, so every time you smile or make a movement, the contraction causes the line to etch a deeper crease or groove.

Surgery, called subcision, can be performed to release these acne scars turned into wrinkles (called fibrous adhesions). Then a filler substance, such as collagen; fat; or a synthetic, such as silicone, Restylane, or Hylaform, is used to fill in the cavity to prevent further wrinkling.

patient history—a perimenopausal woman

Sue is forty-six. She brought in her sixteen-year-old daughter for acne treatment and complained that she had caught it, too, as she pointed to nodules on her chin and jaw. There were several cysts in the same location where she plucked out small black whiskers. She was upset about having to deal not only with a few beard hairs, wrinkles, and gray hair at the same time but now acne!

Sue has classic, perimenopausal mild to moderate acne. We put her on the Rodan & Fields CALM treatment, which includes washing with a cleanser containing sulfur (CALM 1 Wash), followed by an alcohol-free toner with salicylic acid (CALM 2 Prepare). After the toner dries, Sue applies a leave-on lotion with 2.5 percent benzoyl peroxide (CALM 3 Treat). And for extra help with unplugging pores and decreasing inflammation, a prescription retinoid (Tazorac 0.1% cream) is applied five minutes after CALM 3 Treat. Tazorac and retinoids in general are also beneficial for fine lines, postinflammatory hyperpigmentation (brown spots), and, sun damage—all of the aging issues Sue is concerned about.

Sue's skin is now clear and in fact has a youthful luster. This treatment is an excellent combination of prescription and over-the-counter full-face therapy, which Sue will continue to safely maintain for years.

patient history—a menopausal woman

Mary is fifty-eight. After reading about the controversy regarding hormone replacement therapy, she abruptly stopped taking her estrogen and progesterone, which she had been on for ten years. Three months later she started breaking out with pustules and nodules around the nose and lower face. She blamed her breakouts on her makeup and was highly disturbed by this new nuisance. Mary came to us and was shocked to learn that her recurrent red bumps were in fact acne caused by hormone withdrawal.

We put Mary on the Rodan & Fields CALM treatment, which includes washing with a cleanser containing sulfur (CALM 1 Wash), followed by an alcohol-free toner with salicylic acid (CALM 2 Prepare). After the toner dries, Mary applies a leave-on lotion with 2.5 percent benzoyl peroxide (CALM 3 Treat). And once a week, Mary applies a mask with sulfur (CALM Soothe). We also gave Mary the option of using CALM 3 Treat in the morning and Proactiv Solution Clarifying Night Cream at night.

Mary has been using the CALM treatment faithfully, and her acne cleared completely within six weeks. Because acne is not curable, only treatable, Mary's best course of action for the future is to maintain these successful results with the same regimen.

treatments for perimenopausal and menopausal women

Remember, use these products on your *entire face*, not only on acne-prone areas, except where noted.

Every day, you need to clean, tone, and treat your skin, and the products you use contain medicines to unplug pores, remove bacteria, and reduce swelling. The active ingredients in some of these products are applicable in several categories. For example, salicylic acid, which unplugs pores, is often an active ingredient in cleansers, toners, leave-on lotions, and moisturizers, and benzoyl peroxide, which removes bacteria and helps to unplug pores, is often an active ingredient in cleansers and leave-on lotions. This explains why Proactiv Solution Renewing Cleanser and Proactiv Solution Repairing Lotion, which contain benzoyl peroxide, both unplug pores and remove bacteria. However, we are listing cleansers only in Step 1—Unplug Pores and not Step 2—Remove

Bacteria. The reason is simple: Leave-on lotions, such as Proactiv Solution Repairing Lotion, must be applied *after* cleansing and toning.

If you have used Proactiv Solution products, you will notice that the order of the three steps is different for Proactiv Solution products from that for Rodan & Fields CALM products. That's because the formulation in each system is different, although the ingredients are similar and the purpose remains the same. The order of use of ingredients is interchangeable as long as you cleanse, tone, and treat with salicylic acid or glycolic acid, benzoyl peroxide, and sulfur in some combination and end up with a leave-on lotion.

Note: "Apply sparingly" means you should use a dime-sized amount of product. It should be enough to have a thin coat applied over the entire surface of the skin, where needed.

Note: In the Extra Help sections, you may choose more than one product, such as a mask, a microdermabrasion paste, or a moisturizer, if needed.

Acne

TREATMENT 1: RODAN & FIELDS CALM

Start by using this treatment once a day for two weeks, then increase to twice a day. Until you are able to tolerate its use twice a day or if you remain at once a day, use a mild cleanser, such as Cetaphil Gentle Skin Cleanser or Rodan & Fields COMPOUNDS Gentle Wash, when not using Rodan & Fields CALM products.

1. Reduce Swelling—*sulfur*
Rodan & Fields CALM 1   Wash off and pat dry.
  Wash (cleanser)

2. Unplug Pores—*salicylic acid*
Rodan & Fields CALM 2   Apply with gauze or cotton ball. Let dry.
  Prepare (toner)

3. Remove Bacteria—*benzoyl peroxide*
Rodan & Fields CALM 3   Apply with fingertips. Let dry.
  Treat (leave-on lotion)

4. Extra Help
Proactiv Solution Green   Apply sparingly to dry skin.
  Tea Moisturizer

Proactiv Solution Replenishing Eye Cream	Apply with your pinkie finger, gently patting cream on the upper and lower eyelids, including the crow's feet area.
Proactiv Solution Sheer Finish Compact Foundation	Apply sparingly.
Proactiv Solution Sheer Finish Loose Powder	Apply sparingly over foundation.
Proactiv Solution Skin-Clearing Cream to Powder Foundation	Apply sparingly.
Rodan & Fields CALM Soothe (mask)	Mix ingredients into a paste. Apply to face or other affected area. Let dry ten minutes. Peel off. Use once or twice a week or every night for the five nights leading up to menstruation.
Rodan & Fields COMPOUNDS Moisture	Apply to dry skin.
Rodan & Fields COMPOUNDS Moisture Eye	Apply with your pinkie finger, gently patting cream on the upper and lower eyelids, including the crow's feet area.

TREATMENT 2: PROACTIV SOLUTION

Start by using this treatment once a day for two weeks, then increase to twice a day. Until you are able to tolerate its use twice a day or if you remain at once a day, use a mild cleanser, such as Cetaphil Gentle Skin Cleanser or Rodan & Fields COMPOUNDS Gentle Wash, when not using Proactiv Solution products.

1. Unplug Pores—benzoyl peroxide, glycolic acid
a) Renewing Cleanser	Wash off and pat dry.
b) Revitalizing Toner	Apply with gauze or cotton ball. Let dry.

2. Remove Bacteria—benzoyl peroxide
Repairing Lotion	Apply with fingertips. Let dry.

3. Reduce Swelling—sulfur
Concealer Plus	Lightly dot on with applicator. Blend with a concealer brush or fingertips. Use once or twice a day.
Refining Mask	Apply to clean, dry face or other affected area. Let dry ten minutes. Rinse with lukewarm water. Use once or

twice a week for maintenance or every night for the five nights leading up to menstruation.

4. Extra Help—Proactiv Solution

Clarifying Night Cream	Apply sparingly to dry skin. Use only at night.
Daily Oil Control (for slightly oily skin)	Apply to entire face or other affected area with fingertips after toner. Let dry. Use daily or as needed.
Green Tea Moisturizer	Apply sparingly to dry skin.
Mild Exfoliating Peel	Apply thin layer. Let dry one to two minutes. Remove with fingertips. Rinse with lukewarm water. Use once a week.
Oil Blotter Sheets	Use as needed to pat away excess oil.
Sheer Finish Compact Foundation	Apply sparingly.
Sheer Finish Loose Powder	App;y sparingly over foundation.
Skin-Clearing Cream to Powder Foundation	Apply sparingly.

TREATMENT 3: OTHER PRODUCTS

Start by using this treatment once a day for two weeks, then increase to twice a day. Until you are able to tolerate its use twice a day or if you remain at once a day, use a mild cleanser, such as Cetaphil Gentle Skin Cleanser or Rodan & Fields COMPOUNDS Gentle Wash, when not using other products. Remember to pick only one product from each list, except in the Extra Help section, where you may choose more than one product, such as a mask or an eye cream, if needed.

1. Unplug Pores—salicylic acid

Aveeno Acne Treatment Bar	Wash off and pat dry.
L'Oréal Pure Zone Skin Balancing Cream Cleanser	
Neutrogena Multi-vitamin Acne Treatment	
Neutrogena Oil-Free Acne Wash Cream	

2. Remove Bacteria—benzoyl peroxide

Clear By Design Gel 2.5%	Apply with fingertips. Let dry.
Neutrogena On-the-Spot Acne Treatment	

3. Reduce Swelling—sulfur

Clearasil Adult Care Acne Treatment Cream	Apply sparingly with fingertips. Let dry.
Prescriptives Blemish Specialist	

4. Extra Help

Neutrogena Clear Pore Cleanser/Mask	Apply with fingertips. Leave on five to ten minutes. Rinse with lukewarm water. Use once or twice a week or every night for the five nights leading up to menstruation.
Neutrogena Healthy Skin Eye Cream	Apply with your pinkie finger, gently patting cream on the upper and lower eyelids, including the crow's feet area.

Don't Forget the Sunscreen

Applying sunscreen in the morning is the all-important final step for both treatments. Apply after all treatment products have dried.

Clinique Sun Care Face SPF 15

Estée Lauder In the Sun Sunblock for Face SPF 15

Neutrogena Ultra Sheer Dry-Touch Sunblock SPF 30

Olay Complete UV Defense Moisture Lotion

Ombrelle Sunscreen Lotion SPF 30

Prescriptives All You Need Broad Spectrum Oil Absorbing Lotion SPF 15

Proactiv Solution Daily Protection Plus SPF 15

Proactiv Solution Oil Free Moisture SPF 15

Rodan & Fields COMPOUNDS Protect SPF 15

Rodan & Fields RADIANT 4 Protect

Acne and Aging

We devised our Rodan & Fields RADIANT regimen specifically for its antiaging benefits. It helps reduce brown spots and evens out skin tone. A side benefit is that it also works on acne, as the toner contains salicylic acid. So for those

who have both acne and photoaging concerns, we suggest you use the RADI-
ANT treatment in the morning, as it contains a sunscreen, and the CALM
treatment or Proactiv Solution 3-step treatment at night (see pages 123–124
in chapter 5).

Note: As both daytime treatments include a sunscreen in Step 3, no additional sunscreen is needed.

Treatment 1: (a) Rodan & Fields RADIANT

Use only in the morning—start by using this treatment every second or third
day for two weeks, then increase to once a day. Until you are able to tolerate its
use every morning or if you remain at every second or third morning, use a mild
cleanser such as Cetaphil Gentle Cleansing Lotion or Rodan & Fields COM-
POUNDS Gentle Wash, when not using Rodan & Fields RADIANT products.

1. Exfoliate—alpha hydroxy acid

Rodan & Fields
  RADIANT 1 Wash
  (cleanser)

Wash off and pat dry.

2. Fade Brown Spots—hydroquinone

a) Rodan & Fields
   RADIANT 2 Prepare
   (toner)

Apply with gauze or cotton ball. Let dry.

b) Rodan & Fields
   RADIANT 3 Treat
   (leave-on lotion)

Apply with fingertips. Let dry.

3. Protect Skin from Sun—UVA/UVB filters

Rodan & Fields
  RADIANT 4 Protect
(sunscreen)

Apply to face and neck.

4. Extra Help

Start by using once a week. If needed, work up to two or three times a week.

Rodan & Fields RADIANT
  Microdermabrasion
  Paste

Apply to dry skin. Gently massage with fingertips for
one to two minutes. Rinse with lukewarm water.
Pat dry.

Rodan & Fields
  COMPOUNDS
  Moisture

Apply to dry skin.

TREATMENT 1: (B) RODAN & FIELDS CALM

Use only at night—start by using this treatment once every second or third day for two weeks, then increase to once a day. Until you are able to tolerate its use every night or if you remain at every other or third night, use a mild cleanser, such as Cetaphil Gentle Skin Cleansing Lotion or Rodan & Fields COMPOUNDS Gentle Wash, when not using Rodan & Fields CALM products.

Continue to use Rodan & Fields CALM once or twice daily to control break-outs when not using Rodan & Fields RADIANT.

1. Reduce Swelling—sulfur

Rodan & Fields CALM 1 Wash (cleanser)	Wash off and pat dry.

2. Unplug Pores—salicylic acid

Rodan & Fields CALM 2 Prepare (toner)	Apply with gauze or cotton ball. Let dry.

3. Remove Bacteria—benzoyl peroxide

Rodan & Fields CALM 3 Treat (leave-on lotion)	Apply with fingertips. Let dry.

4. Extra Help

Proactiv Solution Green Tea Moisturizer	Apply sparingly to dry skin.
Proactiv Solution Nourishing Eye Cream	Apply with your pinkie finger, gently patting cream on the upper and lower eyelids, including the crow's feet area.
Proactiv Solution Sheer Finish Compact Foundation	Apply sparingly.
Proactiv Solution Sheer Finish Loose Powder	Apply sparingly over foundation.
Proactiv Solution Skin-Clearing Cream to Powder Foundation	Apply sparingly.
Rodan & Fields COMPOUNDS Moisture	Apply to dry skin.
Rodan & Fields COMPOUNDS Moisture Eye	Apply with your pinkie finger, gently patting cream on the upper and lower eyelids, including the crow's feet area.

TREATMENT 2: (A) OTHER PRODUCTS

Use only in the morning—start by using this treatment every second or third day for two weeks, then increase to once a day. Until you are able to tolerate its use every morning or if you remain at every second or third morning, use a mild cleanser, such as Cetaphil Gentle Skin Cleanser or Rodan & Fields COMPOUNDS Gentle Wash, when not using other products. Remember to pick only one product from each list.

1. Exfoliate—alpha hydroxy acid

MD Formulations Face and Body Wash

SkinCeuticals Body Polish

Wash off and pat dry.

2. Fade Brown Spots—hydroquinone

Esoterica Skin Discoloration Fade Cream

MD Forte Skin Bleaching Gel

Porcelana Medicated Fade Cream

Apply with fingertips. Let dry.

3. Protect Skin from Sun—UVA/UVB filters

Clinique Sun Care Face SPF 15

Estée Lauder In the Sun Sunblock For Face SPF 15

Neutrogena Ultra Sheer Dry-Touch Sunblock SPF 30

Olay Complete UV Defense Moisture Lotion

Ombrelle Sunscreen Lotion SPF 30

Prescriptives All You Need Broad Spectrum Oil Absorbing Lotion SPF 15

Apply to face and neck.

4. Extra Help

Start once a week. If needed, work up to twice or three times a week.

Prescriptives Derma-   Apply to dry skin. Gently massage with fingertips for
  polish System   one to two minutes. Rinse with lukewarm water.
                    Pat dry.

TREATMENT 2: (B) OTHER PRODUCTS

Use only at night—start to use this treatment once every second or third day for two weeks, then increase to every day. Until you are able to tolerate its use every night or if you remain at every second or third night, use a mild cleanser, such as Cetaphil Gentle Skin Cleanser or Rodan & Fields COMPOUNDS Gentle Wash, when not using other products. Remember to pick only one from each list, except in the Extra Help section, where you may choose more than one product, such as a mask or an eye cream, if needed.

Continue to use an acne treatment regimen once or twice daily to control breakouts when not using a treatment regimen to brighten skin tone and soften lines.

1. Unplug Pores—salicylic acid

Aveeno Acne Treatment   Wash off and pat dry.
  Bar
L'Oréal Pure Zone Skin
  Balancing Cream
  Cleanser
Neutrogena Multi-
  vitamin Acne
  Treatment
Neutrogena Oil-Free
  Acne Wash Cream
Proactive Solution
  Deep Cleansing Wash

2. Remove Bacteria—benzoyl peroxide

Clear By Design Gel 2.5%   Apply with fingertips. Let dry.
Neutrogena On-the-
  Spot Acne Treatment
Proactive Solution
  Repairing Lotion

3. Reduce Swelling—sulfur

Clearasil Adult Care Acne Treatment Cream	Apply sparingly with fingertips. Let dry.
Prescriptives Blemish Specialist	
Proactiv Solution Refining Masque	Apply to clean, dry face or other affected area. Let dry ten minutes. Rinse with lukewarm water. Use once or twice a week for maintenance or every night for the five nights leading up to menstruation.

4. Extra Help

Neutrogena Clear Pore Cleanser/Mask	Apply with fingertips. Leave on five to ten minutes. Rinse with lukewarm water. Use once a week.
Neutrogena Healthy Skin Eye Cream	Apply with your pinkie finger, gently patting cream on the upper and lower eyelids, including the crow's feet area.

once your acne goes away, you *will* have acne amnesia

No matter what your age, the thrill of seeing acne diminish and disappear can be tremendous. The myth of acne as only a teenage condition has certainly been dispelled. The intrusion of one more annoyance as we age can easily be controlled with an acne regimen designed for adult women. It will not only heal your acne; it will restore the luster of youth to your skin. We urge all women to follow the examples below and enjoy a clear complexion for the rest of their lives.

> "I am seventy-one years old and I have never had a blemish on my skin. All of a sudden I started having these little bumps. I got very upset about it. But after only two weeks using Proactiv Solution, my skin, if you will pardon the expression, was like a baby's butt!"
>
> —*Lucy, age seventy-one*

> "I have been waiting for something like this all my life. I have oily skin and there was always a little something going on with it. No matter what I tried, my face still felt waxy or too dry. I would wash with all these expensive cleansers, and my skin would dry out and then return to its usual weeping-oil state. I couldn't get my makeup to look right—I would have to put it on

too heavy, and then I would feel like I needed to mop it off twenty minutes later because it felt waxy and oily.

"The more I followed your treatment, the better my skin felt, and the waxy feeling went away. Now I can wear just a light powdery base with a little rouge and look soft and smooth. I honestly feel prettier and better, and I don't have to spend as much time on my skin because I don't have to use as much makeup. My skin is much happier about that and less prone to breakouts. Plus I look much younger than my age now."

—Pamela, age sixty-four

"I feel that after a year of following the Rodan and Fields Approach, it's the first time in my sixty years that I really feel confident that my skin is going to be okay from week to week and month to month. I never had a serious acne problem, but it was enough to make me uncomfortable. When you don't feel that you look your best because of acne, it just does something to you. It's particularly nice for more mature women who have skin problems to realize that something can be done about them."

—Julianna, age fifty-eight

"I tried everything—expensive brands, cheap brands—nothing worked. For me Rodan & Fields CALM is the miracle medicine. I thank you because acne was ruining my life.

"Now if you can come up with something for my hot flashes, that would be really, really good!"

—Candace, age forty-nine

chapter eleven
adult men

"As a pastor I have to get up in front of a couple of hundred people every week to speak. Statistically, people fear public speaking more than death, but I have to do it on a regular basis. On top of that, I had acne, which made it really hard to get up in front of my congregation. Plus every week I'd meet new people as they visited our church, so I was constantly making first impressions. The acne problem made it really hard. I could dress up in a nice suit, but I still looked like somebody with bad skin!"

—Eugene, age thirty-six

"I'm a truck driver, and my face is always covered with dirt. Add that to the stress in my life, and my skin was just always a mess."

—John, age thirty-two

the good news for adult men is that acne is much less common for them than it is for adult women. The bad news is that if you've got it, you've probably got it bad—and in some men it can last for decades.

Adult acne is less prevalent in men because they don't have the regular monthly shift in hormones, which trigger outbreaks. Since the testosterone and dihydroxytestosterone levels remain constant after the surges of puberty, most men have entirely outgrown acne by their mid-to-late twenties. It rarely reappears on its own, as it does in women, without some other underlying factors. For example, the causes may be mechanical, such as from rubbing or exposure to the elements (see Cap and Hat Acne on page 246), or from shaving (see page 248). Acne may also appear as a result of prescription drug use, especially steroids; or the use of occlusive pomades (see Pomade Acne on page 262 in chapter 12) or sunscreens. Or it might just be bad genetic luck. We've also found that men who had severe acne as teens are more likely to have it as they grow older than those with mild or moderate cases.

Adult men tend to have scarring, cystic acne. That may be acceptable for men who want to play the heavy in a movie, as most men with pitted acne scars are cast as the bad guys or the tough guys—think Tommy Lee Jones or Edward James Olmos. But it's usually not acceptable for most men; they may kid that acne scars are macho but in truth simply want to have a decent complexion.

Unlike women, men are loath to wear makeup—or to follow a regular skin-care regimen more complicated than a quick wash and a shave. We've found that men with acne are as mortified by it as women, but they pretend to be stoic and try to forget it. They may grow beards (which they often don't really like) to hide it. And they often erroneously assume that their acne can't be helped.

Men usually come to see us at the insistence of their wives or girlfriends. We've had many a wife tell us that it's easier for her spouse to follow through once she makes the appointment. "You don't have to live with this," she'll say to her husband. "I see a dermatologist. You can go see her, too. She'll fix it."

Or men will see us out of necessity, especially if they feel they're not being taken seriously at work. These men have found that many people erroneously assume that acne is a teenage-only disease, which means they also assume that men with acne are not mature or are younger than they really are. For example, we had a patient who was an eminent gynecologist. He told us he was extremely embarrassed whenever his acne was raging: His patients would look at him oddly, and he knew they were wondering just how experienced he was as a physician because his acne was so bad. He didn't feel he would be able to earn their respect, and this had a tremendous negative impact on his self-confidence. It was easier for him to hide, literally, behind his mask.

Sometimes job performance can be compromised because of acne. "I've been troubled with acne for many years and did not do a whole lot to address it until acne began to trouble me in my career," thirty-eight-year-old Gerald explained. "I'm an executive with a certain amount of responsibility, and it became embarrassing to be involved in relatively high-profile business dealings with a fairly obvious outbreak of acne."

Luckily, adult male acne is as treatable as acne in women and teens. Men who do try our Rodan and Fields Approach are usually pleasantly surprised that it takes only minutes and is no more difficult to get used to than brushing their teeth.

"I'm one of those typical guys who, you know, grabs any bar of soap handy

Cap and Hat Acne

Wearing baseball caps too tight can flare acne. Because the brim is often lined in cardboard, they are difficult to wash. The accumulated dirt aggravates acne further. Plus the trend of wearing baseball caps backward leaves a thick plastic strap rubbing against tender forehead skin. Heat plus mechanical friction can flare acne. If you love to wear baseball caps or other hats, feel free to do so, but rotate different ones, never wear them too tight, and wash them by hand whenever they get grimy.

Helmets worn by athletes also trigger acne. Be sure that yours fits properly, which will help reduce breakouts and also provide better safety protection. Keep a baggie of salicylic acid body pads, such as Proactiv Solution Clear Skin Body Pads or Clearasil Pore Cleansing Pads, handy so you can have a quick wipe-down after a sweaty workout.

and scrubs my face, and that's about it," twenty-nine-year-old Jamie says. "So the idea of having to go through a three-step process was just something that I was not looking forward to. You know, who wants to spend all that time? But I was getting a lot of breakouts. I had long hair, and my forehead was the worst from all the grease in my hair. So I started using your products, and within two weeks not only was my skin cleared up but the texture was actually much better. I'm kicking myself for not trying this sooner."

Our patient Toby added, "I'm fifty-two years old and have had acne issues all my life. I had to wear a full beard until recently. A couple of things really help me to make the Rodan and Fields Approach work. First, I take the Proactiv Solution Renewing Cleanser into the shower with me in the morning and use it as a facial scrub. Then I shave. Afterward, I always use the Revitalizing Toner and the Repairing Lotion. That's my system."

It works for Jamie and Toby, and it can work for you.

when should you see a dermatologist?

If you have been following our program religiously and still have not seen any improvement in eight to twelve weeks, we recommend that you see a dermatologist. If you have scarring, we recommend that you see one immediately. Be sure to bring a list of all the supplements you take, as they may contain acneigenic substances. Or you can simply bring your supplements to your appointment. In addition, bring a list of any medicines you are taking and acne treatments you are curently using or have used in the past. Again, you can simply bring these items to your appointment. They will help your dermatologist find the most effective treatment for you.

If your skin is persistently red and flushes easily, you may have rosacea, which we discuss in chapter 13. We see far more adult males for rosacea treatment than we do for acne. If you are unsure as to your condition, make an appointment with a dermatologist.

treatment for adult male acne

Unlike Jamie and Toby, some men we see for acne treatment are not interested in a skin-care routine. They are more likely to be compliant if we prescribe oral medications, such as antibiotics or Accutane. They are, in fact, often ideal candidates for Accutane; after all, they can't get pregnant! Accutane has no effect whatsoever on sperm production or other sexual functions.

For more information about other treatment options, refer to the section on oral antibiotics on page 49 in chapter 2 and the sections on Accutane on page 53 in chapter 2 and page 177 in chapter 8.

acne and stress

Stress is a known promoter of acne, so even men who don't regularly break out may experience acne if their stress levels increase. And as with women, many men have found that their stress levels have *not* decreased as their lives progress and children move out of the house. Stress causes the release of increased levels of cortisol and androgen hormones from the adrenal gland. These hormones have a direct effect on the sebaceous (oil-producing) glands. More hormones can mean more acne, and more acne can mean more stress. In particular, older men often have difficulties expressing their distress with skin problems, thinking either that there are no treatment options or that their pain is not worth discussing. They suffer in silence.

Men can easily learn to use stress-busting techniques to minimize their stress. There is no reason for any man to feel ashamed or embarrassed about having something wonderfully relaxing, like a massage or a facial, to ease his tensions.

For more information on managing stress, see page 98 in chapter 4.

shaving

The act of shaving provides automatic exfoliation, which is a bonus for acne sufferers, but it can also be extremely painful when pimples and cysts are present. It is also very common for men to get shaving bumps, or *pseudofolliculitis barbae,* which is caused by ingrown hairs. As hairs begin to grow back after shaving, they can be trapped inside the follicle, causing irritation and swelling. Not all men get shaving bumps. People with curly hair are most susceptible, which is why *pseudofolliculitis barbae* is often called curly hair disease. It's been estimated that 45 to 80 percent of all African-American men have shaving bumps.

The key to shaving with acne is to first prep the skin with an exfoliant cleanser to lift curly hair; soften the beard with lots of lather and warm water; use a new double or triple blade razor; shave in one direction only; and treat the skin afterward with a leave-on benzoyl peroxide lotion.

Here are more details:

- Change your razor blade more frequently. Once a month is not enough. The duller the blade, the more drag there is on the skin. You'll need to change it as often as every day when you have acne or irritation, as a used blade has microscopic tears in it, which can cut skin. Once your skin has improved, you can change the blade every other day.
- Experiment with double blade or triple blade, sensitive-skin razors, and electric shavers to find the one that creates the least amount of irritation.
- Shave from the chin down your neck. Shaving from the neck up gives a closer shave but causes more skin irritation.
- Have your skin as soft and warm as possible before shaving. Shaving during or after a nice hot shower is a good idea.
- Exfoliating before shaving to lift curly hairs is a great idea to achieve a close shave and to minimize shaving bumps. Try an exfoliating cleanser, such as Proactiv Solution Deep Cleansing Wash or a buff-puff type of cleansing pad, before you shave.

- Use your acne medicines, such as Rodan & Fields CALM 1 Wash, instead of shaving cream. A medicated cleansing product for shaving helps deliver medicine down into the pores because the act of shaving creates exfoliation. Your dermatologist can also prescribe Benzashave, which is a medicated shaving cream containing benzoyl peroxide.
- For bleeding after your shave, apply two seconds of pressure with a clean cotton gauze pad. Tissues and toilet paper, as you know, stick to skin. And styptic pencils sting.
- Many aftershave lotions smell great, but they can cause irritation, especially if they're alcohol-based and heavily fragranced. If you like a scent, try applying some to your wrists or to the pulse points in your neck (away from any breakouts).

For more information about *pseudofolliculitis barbae*, see page 261 in chapter 12.

your aging skin

Men have a thicker dermis than women, so they don't age and wrinkle as quickly. Plus their natural levels of testosterone and masculinizing hormones keep their facial musculature firmer than women's, which begins to sag and atrophy sooner. Men also tend to have oilier skin than women, so they often don't need moisturizers unless they live and work in extremely dry environments.

However, we're starting to see more men interested in cosmetic procedures, such as Botox injections for wrinkles. Facials and other treatments are also becoming appealing to men for their soothing and therapeutic qualities. Men have every right to be concerned about their appearance, especially as they grow older and may worry about competition at work from a younger, eagerly energetic generation. They may even want to investigate supplemental hormones as an option. "What to do to maintain skin quality once hormone levels begin to diminish as men age should be a real issue for men to think about," explains Dr. Natan Bar-Chama, director of the Male Reproductive Medicine and Surgery department at Mount Sinai Hospital in New York. "If their hormone levels are declining, they can discuss options with their urologist and dermatologist and be given supplemental hormones in the form of gel or patches." The actor Dustin Hoffman recently joked about his acne and hormone levels in *People* magazine: "I thank God I still have acne be-cause—may I say this modestly?—that goes hand in hand with a high testos-terone count," he said. "I always hated acne, but now I'll get a pimple and say, 'Stay with me!'"

Men should always use sunscreen—every day, without fail. Using a tinted sunscreen is a great way to achieve photoprotection, with the added bonus of camouflage of the redness caused by acne—no makeup required!

For more information about sunscreen, refer to page 317 in chapter 16. Skin cancer does not differentiate between men and women. It is an equal oppor-tunity disease.

patient history

Trevor is forty-eight. He has a family history of acne and he suffered from se-vere cystic acne in high school. Although his acne started to resolve in his twenties and thirties, he is continually plagued with one to three nodules daily. He is extremely self-conscious. He had dermabrasion twenty years ago for his significant scarring. Unfortunately, he still has many scars today. Trevor shaves with an electric razor because a regular razor seems to make his acne worse, and he continues to have nodules in the beard area.

Trevor has severe acne and is shocked when we tell him that for men, acne is an all-or-nothing phenomenon. Upwards of 90 percent of teen males have acne, but a much smaller percentage continue to have it as adults. For these men, acne becomes a lifetime condition, often continuing into their sixties and seventies.

The stigma that acne carries is literally written over Trevor's face, and no matter what job he has sought out, his acne forever follows him. It has im-peded him socially, and he has even cancelled business meetings in an effort to hide his blemishes.

We put Trevor on the Proactiv Solution full-face treatment, which includes washing with a scrub cleanser containing 2 percent salicylic acid (Proactiv So-lution Deep Cleansing Wash), followed by an alcohol-free toner with glycolic acid (Proactiv Solution Revitalizing Toner). After the toner dries, Trevor applies a leave-on lotion with 2.5 percent benzoyl peroxide (Proactiv Solution Repairing Lotion). And as needed, Trevor uses a mask containing sulfur (Proactiv Solution Refining Mask) to help reduce swelling.

treatments for adult males

Remember, use these products on your *entire face*, not only on acne-prone areas, except where noted.

Every day you need to clean, tone, and treat your skin, and the products you use contain medicines to unplug pores, remove bacteria, and reduce swelling. The active ingredients in some of these products are applicable in several categories. For example, salicylic acid, which unplugs pores, is often an active ingredient in cleansers, toners, leave-on lotions, and moisturizers; and benzoyl peroxide, which removes bacteria and helps to unplug pores, is often an active ingredient in cleansers and leave-on lotions. This explains why Proactiv Solution Renewing Cleanser and Proactiv Solution Repairing Lotion, which contain benzoyl peroxide, both unplug pores and remove bacteria. However, we are listing cleansers only in Step 1—Unplug Pores and not Step 2—Remove Bacteria. The reason is simple: Leave-on lotions, such as Proactiv Solution Repairing Lotion, must be applied *after* cleansing and toning.

Note: "Apply sparingly" means you should use a dime-sized amount of product. It should be enough to have a thin coat applied over the entire surface of the skin, where needed.

Note: In the Extra Help sections, you may choose more than one product, such as a cleansing pad or a leave-on lotion, if needed.

TREATMENT 1: PROACTIV SOLUTION

Start to use this treatment once a day for two weeks, then increase to twice a day. Until you are able to tolerate its use twice a day or if you remain at once a day, use a mild cleanser, such as Cetaphil Gentle Skin Cleanser or Rodan & Fields COMPOUNDS Gentle Wash, when not using Proactiv Solution products.

1. Unplug Pores—salicylic acid, glycolic acid
a) Deep Cleansing Wash   Wash off and pat dry.
b) Revitalizing Toner   Apply with gauze or cotton ball. Let dry.

2. Remove Bacteria—benzoyl peroxide

Repairing Lotion	Apply with fingertips. Let dry.

3. Reduce Swelling—sulfur

Concealer Plus — Lightly dot on with applicator. Blend with concealer brush or fingertips. Use once or twice a day.

Refining Mask — Apply to clean, dry face or other affected area. Let dry ten minutes. Rinse with lukewarm water. Use once or twice a week, more often if needed.

4. Extra Help—Proactiv Solution

ClearZone Body Pads* — Use in place of cleanser.

Daily Oil Control (for slightly oily skin) — Apply to entire face or other affected area with fingertips after toner. Let dry. Use daily or as needed.

Matte Skin Finish (for very oily skin) — Apply sparingly to oily areas. Brush off residue when dry.

Oil Blotter Sheets — Use as needed to pat away excess oil.

Rodan & Fields CLEAN Regimen for Blackhead Extraction — Follow instructions in kit.

* Body pads may be used on the face for a quick midday facial cleansing without a trip to the sink. They can also be used after playing sports.

TREATMENT 2: PROACTIV SOLUTION EXTRA STRENGTH

This treatment includes a 7 percent benzoyl peroxide cleanser and leave-on lotion, which is usually well tolerated by those with extremely oily skin and stubborn acne who have failed treatment with products containing 2.5 percent benzoyl peroxide. Start this treatment once a day for two weeks, then increase to twice a day. Until you are able to tolerate its use twice a day or if you remain at once a day, use a mild cleanser, such as Cetaphil Gentle Skin Cleanser or Rodan & Fields COMPOUNDS Gentle Wash, when not using Proactiv Solution Extra Strength products.

Note that you can also use the regular Proactiv Solution (Treatment 1, above) in the morning and Proactiv Solution Extra Strength at night if you find that the Extra Strength treatment is too drying for your skin when used twice a day.

1. Unplug Pores—salicylic acid

a) Extra Strength
  Cleanser   Wash off and pat dry.

b) Extra Strength Toner   Apply with gauze or cotton ball. Let dry.

2. Remove Bacteria—benzoyl peroxide

Extra Strength Lotion   Apply with fingertips. Let dry.

3. Reduce Swelling—sulfur

Extra Strength Mask   Apply to clean, dry face or other affected area. Let dry
ten minutes. Rinse with lukewarm water. Use once or
twice a week.

4. Fade Brown Spots—hydroquinone

Skin Lightening Lotion   Use at night only. Apply to affected area.

Rodan & Fields RADIANT   Follow directions in kit.
  Regimen

5. Extra Help—Proactiv Solution

ClearZone Body Pads*   Use in place of cleanser.

Daily Oil Control   Apply to entire face or other affected area with
  (for slightly oily skin)   fingertips after toner. Let dry. Use daily or as
                          needed.

Matte Skin Finish   Apply sparingly to oily areas. Brush off residue
  (for very oily skin)   when dry.

Oil Blotter Sheets   Use as needed to pat away excess oil.

Rodan & Fields CLEAN   Follow instructions in kit.
  Regimen for Blackhead
  Extraction

* Body pads may be used on the face for a quick midday facial cleansing without a trip to
the sink. They can also be used after playing sports.

TREATMENT 3: OTHER PRODUCTS

Start to use this treatment once a day for two weeks, then increase to twice a
day. Until you are able to tolerate its use twice a day or if you remain at once a
day, use a mild cleanser, such as Cetaphil Gentle Skin Cleanser or Rodan &
Fields COMPOUNDS Gentle Wash, when not using other products. Remember
to pick only one product from each list, except in the Extra Help section, where
you may choose more than one product, such as cleansing pad or a leave-on
lotion, if needed.

1. Unplug Pores—salicylic acid

Clearasil 3-in-1 Acne   Wash off and pat dry.
Cleanser
L'Oréal Ideal Balance
Foaming Gel Cleanser
Neutrogena Oil Free
Acne Wash
Oxy Oil-Free Maximum
Strength Once A Day
Acne Wash

2. Remove Bacteria—benzoyl peroxide

Clean & Clear Persa-Gel   Apply with fingertips. Let dry.
Fostex 5 Cream
Neutrogena On-the-
Spot Therapy
Oxy 5 Sensitive Skin
Vanishing Lotion
PanOxyl 5 Gel

3. Reduce Swelling—sulfur

Clearasil Adult Care   Apply sparingly with fingertips. Let dry.
Acne Treatment
Cream

4. Extra Help

Clearasil Pore Cleansing   Wipe on. Let dry.
Pads*
Clinique Night   Apply with fingertips. Let dry.
Treatment Gel
Neutrogena Clear Pore
Shine Control Gel
Oxy Daily Cleansing   Wipe on. Let dry.
Pads*
Stri-Dex Sensitive Skin
Triple Action Acne
Pads*

* Body pads may be used on the face for a quick midday facial cleansing without a trip to the sink. They can also be used after playing sports.

Don't Forget the Sunscreen

For all three treatments, applying sunscreen in the morning is the all-important final step. Apply after all treatment products have dried.

Clearasil Acne Treatment Cream SPF 15*
Neutrogena Ultra Sheer Dry-Touch Sunblock SPF 45
Olay Complete UV Defense Moisture Lotion
Ombrelle Sunscreen Lotion SPF 30
Proactiv Solution Daily Protection SPF 15
Proactiv Solution Sheer Tint Moisture SPF 15*
Rodan & Fields COMPOUNDS Protect SPF 15

* These are excellent solutions for men as they're coverups, not makeup, and the slight tint helps camouflage redness while they protect the skin from the sun

once your acne goes away, you *will* have acne amnesia

Acne is every bit as distracting to an adult male as it is to a teenager. Shaving is a daily punishment, and the redness and bumps undermine confidence. A simple treatment program can control the problem and, by doing so, restore self-esteem. Treat acne and you can prevent potential scars as well as years of anguish. Acne will soon be nothing but a fleeting memory.

For example, Eugene, the pastor quoted at the beginning of this chapter, has gotten over his fear of public speaking ever since his acne cleared up. "I have not had one blemish after only one month following the Rodan and Fields Approach. Now when I get up in front of those two hundred people every week, to sing and to speak, I have more confidence than ever before. Having clear skin is a positive asset to my ministry. And there are a lot of other young ministers in the area who have the same problem; they know they have to get up in front of a bunch of people every week, and when there's a blemish, their anxiety is magnified. I'm happy to tell them what I'm doing, and I'm thankful that they listen!"

"I'm thirty-six now and started getting really bad cystic acne when I was thirteen," says David, another patient. "I was on Accutane twice, and it didn't work. I spent a lot of time not wanting to be in public because my face was always blotchy and there were a lot of marks and scars.

"Finally I discovered Proactiv Solution, and now my face has completely cleared up. I mean not a zit, not a mark. Even some of the old stuff that had been discolored finally disappeared. I'm elated!" He adds, "My skin is strong, it looks great, the tone is even, and people compliment me all the time. It doesn't itch and burn when I shave. I know I sound sappy, but when you've dealt with acne all your life and it's always there in the back of your head, you just feel great when you can get up in the morning and don't have to see any of what I call 'visitors in the evening' that just popped up on your face overnight. Using this treatment over the last few months has been a nice step forward for me. It's improved my confidence and made me feel a lot better about myself."

chapter twelve

acne in people of color

"Because I'm a light-skinned African-American woman, my pimples would leave blemishes that stayed on my skin. They looked like dark pores, almost as if I'd been scratched. I was so ashamed that I would wear a facial mask during the evening so the people in my household wouldn't see them. And I would wear it all night until I woke up and put makeup on. I felt like I had a mask on all day. I could never just be free to run out to the grocery store without having to pile on the makeup."

—Janetta, age forty

"My appearance is very important because I am a Chicago police officer. Your face is the first thing people see, but my acne was so bad, people would grimace and ask, 'What's the matter with your skin?' Plus I had a problem with ingrown hairs. I'd get a lot of razor stubble, and, due to my job, I had to shave. My skin was very discolored and dark from shaving scars."

—Antoine, age thirty

Skin is skin—and acne is color blind. The underlying process that causes acne is the same no matter what color your skin, which means that the treatments for acne will be the same as well. One of the comments we've heard most frequently from our African-American, Asian, and Hispanic patients over the years is how surprised they are that the Rodan and Fields Approach is as effective for them as it is for their Caucasian friends. They have erroneously believed that most over-the-counter products are designed only for Caucasians and that dermatologists can't help them. One of the reasons Vanessa Williams has been a powerful spokesperson for Proactiv Solution is she emphasizes that acne is as prevalent in people of color as it is in the white community and that all skin types and colors can be helped by the right acne products and treatments.

Scientists and physicians are studying the differences between pigmented skin and white skin, especially as they relate to the development of acne. According to Dr. Susan Taylor, an assistant clinical professor of dermatology at the College of Physicians and Surgeons at Columbia University and the director of the skin of color center at St. Luke's-Roosevelt Hospital Center in New York City, "further studies of acne in the various ethnic groups are needed."

She added: "A recent study in Singapore found that acne was the second most common dermatologic diagnosis there in patients of Chinese, Malaysian, or Indian descent. A study of Arab patients in Kuwait, where skin tends to be dark, found that acne was the third most common dermatologic diagnosis among the pediatric population." She also found that studies in America and the United Kingdom showed that acne was the most common diagnosis in patients of African ancestry who consulted a dermatologist.

Data from other studies have shown that sebaceous (oil) glands in African Americans tend to be larger and more active than in Asians, Caucasians, and Hispanics. The stratum corneum may also be very slightly thicker. African Americans, however, tend to have less visibly severe acne than Asians, Caucasians, and Hispanics, with fewer cysts. Because darker pigment masks redness, inflammation is not as visible. When we look histologically (by examining biopsied skin samples under a microscope), however, there is plenty of hidden inflammation. Consequently, there is a strong postinflammatory response, which leaves pinkish-brown or dark brown spots, which can persist for months if not years.

In a study of 313 patients (238 African-American, 55 Hispanic, 19 Asian) Dr. Taylor conducted at the skin of color center, she found that African Americans and Hispanics were much more likely to suffer from postinflammatory hyperpigmentation (65.3 percent, 52.7 percent) than scarring (5.9 percent, 21.8 percent). Asians reported 47.4 percent postinflammatory hyperpigmentation and 10.5 percent scarring. Those with lighter skin were also more likely to have numerous cysts and pustules, which can lead to scarring as well.

Because there are African Americans with lighter skin compared with Filipinos, ethnicity is not as important to a dermatologist treating acne as the degree of pigmentation present in the skin. People with dark skin face two specific problems: postinflammatory hyperpigmentation and *pseudofolliculitis barbae,* which for many people are worse than pimples. In fact, some of our patients ignore their pimples and want treatment only for the aftermath—the disfiguring red or brown spots, which are distracting, annoying, and time-consuming to conceal. The good news is that these symptoms are easily treatable.

postinflammatory hyperpigmentation

Skin contains melanocyte cells that produce melanin, the packets of pigment granules that give skin its unique color. The size and quantity of the melanin packets are genetically determined. After acne appears, scavenger cells called melanophages remain behind in the dermis, the second layer of the skin, to clean up the mess left by pimples and pustules. The debris left behind contains melanin granules, which appear as flat red or brown pigmented spots that show up after the pimples have run their course. This is postinflammatory hyperpigmentation. Left untreated, these spots can linger for weeks or months, sometimes even years.

treatment for postinflammatory hyperpigmentation

The most common treatment for postinflammatory hyperpigmentation is bleaching or lightening with an agent called hydroquinone. Many people who have seen how Michael Jackson's skin has been transformed over the years are understandably leery of any lightening products, but they needn't be, as what he most likely used is a drug that is considerably stronger than hydroquinone. Hydroquinone works only by lightening the *abnormally* clumped packets of pigment in your skin; it has no effect whatsoever on the normal color packets, no matter what hue your skin is. It *will not* change your natural skin tone. However, be sure to treat the entire zone with a hydroquinone product, not just the pinkish-brown or brown spots—you may unwittingly create a halo effect, with a new light spot around the old dark spot. Also, if you have any tan whatsoever, as many people do, the hydroquinone will lighten that as well.

One of the reasons we developed our Rodan & Fields RADIANT regimen was to provide relief for postinflammatory hyperpigmentation in African Americans and others with dark complexions. RADIANT is effective for reduc-

ing pinkish-brown spots because the RADIANT products contain hydroquinone, kojic acid, and bearberry extract, which all help fade abnormal pigment. In addition, they contain salicylic acid, retinol, and lactic acid to
enhance penetration into skin pores, promoting more rapid results.

Over-the-counter products, such as Porcelana Medicated Fade Cream, Esoterica Skin Discoloration Fade Cream, and MD Forte Skin Bleaching Gel, which
contain 2 percent hydroquinone, are also effective for reducing postinflammatory hyperpigmentation. They are FDA-approved and safe to use, even by
teenagers. Hydroquinone products should not, however, be used while pregnant or nursing.

If postinflammatory hyperpigmentation persists, we advise you to see
a dermatologist who can treat you in his or her office with a stronger
solution—4 percent or greater—of hydroquinone and can prescribe a topical
retinoid, such as Renova. For faster results, microdermabrasion at a salon or
doctor's office can help with acne and postinflammatory hyperpigmentation.

There is no reason to suffer from postinflammatory hyperpigmentation
when treatments are readily available. Make a resolution to get rid of these
brown spots, today.

pseudofolliculitis barbae, or curly hair disease

Pseudofolliculitis barbae, or curly hair disease, affects from 45 to 80 percent of
men who have curly facial hair. (Women with curly hair can also suffer from it
after shaving in the pubic area, which can be intensely embarrassing.) During
a shave, a razor cuts off curly hair at a sharp angle. The tip of this hair can then
act like a barb, curling back in upon itself and stabbing the skin in the process.
The body reacts to this ingrown hair as if it were a foreign invader, with an inflammatory response. Red and white blood cells flood in, and a painful bump
appears. Because shaving is a daily necessity for men, they can get a new crop
of tiny bumps, pimples, and postinflammatory hyperpigmentation every time
they lather up.

Some also suffer from a condition called acne keloidalis nuchae, which
manifests itself as thick rolled scars at the base of the neck. They're caused by
constant friction at the back of the scalp (usually by the strap of a baseball
cap, a helmet, or a shirt collar) where ingrown hairs form. Those prone to
keloids, particularly African Americans, can develop scars.

Rushawn's Story

"My dad is African-American, and my mom is white, so my skin is medium-toned, and it burns easily. When I hit puberty at twelve, my skin was both oily and sensitive. Around my periods I'd get huge red bumps on my face, which would then fade to a slightly lighter shade of pinky-brown, then turn sort of brown. I tried everything to get rid of the acne and spots, but the products I used only irritated my skin and gave me rashes.

"I got pregnant when I was sixteen, and as for that pregnancy glow—forget it! My friends would say that my face wasn't so bad, that it was all for a good cause, and I would say, 'No way!' It was hard enough to be pregnant so young—still in high school, worrying about everything—and then to have to look at my face! Well, I grew my bangs long so at least I didn't have to see what was going on underneath them on my forehead.

"As for my dating life, I didn't have one! I'd be too embarrassed to go out, and I'd make my excuses, sit at home, and eat popcorn in front of the TV. I'm a really outgoing person, and I was hiding—from what? Acne? I shouldn't have had to be hiding from the world because of pimples and brown spots. What's most upsetting to me now is that I don't have any pictures of me at my daughter's first-birthday party. I was too mortified to have my photo taken. And that's really a shame.

"When I got out of high school, I went to nursing school. I finally summoned up the courage to try the Rodan and Fields Approach and began to use the Proactiv Solution products on my face. After about a week, I noticed the brown bumps were shrinking. Three weeks later, there were hardly any bumps and my skin was much softer. After two months, my skin was completely clear. I couldn't believe it. I used the skin lightening lotion every day and was thrilled when those annoying brown spots disappeared.

"Now I give people travel sizes of Proactiv Solution as gifts. People listen to me talk about my skin because I'm a nurse, and I tell them how awful I felt and looked. I also tell my African-American friends that these products won't bleach them out, dry their skin, sting, or burn. I tell them that they should not be afraid to give it a chance. It's made a world of difference for me. I've got a great boyfriend now, and he loves to touch my skin. I never thought that would happen to me! Proactiv really changed my life."

Treatment for *Pseudofolliculitis Barbae*

We suggest that men with mild cases of *pseudofolliculitis barbae* follow our shaving suggestions on page 248 in chapter 11. You can also try using a bump fighter adjustable razor, whose blade has a silicone coating. Be sure to use a new blade with each shave because even a blade used only once will be microscopically chipped and grow bacteria. The next time you use the razor, it will cut the skin and implant the bacteria. Also, a dermatologist can prescribe a cortisone cream or oral antibiotic for use during the day to reduce inflammation and a topical retinoid cream, which can help release hairs and therefore make shaving easier, to use at night. Finally, ongoing studies are currently looking at the effectiveness of glycolic acid and other alpha hydroxy acids to treat *pseudofolliculitis barbae*. Be sure to make an appointment with your dermatologist to review the latest treatment options.

For moderate to severe cases, hair removal will provide lasting relief. Vaniqa is an effective cream that retards the rate of hair regrowth, although it must be applied every day in order to remain effective. Electrolysis gives permanent results, but be aware that it can be tedious, expensive, and tricky with curly hairs.

Laser hair removal was once more difficult for people of color, because it works by sensing the difference between hair and skin color. Therefore, in people with fair skin and dark hair, it is tremendously effective. For those with dark skin and dark hair, the laser was less able to distinguish between hair and skin. The energy had to be kept very low to avoid burning the skin, which meant it didn't always penetrate all the way down to the hair follicle, so more treatments were required. It was also very expensive.

POMADE ACNE

Pomade acne appears in the form of tiny bumps, sometimes with inflammatory papules (pimples), across the forehead and around the scalp line. It used to be a very common sight among African Americans of all ages or anyone who used thick oily or greasy creams to lubricate their scalps.

Pomades may be great for moisturizing the hair and scalp, but they can be terrible for skin because of their high paraffin and petrolatum content. They are extremely occlusive and pore-clogging.

The best treatment for pomade acne is to discontinue use of all pomade products. Pomade acne, however, is less common than it used to be, as many of the newer products are not as comedogenic. We've found that Finisheen oil sheer or Vita Point products are not occlusive and are safe to use.

If pomade acne persists, try treatment with a topical retinoid such as Differin, Retin-A, or Tazorac.

Now, however, "lasers, especially those with water-cooled hand pieces and longer pulse duration, such as the 1064-nanometer laser, are effective in darker skin as they penetrate deeper with fewer of the side effects of earlier lasers such as blistering and hyperpigmentation," says Dr. Rebat M. Halder, chairman of the dermatology department at Howard University and director of the Ethnic Skin Research Institute. Laser treatments have also come down in price, making them more affordable as a treatment option.

treatment for acne and acne scars

Refer to the appropriate chapter for your age group for more information on acne treatments. For information on the treatment of scarring, see page 62 in chapter 2.

patient history

Leticia is a twenty-two-year-old African-American college student who has moderate acne with pustules and papules over much of her face. The bumps never last long and, indeed, are not that visible. However, after each lesion heals, a dark brown spot is left behind in its place. Leticia is far more bothered by the patchy discoloration that follows than the actual acne breakouts.

We put Leticia on the Rodan & Fields RADIANT and CALM regimens. During the day she uses RADIANT, which includes ingredients to lighten pinkish-brown and brown spots. This regimen includes washing with a mild exfoliating lactic acid cleanser (RADIANT 1 Wash), followed by a toner with hydroquinone, kojic acid, bearberry extract, and salicylic acid (RADIANT 2 Prepare). After the toner dries, Leticia applies a leave-on lotion with hydroquinone, kojic acid, and retinol (RADIANT 3 Treat). She then applies sunscreen with micronized zinc oxide for UVA/UVB protection (RADIANT 4 Protect). Please note: Sunscreen use is critical even for those with dark skin. Most people with dark skin will do fine with this type of sunscreen, as it should not appear too ashy on them. If it does, alternatives are Rodan & Fields COMPOUNDS Protect and Proactiv Solution Daily Protection Plus SPF 15.

At night Leticia uses CALM to manage her acne. This treatment includes washing with a cleanser containing sulfur (CALM 1 Wash), followed by a toner with salicylic acid (CALM 2 Prepare). After the toner dries, Leticia applies a leave-on lotion containing 2.5 percent benzoyl peroxide (CALM 3 Treat).

Leticia followed these treatments daily. Her acne soon healed, and her skin tone was even. Her old brown spots faded, and no new ones appeared. The intense therapy lasted two months. Once she achieved the desired evenness of skin tone, she stopped using RADIANT and continued with CALM once or twice daily to keep her acne under control.

treatment for skin of color

African-American skin can become irritated by prescription acne medications. Patients should use low-strength benzoyl peroxide and retinoids for acne treatment. See page 115 for the low-strength benzoyl peroxide Proactiv Solution treatment. See page 56 for more information about retinoids.

postinflammatory hyperpigmentation

Remember, use these products on your *entire face,* not only on acne-prone areas, except where noted.

If you have postinflammatory hyperpigmentation as well as acne, use either of these treatments *in the morning only* and then the appropriate acne treatment from the treatments listed in chapters 7–11 *at night only.*

Note: As both treatments include a sunscreen in Step 3, no additional sunscreen is needed.

Treatment 1: Rodan & Fields RADIANT
Use only in the morning—start to use this treatment every second or third day for two weeks, then increase to once a day. Until you are able to tolerate its use every morning or if you remain at every second or third morning, use a mild cleanser such as Cetaphil Gentle Cleansing Lotion or Rodan & Fields COMPOUNDS Gentle Wash, when not using Rodan & Fields RADIANT products.

1. Exfoliate—alpha hydroxy acid
Rodan & Fields   Wash off and pat dry.
 RADIANT 1 Wash
 (cleanser)

2. Fade Brown Spots—hydroquinone

a) Rodan & Fields   Apply with gauze or cotton ball. Let dry.
   RADIANT 2 Prepare
   (toner)

b) Rodan & Fields   Apply with fingertips. Let dry.
   RADIANT 3 Treat
   (leave-on lotion)

3. Protect Skin from Sun—UVA/UVB filters

Rodan & Fields   Apply to face and neck.
   RADIANT 4 Protect
   (sunscreen)

4. Extra Help

Start once a week. If needed, work up to twice or three times a week.

Rodan & Fields RADIANT   Apply to dry skin. Gently massage with fingertips for
   Microdermabrasion   one to two minutes. Rinse with lukewarm water.
   Paste   Pat dry.
Rodan & Fields   Apply to dry skin.
   COMPOUNDS Moisture

TREATMENT 2: OTHER PRODUCTS

Use only in the morning—start to use this treatment every second or third day for two weeks, then increase to once a day. Until you are able to tolerate its use every morning or if you remain at every second or third morning, use a mild cleanser, such as Cetaphil Gentle Skin Cleanser or Rodan & Fields COMPOUNDS Gentle Wash, when not using other products. Remember to pick only one product from each list.

1. Exfoliate—alpha hydroxy acid

MD Formulations Face   Wash off and pat dry.
   and Body Wash
SkinCeuticals Body
   Polish

2. Fade Brown Spots—hydroquinone

Esoterica Skin Discol-   Apply with fingertips. Let dry.
   oration Fade Cream
MD Forte Skin
   Bleaching Gel

Porcelana Medicated
  Fade Cream

3. Protect Skin from Sun—UVA/UVB filters

Clinique Sun Care Face   Apply to face and neck.
  SPF 15
Estée Lauder In the Sun
  Sunblock For Face
  SPF 15
Neutrogena Ultra Sheer
  Dry-Touch Sunblock
  SPF 30
Olay Complete
  UV Defense Moisture
  Lotion
Ombrelle Sunscreen
  Lotion SPF 30
Prescriptives All You
  Need Broad Spectrum
  Oil Absorbing Lotion
  SPF 15

4. Extra Help

Start by using once a week. If needed, work up to two or three times a week.

Prescriptives Derma-   Apply to dry skin. Gently massage with fingertips for
  polish System   one to two minutes. Rinse with lukewarm water.
                           Pat dry.

all people of color need sunscreen, too

The key to successfully treating acne in skin of color is to pay attention to pinkish-brown and brown spots left by postinflammatory hyperpigmentation and to treat them immediately. Being out in the sun without protection most definitely makes these spots darker. Plus they persist longer. Therefore, no matter what your skin tone, you should protect yourself from getting darker due to sun exposure. People of color, especially African Americans, are rarely told that they need sunscreen, as their risk factors for sunburn, skin cancer, and wrinkles are not as great as those of Caucasians. But this is a dangerous fallacy. Anyone can get skin cancer or premature aging changes from excessive sun exposure.

A UVA/UVB-blocking sunscreen is a must. Be aware that some of those containing zinc may look ashy on very dark complexions. If this is the case, look for sunscreens containing avobenzone (Parsol 1789). Be diligent about using sunscreen every day, rain or shine, summer or winter.

For more information on sunscreen, see page 317 in chapter 16.

once your acne goes away, you *will* have acne amnesia

In general, while we say that acne affects all people and all skin colors, the type of acne does seem to vary from one ethnic group to another. Cystic acne is more prevalent in Caucasians and Hispanics, Asians tend to scar more easily from acne, and African Americans tend to have fewer cysts but more widespread small inflammatory acne lesions.

The common denominator in those African Americans with acne is the propensity for postinflammatory hyperpigmentation. Our patients are as troubled by the dark spots on their skin that follow a healed pimple as they are by the pimple itself. Therefore, controlling the acne and fading the dark marks are equally important missions. A new treatment regime, whether for acne or postinflammatory hyperpigmentation, can quickly bring results and ecstatic satisfaction when brown spots fade forever! Here are a few examples of transformed patients:

"As soon as I started using Proactiv Solution, I was in a totally different world," Antoine, the Chicago police officer we quoted at the beginning of this chapter, happily told us. "I was getting compliments, and people approached me differently. Since I'm a public servant, I also believe this enhanced my relationships with people, helping me do a better job.

"This new treatment put the icing on my pound cake. I have a different walk and a different attitude. I feel great about myself. I hold my head up higher. And I'm glad when people look at my face, because the pimples, spots, and bumps are gone."

"My skin is clear now, and everyone notices it," Janetta, also quoted at the beginning of this chapter, adds. "I coach women's basketball, and now I have no problem going to practice with no makeup on my face. I used to have to cover up everything, and after a long practice or game, all that makeup would be all over my uniform and shirts. Now my self-esteem is higher and my confidence level is up."

"I always thought that when I saw Caucasians talking about acne, they weren't talking about me. I thought that black skin was totally different and that what works for them wouldn't work for us," admits Sylvia, age forty-eight. "I was one who never went out of the house without makeup. Now, honey, I get my little happy hips in some jeans and go right on outside that door without any makeup on. And that's a change for me!"

chapter thirteen

rosacea

"My husband and I are health nuts, but my husband started breaking out with rosacea when he turned sixty-eight. He didn't want to take antibiotics, so we did everything else we could to find an effective treatment, but nothing worked. I mean, nothing. Even his being very careful about what he ate didn't help. He's a sales representative and out in the public all the time, so this was a real problem for him."

—Josephine, age seventy-two

"Every time I had my menstrual cycle or when I ovulated, that patch of rosacea on my cheeks would become inflamed. I would have red bumps on it, which were very unsightly and uncomfortable, too. My friends told me I was lucky I didn't have pimples, but I didn't feel lucky. I felt splotchy and red and old!"

—Nicole, age forty-five

most notably, W. C. Fields had it. Princess Diana had it, too. And Bill Clinton and George W. Bush have it.

Rosacea is an extremely common skin disease, often referred to in the press as the new red menace. Several studies estimate that seventeen million Americans have it; we'd say that figure is probably closer to twenty to thirty million. Some dermatologists estimate that over half of their adult acne patients come in because of rosacea. Yet this disease is grossly misunderstood (leading to accusations of alcoholism), is often misdiagnosed as contact dermatitis and improperly treated, and is as conspicuous and embarrassing to its sufferers as a face full of pimples.

Rosacea itself is not acne, although it is usually erroneously referred to as adult acne. There are no plugged pores or excess oil, which, as you know, cause acne. Rosacea is its own skin disease, a vascular condition that classically appears as a flush or blush on the face and sometimes the sides of the neck and chest. It is a common reaction to many stimulants, including embarrassment, exercise, stress, temperature changes, heat, alcohol, and a long list of foods (see below). In addition, we believe there is a genetic component to rosacea. It's most noticeable in Caucasians, especially those of Celtic or Scandinavian ancestry, whose fair skin cannot hide the redness. (In fact, children with delicious apple pink cheeks often develop rosacea in adulthood.) Rosacea also affects people of color, although it may be less visible on their dark skin. "I'm in my thirties and have an olive complexion," Rosita told us. "People think because I have a dark complexion that my skin isn't sensitive or I can't possibly have rosacea, but I do. My skin can get as bright as cherries."

The exact trip wire that starts the rosacea response is unknown. Many studies have been conducted, as scientists and doctors try to understand this disease. Some doctors have suggested that the demodex mite, which lives on the skin, the *p. acnes* bacteria, or a gastrointestinal organism triggering an autoimmune disorder may be the cause of rosacea. But none of these theories have held up, and the cause of rosacea remains obscure.

With rosacea, the constant dilation or constriction of the blood vessels in your face—the same vessels that allow you to blush—become overstimulated. The flush may stay this way for minutes or hours. Over time, the redness deepens and may evolve into persistent pink patches. It can lead to permanent capillary damage, which becomes visible as red or purplish threads, usually on the cheeks and nose. Rosacea is also exacerbated by sun exposure. What look like broken blood vessels on the face are actually new and dilated capillaries formed in response to the sun's harmful rays.

Rosacea is also associated with central face acne-like bumps. These are often red papules and pustules on the cheeks and nose, without blackheads. In rare cases, the skin thickens. The nose can become large and bulbous (called rhinophyma), like the one W. C. Fields was known for.

In a recent survey by the National Rosacea Society, 44 percent of the respondents said rosacea symptoms first appeared when they were in their thirties or forties, and 43 percent first experienced rosacea after age fifty. It can also be hormonally triggered—yet another aggravation for perimenopausal women who already have red faces from hot flashes!

Rosacea is a progressive condition. Left untreated, it will not spontaneously resolve. It simply worsens. Because rosacea is incurable, suppressive therapy is required. There are currently no FDA-approved over-the-counter treatments specifically targeting rosacea.

Acne and rosacea often overlap, with many adults having a little bit of both—an acne component and a rosacea component. For example, adults who have suffered on and off with acne for years may develop the flush/blush response associated with rosacea in their thirties. The final picture is a red-hot face studded with pustules, thanks to rosacea and occasional nodules, premenstrual flares, and blackheads, all signs of acne. Fortunately, most medications that treat and control acne are helpful for rosacea. However, because rosacea is associated with skin sensitivity, avoiding strong, potentially irritating acne medications is critical.

rosacea triggers

Before we move on to treatments for acne and rosacea, remember that because rosacea is a chronic condition, it's extremely important to figure out what your specific trigger factors are and do your best to avoid them. These triggers may include:

Beverages

Alcohol, especially red wine, beer, bourbon, and champagne; hot-temperature drinks; caffeinated beverages.

Cosmetics and Skin-Care Products

Any product that causes redness or stinging when applied; any product containing high levels of alcohol or acetone; some heavily fragranced products.

Drugs

Heart and blood pressure medications, such as calcium channel blockers; opiates, tamoxifen, topical steroids, and vasodilators.

Emotional Conditions

Anxiety; embarrassment; rage; stress.

Foods

Avocados, bananas, cheese (especially aged cheeses, such as parmesan, blue cheese, and brie—but not cottage cheese), chocolate, citrus fruits, eggplant, figs, lima beans, liver, navy beans, raisins, red plums, sour cream, soy sauce, spicy foods, spinach, tomatoes, vanilla, vinegar, yeast extract, and yogurt. Foods and beverages served hot can trigger a flush/blush reaction because heat applied to the soft palate of the mouth may trigger dilation of facial capillaries. Also, foods high in histamines and large meals heavy with carbohydrates can trigger rosacea.

Medical Conditions

Caffeine withdrawal; chronic cough; high blood pressure; menopause.

Physical Exertion

Exercise; lifting and loading; straining.

Temperature

Exercise; hot or steam baths; radiant heat; saunas; warm environments.

Weather

Cold, strong winds; direct sun; hot, humid temperatures.

To establish proper treatment, it is also vital to learn to recognize the differences between acne and rosacea. (See table on page 273.)

emotional effects of rosacea

The response to rosacea by friends and strangers is often just as embarrassing as the redness itself. Because faces can remain deeply flushed, the inevitable response is that the rosacea sufferer has a drinking problem or is an outright alcoholic. This is one of the unfounded and unfair myths about rosacea; the irony is that many people with rosacea know they must avoid drinking alcohol.

Rosacea can also create mortifying situations at work. "Never let them see

THE DIFFERENCES BETWEEN ACNE AND ROSACEA

	Acne	Rosacea
age	ten and up	twenty-five to sixty.
gender	equal distribution	more women than men
frequency	very common	common
affected areas	face, body	central face, neck, central chest
ethnicity	less common in African Americans, Asians	more common in people of Celtic or Scandinavian descent
primary	comedones, papules, pustules, nodules, and cysts on full face or just chin	no comedones; sometimes papules and pustules, on central face, midforehead, midcheek, midchin
contributing factors	picking, rubbing, pressure, stress, comedogenic products	see Rosacea Triggers, page 271
cause	many different factors	unknown
organisms	*p. acnes* bacteria	none proven
medication triggers	corticosteroids, oral contraceptives, antidepressants, antiepileptics	topical corticosteroids, vasodilators
hereditary	yes	yes
ocular involvement	no	common
rhinophyma	no	yes
flushing/blushing	no	yes
postinflammatory hyperpigmentation	yes	no
scarring	yes	rare
psychosocial effects	yes	yes

you sweat," the saying goes. It could just as easily be "Never let them see you blush." You may be able to hide your perspiration, but you can't put a bag over your face and hide the red component. Particularly when colleagues remark, "Are you warm? You're blushing," right before you're about to give an important presentation. This can be devastating to self-esteem, credibility, and professional standing.

One study conducted by the National Rosacea Society had stunning figures for the emotional toll rosacea takes on its sufferers. These include:

- low self-esteem (75 percent)
- embarrassment (70 percent)
- frustration (69 percent)
- negative impact on professional interactions (60 percent)
- interference with social life (57 percent)
- feeling robbed of pleasure and happiness (56 percent)
- adverse impact on ability to establish new relationships (39 percent)

As you can see, these feelings are as common to those with rosacea as they are to those with acne. Finding emotional support is crucial, as is the management of stress (see page 98 for the Rodan and Fields Stress-Busting Program).

It can often be a relief to many when they are finally diagnosed, because they now realize that they are suffering from a condition and that their symptoms and distress are real and should be taken seriously. If you suspect that you have rosacea, don't delay seeing a dermatologist for diagnosis and treatment.

about sensitive skin

Over 70 percent of consumers believe they have sensitive skin. Some are correct, but most are not. Because sensitive skin often produces a feeling of stinging or burning rather than physical evidence, it is difficult for dermatologists to study it precisely. "Sensitive" is a word commonly voiced by consumers who have experienced some form of irritation from a skin-care product, and it is egregiously overhyped as a category by skin-care companies.

There is tremendous variability in how sensitive skin reactions appear. There may be redness, tightness, dryness, and blemishes. There may also be blotchiness, dry patches, itching, and stinging.

A study by the Epidermal and Sensory Research and Investigation Center in Paris reported in May 2000 classified sensitive skin into four general categories:

Type 1

Redness associated with diet, alcohol, stress, emotion, and temperature changes (in other words, rosacea).

Type 2

Redness, scaling, and tightness associated with environmental factors, such as cold, wind, air conditioning, and excessive heat.

Type 3

Redness, tightness, stinging, and small papules associated with cosmetic use, soap and detergents, and hard water.

Type 4

Red patches associated with hormonal changes, such as the menstrual cycle.

Rosacea sufferers may have sensitive skin of all four types and therefore must adjust their skin-care routines to assist healing and avoid continuous irritation. However, you do not need to discontinue the use of all acne medicines, moisturizers, and cosmetics when you have rosacea. You simply have to find the products that work best for you.

As we all know too well, our skin changes over time from the inevitable aging process and hormonal influences on the skin. Unfortunately, as we age our immune systems begin to weaken as well, making us more susceptible to the environment—most notably sun exposure—and potentially irritating substances. This means you should use common sense about skin care, especially when selecting and applying sunscreen. So, be savvy about claims that a specific product is needed if you have rosacea.

Many cosmetic companies have created successful lines of sensitive-skin products, which do not contain well-known irritating agents. While these cosmetics can be wonderful, overuse of any product is a common cause of sensitivity. Studies in Japan have found that because Japanese women are overzealous in their cleansing regimens and use ten or more different products, their skin often rebels and reacts. By using harsh cleansers that strip off the barrier layer of skin, then layering on several different toners, creams, and moisturizers, a woman can inadvertently contribute to her own skin sensitivity.

If you believe your skin is sensitive, read labels and proceed cautiously whenever trying anything new. Use fragrance-free and hypoallergenic products with the fewest number of ingredients on the label. Almay, Aveeno, and Physicians Formula are well-tested and worth exploring. If a cream or moisturizer has an ingredient that you know produces irritation as one of the first four ingredients on the label, you may want to avoid it. If it's listed near the bottom, it may still be worth trying. Ingredients on cosmetic labels are listed in descending order by quantity of ingredient, usually beginning with water and ending with preservatives and fragrance. Be sure to do a patch test for sensitivity first. (See page 308 in chapter 15 for more information about patch testing for sensitivity. For information on cosmetic comedogenicity and irritation, see page 303 in chapter 15, and chapter 17.)

ROSACEA IRRITANTS

Many of these ingredients are particularly irritating to rosacea-sensitized skin. Read the labels carefully.

acetone	alcohol (especially benzyl)	alpha hydroxy acids
benzoyl peroxide (5 percent and 10 percent)	cinnamates	ethanol
formaldehyde	glycerin	isopropyl palmitate
menthol	mica	polyethylene beads
propylene glycol	sodium laurel sulfate	sorbic acid
tretinoin	urea	

People allergic to sulfur taken orally will usually tolerate topical sulfur and sodium sulfacetamide—active ingredients found in prescription and non-prescription medications. Discuss your ingredient sensitivities and options with your dermatologist so potential irritants can be avoided, and do patch testing with any new skin-care product (see page 308 in chapter 15).

ocular, steroid, and toothpaste rosacea

Ocular Rosacea

One of the most common adjuncts to rosacea on the skin is ocular rosacea, or rosacea of the eye. It is extremely easy to misdiagnose as irritation from contact lenses, smoking, air pollution, or as pink eye (conjunctivitis), a highly contagious virus.

Ocular rosacea sometimes appears as a precursor to skin rosacea. It produces redness of the eyeball and often feels as if particles of grit or sand are under the eyelids. It may be associated with blurred vision and photosensitivity.

As many patients with ocular rosacea have no idea that this is a sign of rosacea, they don't mention eye symptoms to their dermatologist, seeking treatment from their ophthalmologist instead. Be sure to mention persistent eye redness or irritation to your doctor so it can be treated appropriately.

Dr. Rona Silkiss, the chief of ophthalmic plastic reconstructive and orbital surgery at the California Pacific Medical Center in San Francisco, treats ocular rosacea with oral tetracycline or doxycycline until clear. She recommends gentle eye scrubs on the eyelid or lash line with no-tears baby shampoos and occasional erythromycin drops on the eyeball itself.

Steroid Rosacea

Fluorinated steroids are potent topical anti-inflammatory medications. Because use on the face for more than a few days can precipitate rosacea, fluorinated steroids are meant for rashes on the body. Only mild cortisone creams are prescribed for facial use. Once treatment with steroids is stopped, symptoms of steroid-induced rosacea frequently become worse before they improve. Rosacea treatment medications, such as sulfur and antibiotics, may be prescribed to alleviate rosacea flares from steroid use.

Toothpaste Rosacea

Rosacea may appear around the mouth from a sensitivity to the fluorinated products often found in toothpaste. Fluoride is great for cavity protection, but it's not so great for rosacea. Always be sure to clean any excess toothpaste from the skin around the mouth after brushing, and ask your dentist or pharmacist for recommendations for nonfluorinated toothpastes effective for your dental needs.

treatment for rosacea

Unfortunately, there are no FDA-approved over-the-counter drugs to treat rosacea, only prescription medications. Because the exact cause of this disease is unknown, a single medicine to treat it has yet to be found. And since the cost of developing and launching new drugs is extraordinarily high, drug companies do not seem to be in hot pursuit of novel therapies to address the needs of what is misperceived as a condition that affects a relatively small number of people.

Over-the-counter acne therapy can be used to treat the acne component of rosacea. We developed Rodan & Fields CALM with sulfur and low-strength benzoyl peroxide to treat the acne component of rosacea, as well as with azelaic acid to help minimize the redness component of rosacea. While it is not specifically an antirosacea treatment system, many of our customers and patients have told us that it significantly reduced rosacea's symptoms. It may be worth trying, but be sure to patch-test the products first (see page 308 in chapter 15).

Here are some other tips for treating rosacea:

- Even though rosacea is not acne, mild over-the-counter acne products may help counteract redness and breakouts.
- Use a mild soap, such as Cetaphil Gentle Skin Cleanser, which tests have shown to be the least irritating cleanser available. Dove soap may also be used. Mildly medicated cleansers with sulfur (Rodan & Fields CALM 1 Wash) or 2.5 percent benzoyl peroxide (Proactiv Solution Renewing Cleanser) used once daily may help combat the *p. acnes* bacteria, a culprit in acne.
- It's best to apply cleanser with clean fingers rather than with an abrasive washcloth. Never wash more than twice a day. More frequent washing will result in dry, irritated skin from the stripping of the stratum corneum. Also remember to use tepid water to avoid stimulating and dilating facial blood vessels.
- Avoid isopropyl alcohol–based toners and aggressive scrubs.

- Always wear a broad-spectrum sunscreen (with zinc oxide or avobenzone) to provide protection from UVA/UVB radiation. Sunscreens with physical blockers, such as zinc oxide or titanium dioxide, are less irritating for those with sensitive skin.
- Taking an aspirin or ibuprofen one hour before a dinner party or lunch meeting may stave off the flush response. (Note: If you have any medical condition that precludes the use of aspirin, do not take it without the advice of your doctor.)
- Cool yourself down whenever possible, but never apply ice directly to your face. This can cause partial freezing and will exacerbate rosacea, not diminish it. Try sucking on ice chips, instead. (Sucking on ice chips can be especially useful right before an important meeting or event.) Or, apply freezer cool packs, carefully wrapped in several layers of towel, to the face or neck. Sporting goods stores also sell some clever devices that retain their cold temperature after being soaked in water. These are great for draping around the neck after you get into a hot car. Finally, an old southern belle's trick is to hold an iced drink against the pulse points in your wrists. It provides immediate cooling to the entire body.
- Use camouflaging makeup. Any cover-up or foundation containing green will help counteract redness. Physicians Formula has a green-based noncomedogenic cover-up. Use it under your regular foundation, and apply it sparingly only to affected areas. We also like crushed powder mineral-based makeups from Bare Escentuals, Belladonna, or Proactiv Solution (Sheer Finish Loose Powder or Sheer Finish Translucent Pressed Powder), which are available in a broad color spectrum.

  Men can try using a tinted moisturizer with sunscreen, such as Proactiv Solution Sheer Tint Moisture with SPF 15. Those men who are brave enough can use the green cover-ups underneath it as well.

  For more information on camouflaging techniques, see chapter 17.

when to see a dermatologist

Anyone who has rosacea should see a dermatologist, as the disease is both incurable and progressive. The red component of rosacea and the flush/blush reaction are difficult to treat, and your dermatologist will help you manage your condition much more effectively than you can on your own. No matter what your skin tone, suggested treatments will be the same. These include, in order of the most commonly prescribed, topical creams, oral antibiotics, Accutane, hormone therapy, and intense pulse light treatment. (Note that none of these oral or topical medications or other treatments completely resolve this condition for all patients.)

Topical Creams

Metronidazole

The most commonly prescribed topical medication for rosacea is metronidazole, available as MetroCream, MetroGel, MetroLotion, and Noritate. Your dermatologist will prescribe one according to the oil content of your skin. How metronidazole works is not completely understood, but it may help rosacea by killing the demodex mite, which lodges inside pores, thereby decreasing inflammation.

Azelaic Acid

Azelaic acid is an anti-inflammatory, antibacterial topical medication that may also unplug pores. Dr. Diane M. Thiboutot, associate professor of medicine/dermatology at Pennsylvania State University College of Medicine and one of the principal investigators in the clinical trials of this product, claimed in a report published in *Dermatology Times* in June 2003 that data from two double-blind studies showed that a 15 percent azelaic acid gel (Finacea) was more effective than metronidazole for treating rosacea. Combining both topicals, for example, metronidazole in the morning and azelaic acid in the evening, may provide effective control for rosacea symptoms.

Benzoyl Peroxide

New research implicates the *p. acnes* bacteria as a cause of rosacea and finds benzoyl peroxide effective in treating the acne component of the condition. One promising study conducted by dermatologists in Cincinnati showed that a combination of a low-dose benzoyl peroxide (1 percent) with the antibiotic clindamycin gel (5 percent) had good results. It's too soon to know if this will translate to a regularly prescribed treatment for rosacea, but these two medications may be worth trying.

Vitamin Creams

Ongoing studies are also looking at the use of topical Vitamin C, zinc, and niacinamide for the treatment of rosacea. While results are not expected to be dramatic, these ingredients may be a helpful adjunct.

Oral Antibiotics

As with acne, tetracycline and its derivatives, doxycycline and minocycline, can produce dramatic reduction of the symptoms of rosacea. These oral antibiotics are often combined with topical creams for fairly immediate relief of rosacea symptoms. Once the rosacea is controlled, the patient is weaned from the oral antibiotics and maintained on topical creams.

One possible breakthrough in the oral antibiotic treatment of rosaca is the use of zithromycin (sometimes in the form of Zithromax Z-Pak), a derivative of erythromycin, instead of the tetracyclines or other antibiotics. The Zithromax Z-Pak is used until a patient's skin is clear, then the patient is treated with it only once a month or as needed—no topical creams are required.

Accutane

Accutane may be an option for those with severe rosacea. Because Accutane causes birth defects if taken during pregnancy, birth control should be prescribed for all women of childbearing age who are taking this drug. For more information about how Accutane works and a full account of its side effects, please turn to page 53 in chapter 2.

Hormone Therapy (Women Only)

Just as fluctuating levels of feminizing hormones can cause hot flashes, so they can exacerbate rosacea. Using hormone therapy (HT) or taking birth control pills to treat rosacea are viable options women should discuss with both their dermatologist and gynecologist. (Note that long-term hormone therapy may be inappropriate for postmenopausal women.)

Intense Pulse Light Treatment

One of the most promising treatments for the red reactions and permanent visible blood vessels of rosacea is called intense pulse light, or IPL. IPL delivers multiple wavelengths of light to the skin to treat both red and brown pigmentation. Four to six treatments at monthly intervals help to eradicate the tiny matted vessels across the nose, cheeks, and chin. Also, with each treatment, the redness diminishes and brown age spots may crust over and fall off. The benefits from a series of IPL treatments may last a year or more; nevertheless, it is recommended to use topical medications daily to help maintain results, since without some form of ongoing therapy rosacea will recur.

The downside of IPL treatments include the out-of-pocket cost of $2,000–$3,000 for four to six treatment sessions; possible lack of response; potential blistering; swelling, which can last a week or more; and, rarely, scarring. Also, IPL is most effective for those with lighter skin tones. However, as these sophisticated light sources continue to be developed and refined, IPL will become a more available option for everyone.

patient history

Sister Marie O'Riley is forty-six and has never had a drink in her life, but she does remember burning miserably in the hot sunshine as a child. She came to see us with a red face, fine capillaries on the nose and cheeks, and a few small nodules on the nose. She explained that her face became worse with exercise, sun, spicy foods, hot foods, and even tea. She is highly embarrassed by her rosacea and willing to try anything to rid herself of the troublesome redness.

We put Sister Mary on the Rodan & Fields CALM regimen, which includes washing with a cleanser containing sulfur (CALM 1 Wash), followed by an alcohol-free toner with salicylic acid (CALM 2 Prepare). After the toner dries, Sister Mary applies a leave-on lotion with 2.5 percent benzoyl peroxide (CALM 3 Treat). As needed, she uses a mask with sulfur (CALM Soothe).

Sister Mary tolerated the treatment well, with no reaction to the sulfur, and showed improvement after three weeks. Optional advanced therapy for Sister Mary includes IPL therapy to reduce the size and number of blood vessels. She has also stopped drinking hot tea, which, she explained, was a small price to pay for having clear skin. Because rosacea is not curable, Sister Mary's maintenance treatment is the same as her initial treatment.

treatment for the acne component of rosacea

There is no FDA-approved over-the-counter therapy for rosacea, but you can use mild acne products to treat the acne component of this condition.

Remember, use these products on your *entire face*, not only on acne-prone areas, except where noted. The sensitive eye area should be avoided, of course, except where eye creams are indicated.

Every day you need to clean, tone, and treat your skin. The products you use need medicines to unplug pores, remove bacteria, and reduce swelling. The active ingredients in some of these products are applicable in several categories. For example, salicylic acid, which unplugs pores, is often an active ingredient in cleansers, toners, leave-on lotions, and moisturizers: and benzoyl peroxide, which removes bacteria and helps to unplugs pores, is often an active ingredient in cleansers and leave-on lotions. This explains why Proactiv Solution Renewing Cleanser and Proactiv Solution Repairing Lotion, which contain benzoyl peroxide, both unplug pores and remove bacteria. However, we are listing cleansers only in Step 1—Unplug Pores and not Step 2—Remove Bacteria. The reason is simple: Leave-on lotions, such as Proactiv Solution Repairing Lotion, must be applied *after* cleansing and toning.

You will also notice that the order of the three steps is different for Proactiv Solution products from that for Rodan & Fields CALM products. That's because the formulation in each system is different, even though some ingredients are similar and the purpose remains the same. The order of use of ingredients is interchangeable as long as you cleanse, tone, and treat with salicylic acid or glycolic acid, benzoyl peroxide, and sulfur in some combination and end up with a leave-on lotion.

Note: "Apply sparingly" means you should use a dime-sized amount of product. It should be enough to have a thin coat applied over the entire surface of the skin where needed. It is always better to use less product rather than more!

Note: In the Extra Help sections, you may choose more than one product, such as a mask, a leave-on lotion, or a moisturizer, if needed.

Note: For photographic examples, go to www.unblemished.com.

Treatment 1: Rodan & Fields CALM

Start to use this treatment once a day for two weeks, then increase to twice a day. Until you are able to tolerate its use twice a day or if you remain at once a day, use a mild cleanser, such as Cetaphil Gentle Skin Cleanser or Rodan & Fields COMPOUNDS Gentle Wash, when not using Rodan & Fields CALM products.

1. Reduce Swelling—sulfur

Rodan & Fields CALM 1 Wash (cleanser)	Wash off and pat dry.

2. Unplug Pores—salicylic acid

Rodan & Fields CALM 2 Prepare (toner)	Apply with gauze or cotton ball. Let dry.

3. Remove Bacteria—benzoyl peroxide

Rodan & Fields CALM 3 Treat (leave-on lotion)	Apply with fingertips. Let dry.

4. Extra Help

Proactiv Solution Green Tea Moisturizer	Apply sparingly to dry skin.
Proactiv Solution Replenishing Eye Cream	Apply with your pinkie finger, gently patting cream on the upper and lower eyelids, including the crow's feet area.
Proactiv Solution Sheer Finish Compact Foundation	Apply sparingly.
Proactiv Solution Sheer Finish Loose Powder	Apply sparingly over foundation.
Proactiv Solution Skin-Clearing Cream to Powder Foundation	Apply sparingly.
Rodan & Fields CALM Soothe (mask)	Mix ingredients into a paste. Apply to face or other affected area. Let dry ten minutes. Peel off. Use once or twice a week or every night for the five nights leading up to menstruation.
Rodan & Fields COMPOUNDS Moisture	Apply to dry skin.

| Rodan & Fields COMPOUNDS Moisture Eye | Apply with your pinkie finger, gently patting cream on the upper and lower eyelids, including the crow's feet area. |

TREATMENT 2: PROACTIV SOLUTION

Start by using this treatment once a day for two weeks, then increase to twice a day. Until you are able to tolerate its use twice a day or if you remain at once a day, use a mild cleanser, such as Cetaphil Gentle Skin Cleanser or Rodan & Fields COMPOUNDS Gentle Wash, when not using Proactiv Solution products.

1. Unplug Pores—benzoyl peroxide, glycolic acid

| a) Renewing cleanser | Wash off and pat dry. |
| b) Revitalizing toner | Apply with gauze or cotton ball. Let dry. |

2. Remove Bacteria—benzoyl peroxide

| Repairing Lotion | Apply with fingertips. Let dry. |

3. Reduce Swelling—sulfur

| Concealer Plus | Lightly dot on with applicator. Blend with concealer brush or fingertips. Use once or twice a day. |
| Refining Mask | Apply to clean, dry face or other affected area. Let dry ten minutes. Rinse with lukewarm water. Use once or twice a week for maintenance or every night for the five nights leading up to menstruation. |

4. Extra Help—Proactiv Solution

Clarifying Night Cream	Apply sparingly to dry skin. Use only at night.
Daily Oil Control (for slightly oily skin)	Apply to entire face or other affected area with fingertips after toner. Let dry. Use daily or as needed.
Green Tea Moisturizer	Apply sparingly to dry skin.
Mild Exfoliating Peel	Apply thin layer. Let dry one to two minutes. Remove with fingertips. Rinse with lukewarm water. Use once a week.
Oil Blotter Sheets	Use as needed to pat away excess oil.
Sheer Finish Compact Foundation	Apply sparingly.
Sheer Finish Loose Powder	Apply sparingly over foundation.
Skin-Clearing Cream to Powder Foundation	Apply sparingly.

Treatment 3A: Other Products—for Women

Start to use this treatment once a day for two weeks, then increase to twice a day. Until you are able to tolerate its use twice a day or if you remain at once a day, use a mild cleanser, such as Cetaphil Gentle Skin Cleanser or Rodan & Fields COMPOUNDS Gentle Wash, when not using other products. Remember to pick only one product from each list, except in the Extra Help section, where you may choose more than one product, such as a mask, or an eye cream, if needed.

1. Unplug Pores—salicylic acid

Aveeno Acne Treatment   Wash off and pat dry.
  Bar
L'Oréal Pure Zone Skin
  Balancing Cream
  Cleanser
Neutrogena Multi-
  vitamin Acne
  Treatment
Neutrogena Oil-Free
  Acne Wash Cream

2. Remove Bacteria—benzoyl peroxide

Clear By Design Gel 2.5%   Apply with fingertips. Let dry.
Neutrogena On-the-
  Spot Acne Treatment

3. Reduce Swelling—sulfur

Clearasil Adult Care   Apply sparingly with fingertips. Let dry.
  Acne Treatment Cream
Prescriptives Blemish
  Specialist

4. Extra Help

Neutrogena Clear Pore   Apply with fingertips. Leave on five to ten minutes.
  Cleanser/Mask   Rinse with lukewarm water. Use once or twice a week
                            or every night for the five nights leading up to
                            menstruation.
Neutrogena Healthy   Apply with your pinkie finger, gently patting cream on
  Skin Eye Cream   the upper and lower eyelids, including the crow's feet
                            area.

Don't Forget the Sunscreen

For all three treatments, applying sunblock in the morning is the all-important final step. Apply after all treatment products have dried.

Clinique Sun Care Face SPF 15
Estée Lauder In the Sun Sunblock For Face SPF 15
Neutrogena Ultra Sheer Dry-Touch Sunblock SPF 30
Olay Complete UV Defense Moisture Lotion
Ombrelle Sunscreen Lotion SPF 30
Prescriptives All You Need Broad Spectrum Oil Absorbing Lotion SPF 15
Proactiv Solution Daily Protection Plus SPF 15
Proactiv Solution Oil Free Moisture SPF 15
Rodan & Fields COMPOUNDS Protect SPF 15

TREATMENT 3B: OTHER PRODUCTS—FOR MEN

Start to use this treatment once a day for two weeks, then increase to twice a day. Until you are able to tolerate its use twice a day or if you remain at once a day, use a mild cleanser, such as Cetaphil Gentle Skin Cleanser or Rodan & Fields COMPOUNDS Gentle Wash, when not using other products. Remember to pick only one product from each list, except in the Extra Help section, where you may choose more than one product, such as a cleansing pad or a leave-on lotion, if needed.

1. Unplug Pores—salicylic acid

Clearasil 3-in-1 Acne   Wash off and pat dry.
  Cleanser
L'Oréal Ideal Balance
  Foaming Gel Cleanser
Neutrogena Oil-Free
  Acne Wash
Oxy Oil-Free Maximum
  Strength Once A Day
  Acne Wash

2. Remove Bacteria—benzoyl peroxide

Clean & Clear PersaGel   Apply with fingertips. Let dry.
Clinique Emergency
  Lotion

Neutrogena On-the-
  Spot Therapy

3. Reduce Swelling—sulfur

Clearasil Adult Care   Apply sparingly with fingertips. Let dry.
  Acne Treatment Cream

4. Extra Help

Clearasil Pore Cleansing   Wipe on. Let dry.
  Pads*

Clinique Night   Apply with fingertips. Let dry.
  Treatment Gel

Neutrogena Clear Pore
  Shine Control Gel

Oxy Daily Cleansing   Wipe on. Let dry.
  Pads*

Stri-Dex Sensitive Skin
  Triple Action Acne
  Pads*

* Body pads may be used on the face for a quick midday facial cleansing without a trip to
the sink. They can also be used after playing sports.

Don't Forget the Sunscreen

For all men with rosacea, applying sunscreen in the morning is the all-
important final step. Apply after all treatment products have dried.

  Clearasil Acne Treatment Cream SPF 15*
  Neutrogena Ultra Sheer Dry-Touch Sunblock SPF 45
  Olay Complete UV Defense Moisture Lotion
  Ombrelle Sunscreen Lotion SPF 30
  Proactiv Solution Daily Protection SPF 15
  Proactiv Solution Sheer Tint Moisture SPF 15*
  Rodan & Fields COMPOUNDS Protect SPF 15

* These are excellent solutions for men as they're cover-ups, not makeup, and the slight tint
helps camouflage redness while they protect skin from the sun.

once your rosacea goes away, you *will* have rosacea amnesia

The persistent redness and facial flushing associated with rosacea make it a stigmatizing disease. The sufferer is often perceived to be an alcoholic because of the permanent facial redness or as insecure or highly embarrassed because of the flush response in social situations. Though the causes of acne and rosacea are entirely different, most of the treatments for acne help rosacea. Because sensitive skin may be a component of rosacea, using mildly medicated, less irritating products help give the best results with the fewest side effects.

Josephine's husband, quoted at the beginning of this chapter, began using our CALM treatment once a day. Within a month, his rosacea had diminished considerably. "The other day, for the first time in a long, long time, he had a couple of glasses of red wine when we were out to dinner, and he didn't turn red. We were both amazed and very happy. This has helped his entire demeanor," Josephine reported.

Tina, age forty-nine, told us, "I grew my hair longer and would always hide my face by pushing my hair in front of it. I was embarrassed and couldn't look people in the eye because I knew as soon as they looked at me, they'd be staring at the ugly redness on my cheeks. I was miserable until I tried CALM. People who saw me when the rosacea was active cannot believe that I still have it, because my skin looks so good. Once I realized your products were definitely working, I even got bold enough to cut my hair short. Proper treatment for my rosacea has been a lifesaver."

Don't delay treatment. See a dermatologist and explore the many options available, and your rosacea will be helped much sooner than you thought possible. Then you can revel in your own case of rosacea amnesia.

chapter fourteen
acne on the body

"I started taking estrogen as part of the hormone replacement therapy recommended by my gynecologist when I hit menopause. It was a great help with eliminating my hot flashes, but I suddenly developed acne on my buttocks and back. It was not attractive, to put it mildly. Frankly, it was pretty mortifying. I sure didn't want my husband to see it!"

—**Susan, age forty-nine**

"I've been getting huge pimples on my back and chest for years. They really hurt, and they seemed to last for weeks. I was too embarrassed to go to the beach, and as for dating, forget it. What girl would touch my skin when it was covered with huge zits? I mean, *I* didn't want to touch it! I was getting desperate."

—**Diego, age nineteen**

as many people know only too well, acne can make a highly unwelcome appearance on different parts of the body, usually the neck, shoulders, back, chest, and buttocks. And it can cause as much acute mortification as a huge red pimple on a prom queen's cheek. Yet because many people don't know how common body acne is and because it can be difficult to mention the presence of acne in unmentionable places, they often don't seek out treatment. For example, we've had patients come to us to discuss treatment of facial acne without mentioning that they had body acne until they were walking out the door. No one should ever be too embarrassed to tell a doctor where acne has sprouted.

Acne on the body occurs for the same reasons as acne occurs on the face—any pore on the body is fair game for acne. On the body, the greatest density of hair follicles and sebaceous (oil) glands occurs on the chest, shoulders, upper arms, and buttocks. Plus body acne is often exacerbated by sweat, heat, and mechanical friction, such as clothing or backpacks rubbing and pressing against your skin. We tend to see severe acne on the body more in men than in women.

Body acne rarely goes away spontaneously. It can be vicious, with large, painful cysts that heal leaving thick scars or dark brown stains. It can be stubborn to treat, so it's important to seek help from a dermatologist. In addition, many other skin conditions, such as folliculitis, resemble body acne. A dermatologist will be able to identify such conditions, which require different treatment. For more information on acne imposters, see chapter 15.

For photographic examples of body acne, go to www.unblemished.com.

buttock acne

When athletes come to see us, we often make them laugh by referring to buttock acne as biker's butt. Red bumps and pimples appearing on the buttocks are not a surprise—and are surprisingly typical, even if you aren't an athlete. There *are* sebaceous (oil) glands on the buttocks, and although they are less dense than elsewhere on the body, they are more deep-seated. So, for example, when cyclists go for exhilarating long rides and stew for hours in their sweat, acne can sprout. Other athletes are equally susceptible if they run, jog, or participate in other sports in the heat while wearing close-fitting workout clothes that keep moisture close to the body. And surfers and swimmers can literally marinate bacteria in wetsuits and bathing suits for hours on end, creating a breeding ground for acne.

Fortunately, buttock acne is easily treatable with the same medications used on facial acne: benzoyl peroxide, salicylic acid, and sulfur. Here are some tips:

- Follow the recommendations in the section on Torso Acne on page 296 or a treatment plan in whichever chapter is appropriate for your gender and age group. *Never spot-treat. Always apply medication to the entire area.*
- Using large pads containing salicylic acid, such as Proactiv Solution Clear-Zone Body Pads, right after a workout will remove most of the sweat even if you are unable to take a shower. Keep some in a Ziploc bag so they're always handy.

- Benzoyl peroxide products can bleach underwear and T-shirts, so always wear white undergarments when using these products. If you like to sleep in the buff, it's probably best to use white bedding.
- Work out in clothing that has a high wicking quotient to pull moisture away from the skin. There are many new synthetic fabrics specifically designed for athletes with this purpose. They are available in underwear and outerwear. Ask for recommendations in a sporting goods store.
- For regular daily use, wear either 100 percent cotton underwear or the newer wicking synthetics. Old-fashioned polyester undies may feel good and look lovely, but they do not breathe. Women can also try wearing thongs.

ear acne

Pimples, cysts, and blackheads can appear inside and behind the ears, and they are often very painful. "I fly in the navy and have to deal with an oxygen mask every time we're airborne," a thirty-five-year-old pilot explained. "That causes the acne behind my ears to flare up, and it can be very painful."

A thirty-seven-year-old female patient saw her mild case of facial acne gradually shift and become more intense: Large cysts appeared inside and behind her ears and on the back of her neck. "I grew my hair long, even though I didn't really want to, and the reason was to cover up the pimples and cysts I always had," she told us.

Ear acne should be treated by a dermatologist, as it tends to be severe and can leave permanent scars that can be as disfiguring as the cysts. If you have ear acne, make an appointment with a dermatologist right away.

exercise acne

As we said in the section above on buttock acne, biker's butt is a common side effect of exercising. Exercise can also lead to acne appearing on other parts of the body. For example, many people like to work out with friends, perhaps on a team, and go out to eat afterward without taking a quick shower. Indeed, shower facilities often aren't even available. This can leave you soaking in your own sweat, a breeding ground for acne all over the body.

We never want to discourage anyone from exercising or participating in team sports. For the health of your skin, however, follow whatever cleansing routine works for you immediately after an exercise session, then apply your topical acne medicines after cleansing. You can pour small amounts of your medicines into travel-size bottles for easy portability. These are inexpensive and available at most drugstores. Also, if showers are not available, pack medicated wipes in your gym bag and use them for a quick wipe-down after your workout.

"My son is a football player," one mother told us. "The chinstrap used to make his neck and chin break out, and the helmet made his face break out. He had red marks all over his face. But once he started using Proactiv Solution, it worked like magic. What amazes me is that he uses it the way it's supposed to be used. He takes it with him everywhere. It excites me because he feels good about himself now and maintains his treatment accordingly. Before he would just give up and let it go. I am so happy for him that this system is working. He hasn't had any pimples for months."

groin and underarm acne

Groin and underarm acne is a rare acne condition called *hidradenitis suppurativa*. It causes pimples and an extensive network of cysts and nodules that can leave scarring and hyperpigmentation in their wake. It is painful, often has a terrible smell, and is distressing to anyone unlucky enough to have it.

Anyone with groin or underarm acne should see a dermatologist right away. Surgery is often necessary to excise the persistent cysts. Antibiotics or Accutane may be tried, although Accutane is not nearly as successful with this problem as it is for other forms of acne.

scalp acne

"I've been to every kind of doctor imaginable—from a cancer specialist to an infectious disease specialist to local dermatologists—and the best they can figure is that I have a severe case of acne on my scalp. It's the only place I have it," thirty-two-year-old Winston told us. "The pimples are filled with green pus, and they smell bad when they pop. There's also a lot of redness and inflammation. It looks terrible, and it's really, really painful. Plus I can't stop picking at the pimples, and that's upsetting me and my wife."

Scalp acne with tender red bumps is common. The scalp is loaded with se-

ALL ABOUT DANDRUFF

For reasons yet unknown to science, dandruff often accompanies facial acne, especially in adolescents. It's not a result of too much hair washing. Instead, for dandruff sufferers, the natural process of scalp-cell renewal is accelerated when fighting off *p. ovale*, a yeast found normally on every human head. In response, dead skin cells slough off more quickly, creating flaking, scaling, and itching. Dandruff is also associated with tiny papules and bumps on the scalp. Climate, heredity, diet, hormones, and stress can affect dandruff. It can also worsen with heat and humidity, infrequent shampooing, and illness. Most cases can be managed with nonprescription medicated shampoos containing zinc, selenium sulfide, coal tar, or salicylic acid. Stronger shampoos and topical medications containing steroids or tar can be prescribed by your dermatologist if the condition persists. Try to keep your hands away from your head, as scratching or picking the scalp can worsen dandruff.

baceous (oil) glands, which explains why your hair becomes oily, requiring you to wash it regularly. Many people with acne on their faces also have a few pimples on their heads, but unless they run their fingers over their scalps regularly, they may have no idea that acne is hiding there. Scalp acne can be painful, and unlike acne on other parts of the body, it's often itchy, causing people to pick at it incessantly. Running your hands through your hair in search of more bumps can become a difficult habit to break. And when you do so, the scalp becomes more inflamed and acne worsens, creating a vicious cycle.

Frequent hair brushing and the use of hair-styling products can inflame scalp acne. Scalp acne is also exacerbated by the natural oils present on the scalp, by stress, and by wearing close-fitting caps or sweatbands during exercise (such as tennis bands). Blow-drying your hair has no effect on scalp acne, but excess heat can increase scalp itching, so always use the lowest setting on your dryer.

Dermatologists treat scalp acne with prescription shampoos containing cortisone, ketoconazole, salicylic acid, or tar, and with oral tetracycline antibiotics. Treatment typically lasts one to two months.

Over-the-counter treatment for scalp acne is one of the few exceptions to the typical acne treatment rule, as we recommend spot treatment rather than full-head treatment. The pHisoderm Clear Confidence Skin Care Clear

Swab comes with handy applicators that are terrific for this purpose. Topical hydrocortisone in a 1 percent formulation can also be helpful.

Most red bumps on the scalp are acne, but if a "pimple" persists longer than a month, have it checked by a dermatologist. The scalp is a common area for skin cancer, especially in those who have had significant hair loss. Melanomas are asymptomatic. Also, many skin conditions, such as seborrheic dermatitis, a dandrufflike condition, can mimic scalp acne. It is imperative to have a proper diagnosis made by a dermatologist so appropriate treatment can be prescribed. For more information on acne imposters, see chapter 15.

How to Wash Your Scalp and Hair

"Hair produces no sebum," says Dr. Zoe D. Draelos, a clinical associate professor of dermatology at Wake Forest University School of Medicine. "The hair simply wicks the oil away from the scalp. The key to controlling oily hair is to remove the sebum adequately from the scalp."

Shampoos are designed to work on the scalp, not the hair. Few people, especially teenage girls with long hair, understand this principle. They use copious amounts of shampoo and conditioner, then can't understand why their scalps are still greasy just a few hours later.

You need to use only about a quarter-sized dollop of shampoo applied directly to the scalp to properly cleanse oils away. Massage the shampoo vigorously into your scalp with your fingertips. There is no need to add shampoo to the hair itself, as rinsing will send the shampoo down the hair, cleansing it along the way. Note: The cleansing ability of a shampoo is not indicated by whether it foams or lathers; medicated dandruff shampoos often do not foam or lather well.

Conditioner, particularly for those with oily scalps, should *never* be applied to the scalp. Sebum, as you know, is oil, so it is already conditioning the base of the hairs themselves. Conditioning for detangling or dry ends should be applied only to hair below the neck.

If you have scalp acne, we recommend the use of shampoos for oily hair or clarifying shampoos, which remove styling products and contain no conditioning agents. You can try Proactiv Solution Gentle Formula Anti-Dandruff Shampoo and Conditioner. We also like the Philip B Anti-Flake Relief Shampoo, available in department stores and salons, and Nizoral and Head and Shoulders shampoos, available in drugstores.

torso acne—back, chest, and shoulders

"My brother-in-law was getting married, and when his bride asked me to be in the wedding, I accepted," twenty-seven-year-old Amelia told us. "But then she told me I'd be wearing a strapless dress. She had no idea I had acne on my shoulders and neck! I almost backed out of the wedding because I was just too embarrassed."

As with acne on other parts of the body, torso acne is very common and equally devastating. It's bumpy, it feels awful, and it rubs against clothing. Teenage girls won't wear the spaghetti strap tops all their friends are enjoying, and teenage boys can't reveal their torsos. It means people of all ages resist swimming, too embarrassed to be seen in revealing bathing suits. Moreover, torso acne can have a profound effect on a sufferer's emotional life, as anyone contemplating intimacy with either a new partner or an old one is justifiably inhibited about disrobing.

Some people with acne on their torsos believe it's their fault, stemming from using the wrong kind of hair conditioner or styling product. They're wrong. The acne on your torso is caused by the same hormones, plugged pores, and proliferation of bacteria as any other acne. It's not your fault. Your torso just happens to be your acne trigger site.

Severe cystic acne on the torso seems to be more prevalent in males. Chest or shoulder acne is more prevalent in females. Acne in these areas is worsened by chronic rubbing from shoulder straps on bras or backpacks and from the friction from athletic equipment, such as football shoulder pads.

Torso acne tends to be stubborn and is more challenging to treat than facial acne. Skin on the torso, especially the back, is many times thicker than facial skin and therefore requires higher doses of medication over a longer period of time to penetrate the pores effectively.

Torso acne also tends to scar more easily, producing thick red scars, called keloids. The sternal area of the chest is, for some unknown reason, a danger zone for the development of keloidal scars, which can be impossible to remove. (For more information about keloids, see page 35 in chapter 1.) Torso acne can also leave behind red and brown spots known as postinflammatory hyperpigmentation, which can linger for months, even years. Postinflamma-tory hyperpigmentation is often as distressing as the actual pimples or cysts that caused it in the first place. (For more information about postinflamma-tory hyperpigmentation, see page 259 in chapter 12.)

It *is* possible to treat torso acne with over-the-counter products, but as it tends to be more intractable, we suggest that everyone with moderate to se-vere torso acne be seen by a dermatologist.

Dermatologist Treatment for Torso Acne

Dermatologists can prescribe a combination of antibiotic body pads (erythro-mycin or clindamycin), benzoyl peroxide lotion, and topical retinoids or a retinoid body pad (Differin body pads) for torso acne. For example, you might be given antibiotic Cleocin-T pads along with either the topical retinoid lotion (Retin-A Micro) or retinoid pad (Differin). Or you might be prescribed benzoyl peroxide lotion in any of a variety of strengths. Benzoyl peroxide lotion is best used at night, worn under an old white tee-shirt, because it can bleach cloth-ing. For this reason, we often prescribe a backward routine for treating torso acne: Instead of applying a retinoid medication at night, apply it in the morn-ing—it will not stain clothing, and your skin will be hidden from sun exposure by your clothing. Use a benzoyl peroxide lotion at night.

Severe cases of torso acne may require treatment with oral antibiotics or Accutane. However, antibiotics and Accutane may take longer to work and are sometimes less effective for torso acne than they are for facial acne. In con-trast, exfoliating treatments for the face, such as microdermabrasion or gly-colic acid peels, can be successfully used on the torso. Go ahead and give them a try.

It is also very common to see blackheads on the torso, in particular on the back. These blackheads can be removed with a comedone extractor. This can be done by a family member using our comedone extractor or by a dermatol-ogist or esthetician.

patient history

Max is eighteen and an all-around athlete. He plays football, soccer, and golf. He is in excellent shape and does not take any protein supplements or ana-bolic steroids. (He knows friends who do, and their acne looks far worse.) Max has papules and nodules over the upper chest and much of his back. He finds that the acne is aggravated when he wears sports equipment, especially in the summer, when he sweats more than he does in the spring and fall.

Max's treatment includes using better-fitting sports equipment, purchasing clothing made from fabrics that wick moisture away from the body, showering immediately after a workout, and applying topical antibiotic body pads.

His prescription medications include Differin pads to unplug pores, followed by clindamycin pads (Clindets or Pledgets) as an antibacterial applied every morning. An over-the-counter salicylic acid pad, such as Clearasil Pore Cleansing Pads, Stri-Dex Triple Action Acne Pads, or Proactiv Solution Clearzone Body Pads, was used to clean the skin and unplug pores after exercise. Max used a 7 percent benzoyl peroxide lotion (Proactiv Solution Extra Strength Lotion) at night and wore an old T-shirt to prevent bleaching of sheets since benzoyl peroxide used topically can bleach fabric.

In Max's case, he was able to apply the pads twice a day and the lotion every night, with significant clearing as a result. However, had his topical therapy failed, he would've been placed on oral tetracyclines.

Max's intense treatment lasted one month, and his maintenance treatment lasted six months. His maintenance treatment included washing daily in the shower with an exfoliant cleanser containing salicylic acid (like Proactiv Solution Deep Cleansing Wash), then application of Differin pads in the morning and a 2.5 percent benzoyl peroxide lotion (Proactiv Solution Repairing Lotion) at night. He will continue this treatment for as long as it is necessary.

Over-the-Counter Treatment for Torso Acne

Please note that body pads saturated with medication are easier to apply to broad areas of the body, but it still might be difficult to apply other medications to your back. You'll need to ask for help from a family member at home or a trusted friend, particularly with masks or peels. Alternatively, drugstores carry applicators that resemble sponges on a long stick. With one of these applicators, you can pour a small amount of medication on the sponge and apply it wherever needed.

Loofahs or sponges that sit in the shower collect mildew and molds. Throw them away. For cleansing in the shower, use either a disposable sponge or a soft cotton washcloth that can be laundered in hot water.

And remember, excess scrubbing will not scrub the pimples away. Be gentle. Torso skin is thicker than facial skin, but you still don't have a rhino's hide on your back.

TREATMENT 1: PROACTIV SOLUTION

Start to use this treatment once a day for two weeks, then increase to twice a day. Until you are able to tolerate its use twice a day or if you remain at once a day, use a mild cleanser, such as Cetaphil Gentle Skin Cleanser or Rodan & Fields COMPOUNDS Gentle Wash, when not using Proactiv Solution products.

1. Unplug Pores—salicylic acid, glycolic acid

a) Deep Cleansing Wash	Wash off and pat dry.
b) ClearZone Body Pads or ClearZone Body Lotion	For pads, wipe on. Let dry. Or apply lotion with fingertips to full area of chest, back, and shoulders. Let dry.

2. Remove Bacteria—benzoyl peroxide

Repairing Lotion	Apply with fingertips. Let dry.

3. Reduce Swelling—sulfur

Concealer Plus	Lightly dot on with applicator. Blend with concealer brush or fingertips. Use once or twice a day.
Refining Mask	Apply to clean, dry skin. Let dry ten minutes. Rinse with lukewarm water. Use once or twice a week, more often if needed.

4. Extra Help—Proactiv Solution

Daily Oil Control (for slightly oily skin)	Apply to entire affected area with fingertips after toner. Let dry. Use daily or as needed.
Matte Skin Finish (for very oily skin)	Apply sparingly to oily areas. Brush off residue when dry.
Mild Exfoliating Peel	Apply thin layer. Let dry one to two minutes. Remove with fingertips. Rinse with lukewarm water. Use once a week.
Rodan & Fields CLEAN Regimen for Blackhead Extraction	Follow instructions in kit.

TREATMENT 2: PROACTIV SOLUTION EXTRA STRENGTH

This treatment includes a 7 percent benzoyl peroxide cleanser and leave-on lotion, which is usually well tolerated by those with extremely stubborn torso acne and who have failed treatment with products containing 2.5 percent benzoyl peroxide.

Use this treatment at night only. (Use regular strength Proactiv Solution in the morning.) Start to use this treatment every second night for two weeks, then increase to every night. If irritation occurs, return to using Proactiv Solution Repairing Lotion. Until you are able to tolerate its use every night or if you remain at every second night, use a mild cleanser, such as Cetaphil Gentle Skin Cleanser or Rodan & Fields COMPOUNDS Gentle Wash, when not using Proactiv Solution Extra Strength products.

1. Unplug Pores—salicylic acid

a) Extra Strength Cleanser	Wash off and pat dry.
b) Extra Strength Toner or ClearZone Body Pads or ClearZone Body Lotion	Apply toner/lotion with gauze or cotton ball. Let dry.

2. Remove Bacteria—benzoyl peroxide

Extra Strength Lotion	Apply with fingertips. Let dry.

3. Reduce Swelling

Extra Strength Mask	Apply to clean, dry skin. Let dry ten minutes. Rinse with lukewarm water. Use once or twice a week.

4. Fade Brown Spots—hydroquinone

Skin Lightening Lotion	Use at night only. Apply to affected area.
Rodan & Fields RADIANT Regimen	Follow instructions in kit.

5. Extra Help—Proactiv Solution

Matte Skin Finish (for very oily skin)	Apply sparingly to oily areas. Brush off residue when dry.
Rodan & Fields CLEAN Regimen for Blackhead Extraction	Follow instructions in kit.

TREATMENT 3: OTHER PRODUCTS

As with Treatment 2, we suggest that those with extremely stubborn torso acne may need a higher strength of benzoyl peroxide, such as 5 or 10 percent, which is usually well tolerated by those with extremely oily skin and who have failed treatment with products containing 2.5 percent benzoyl peroxide. If irritation occurs, return to 2.5 percent.

Start to use this treatment once a day for two weeks, then increase to twice a day. Until you are able to tolerate its use twice a day or if you remain at once a day, use a mild cleanser, such as Cetaphil Gentle Skin Cleanser or Rodan & Fields COMPOUNDS Gentle Wash, when not using other products. Remember to pick only one product from each list, except in the Extra Help section, where you may choose more than one product, such as a cleansing pad or a leave-on lotion, if needed.

1. Unplug Pores—salicylic acid

Clearasil 3-in-1 Acne Cleanser — Wash off and pat dry.
L'Oréal Ideal Balance Foaming Gel Cleanser
Neutrogena Oil-Free Acne Wash

2. Remove Bacteria—benzoyl peroxide

Clean & Clear Persa-Gel 5 — Apply with fingertips. Let dry.
Fostex 5 Cream
Neutrogena On-the-Spot Therapy
Oxy 5 Sensitive Skin Vanishing Lotion
Oxy Balance Maximum Strength Acne Treatment
PanOxyl 5 Gel

3. Reduce Swelling—sulfur

Clearasil Adult Care Acne Treatment Cream — Apply sparingly with fingertips. Let dry.

4. Extra Help

Clearasil Pore Cleansing Pads — Wipe on. Let dry.
Nature's Cure Body Acne Treatment System — Spray on, using the upside-down pump. Let dry. Do not rinse.

Neutrogena Clear Pore Shine Control Gel	Apply with fingertips. Let dry.
Oxy Daily Cleansing Pads	Wipe on. Let dry.
Stri-Dex Triple Action Acne Pads	

Don't Forget the Sunscreen

Always apply sunscreen to exposed areas of the chest and arms. It is just as crucial to protect all exposed areas of the body from the sun as it is vital to shield your face. For all three treatments, applying sunscreen in the morning is the all-important final step. Apply after all treatment products have dried.

Clearasil Acne Treatment Cream SPF 15*
Neutrogena Ultra Sheer Dry-Touch Sunblock SPF 45
Olay Complete UV Defense Moisture Lotion
Ombrelle Sunscreen Lotion SPF 30
Proactiv Solution Daily Protection Plus SPF 15
Proactiv Solution Sheer Tint Moisture SPF 15*
Rodan & Fields COMPOUNDS Protect SPF 15

* These are excellent solutions for boys and men as they're cover-ups, not makeup, and the slight tint helps camouflage redness while they protect skin from the sun.

Body acne, though easily hidden by clothing, can lead to scarring more frequently than facial acne. A diligently used combination of topical medications applied daily, especially immediately after exercising, is critical to bring body acne under control.

not just acne: acne imposters

many skin diseases mimic acne. Almost impossible to self-diagnose, these conditions warrant advice from a dermatologist. Treatments can vary tremendously, and only a dermatologist can make a conclusive diagnosis and prescribe the proper treatment.

For photographic examples, go to www.unblemished.com.

chloracne

Chloracne is a severe skin reaction to chemicals called dioxins, which are found in herbicides. Dioxins were used in Agent Orange (a chemical defoliant) and are still used in chemical warfare. These chemical pollutants are stored in body fat and cause devastating trauma to the skin, with permanent, irreversible scarring.

Unless there is a toxic spill of dioxins in your neighborhood, there is no reason to worry about chloracne. It is extremely rare. However, if you suspect you've had exposure to dioxins and are experiencing skin outbreaks, see a dermatologist.

cosmetic acne, or *acne cosmetica*

Cosmetics can cause acne. Tiny pink bumps blossom when hair follicles are chemically irritated by skin-care products and makeup. Cosmetic acne can affect anyone, especially someone with sensitive skin. It can occur in those not normally prone to breakouts. Small pink bumps on the cheeks, chin, and forehead, which may itch or look like a rash, usually develop gradually over a few weeks or months. They may persist until treatment is sought, but they rarely result in scars. Cosmetic acne should completely resolve if use of the offending product is stopped.

One study found that as much as 50 percent of cosmetic ingredients are potentially comedogenic, which means they can clog pores. The presence of individual comedogenic ingredients does not mean, however, that the final formulation clogs pores and causes breakouts.

How do you avoid comedogenic products? Look for the word "noncomedogenic" when shopping for skin-care products and makeup. The label "noncomedogenic" is given to products that have undergone laboratory tests demonstrating that the final product formulation does not cause blackheads and whiteheads, even with prolonged use.

Specifically, cosmetic acne may be triggered by the improper use of oily makeup remover. Small amounts will often remain around the eye area and cascade down the cheeks, causing acne. Oily makeup removers are best avoided and are rarely needed, as most mascara and eye shadows are water-soluble. Many non-soap cleansers like Cetaphil Gentle Skin Cleanser or Rodan & Fields COMPOUNDS Gentle Wash are safe for use on the eyes as a makeup remover, and they better solubilize facial makeup in general compared to soap-based cleansers.

For more information on the proper use of cosmetics, see chapter 17.

dandruff

For information about dandruff, see page 294 in chapter 14.

dermatitis

Dermatitis means inflammation of the skin. Many substances can cause this condition, and most people experience it at some point in their lives, either from allergens (substances to which you are allergic), irritants (detergents or harsh chemicals), or a genetic predisposition to a skin problem like eczema. Because dermatitis causes small itchy bumps, it can resemble acne. Dermatitis can appear once or come and go throughout people's lives. It comes in

The Most Highly Comedogenic and Irritating Cosmetic Ingredients

Comedogenicity and irritancy are rated on a scale of zero to five. In this list we're including ingredients which are rated four or higher for comedogenicity. Avoid these ingredients whenever possible, but remember that it is the final formulation of a product that determines comedogenicity, not the presence of one or two comedogenic ingredients. If the ingredient in question appears in the lower half of the ingredient list, the actual amount may be very low and unlikely to cause problems. Always patch-test before using if you have any doubts (see page 308).

Ingredient	Comedogenicity	Irritancy
acetylated lanolin	4	0
acetylated lanolin alcohol	4	2
cetearyl alcohol + cetearath 20	4	1
cocoa butter	4	0
coconut butter	4	0
glyceryl stearate SE	3	2
isopropyl isostearate	5	0
isopropyl myristate	5	3
isostearyl isostearate	4	1
laureth-4	5	4
lauric acid	4	1
myristyl lactate	4	2
myristyl myristate	5	2
oleth-3	5	2
PEG 16 lanolin	4	3
stearic acid:TEA	3	2
stearyl heptanoate	4	0

several different forms: atopic dermatitis (excema); contact dermatitis, including allergic and irritant contact dermatitis; perioral dermatitis; and seborrheic dermatitis. We will take a closer look at each of these forms of dermatitis below.

Atopic Dermatitis (Eczema)

Atopic dermatitis is commonly known as eczema. It is characterized by a rapidly spreading red rash, sometimes appearing in patches, which are itchy, blistered, or swollen. It occurs in 20 percent of children, with onset in the first year of life, generally resolving by age twelve. Children with a genetic predisposition to asthma and hay fever types of allergies are most likely to have eczema.

In adults, eczema appears as thickened, heavily lined, elephant-like skin with a pink background. Adults with eczema tend to have dry, sensitive skin. And, as with children, adults with a predisposition to asthma and hay fever types of allergies are more likely to have eczema.

Dermatologist treatments for eczema include a combination of oral antihistamines, topical steroid creams, and topical medications that treat the skin's immune response, such as Elidel or Protopic. Over-the-counter 1 percent hydrocortisone cream can be helpful, too. A course of oral antibiotics is necessary if the skin is secondarily infected. Soap and hot baths sap moisture from the skin and should be limited. Instead, daily soap- and water-free cleansers, such as Cetaphil or Aquanil, used over the entire body and wiped away, can provide hydration while cleansing. Avoid all known comedogenic and irritating cosmetic ingredients, including fragrance (see page 305), and use products with a minimum of ingredients, ideally fewer than ten.

Contact Dermatitis

Contact dermatitis is a skin reaction to anything touching your face or body. The possibilities are endless. The hallmark of dermatitis is itching and redness. True acne is rarely itchy and has comedones, papules, and pustules, which helps us differentiate between contact dermatitis and acne. There are two types of contact dermatitis: allergic and irritant.

Allergic Contact Dermatitis

Anyone who's ever had poison ivy or poison oak knows exactly what allergic dermatitis feels like, and it's no fun. The allergic response is individualized, so something that might cause a breakout in your sister may have no effect whatsoever in your brother. Allergic reactions are much less common than true contact irritant reactions (see below), but they may appear similar. Allergic contact dermatitis reactions surface seven to twenty-one days following the initial exposure. Reexposure provokes redness, itching, and a bumpy rash within one to three days. Also, allergic contact dermatitis spreads. For example, if your hands come in contact with an allergen, the rash will spread over your face and the rest of your body before you know it. Once you have removed the offending allergen from your skin by thorough cleansing, the rash can continue to spread via an allergic response mounted by your body, not from a continued spreading of the chemicals over your skin by touching affected areas.

Fragrance is the number one cause of allergic skin reactions, followed by preservative agents. Even nail polish, which contains formaldehyde, a common allergen, can trigger allergic skin reactions, first on delicate eyelid skin following the transfer of the allergen to the face by the fingertips. If you know you are susceptible to certain allergens, learn to read labels diligently and avoid allergenic substances.

If you're treating your acne with medications and it's getting worse, particularly if you experience redness and itching, you may be allergic to your acne medicine. For example, benzoyl peroxide causes an allergic reaction in 1 to 3 percent of users. If you experience an allergic reaction to your acne medications, discontinue their use and consult your dermatologist. Mild cases of allergic contact dermatitis can be treated with over-the-counter topical 1 percent hydrocortisone cream, which is an anti-inflammatory. But for severe reactions you may need systemic steroids, orally or by injection.

Irritant Contact Dermatitis

An irritant dermatitis appears only in the areas of skin with which the irritant has come into contact. Reactions include dry, red, itchy patches, and chapped skin.

We are all susceptible to irritant dermatitis from the many chemicals used in everyday products, such as soaps, laundry detergents, and household cleaning products. High enough levels of a potentially irritating substance will provoke a response in everyone. A perfect example is benzoyl peroxide. Many people who have used it at the higher 5 percent or 10 percent levels experienced dry, red patches, assumed they were an allergy, and discontinued benzoyl peroxide use. In truth, they were only irritated by the high concentration and may have no reaction to a lower-strength benzoyl peroxide, such as 2.5 percent.

Patch Tests

Patch testing is a simple way to identify allergens. Dermatologists routinely perform these tests by isolating common allergen ingredients in preservatives. A tiny amount of these allergens is then applied in small patches to the back of the body and covered with tape. After forty-eight hours, the skin is inspected for redness, inflammation, and itching. If an allergen is identified, the main course of action is its avoidance.

A single at-home patch test is easy to do. Apply a small amount of a suspect product, such as a sunscreen or moisturizer, to the side of your neck or the inside of your arm. Repeat each day for several days. Look for an adverse reaction. If no reaction occurs, you should be safe applying whatever was tested to other parts of your body.

More specifically, athletes can suffer from irritant dermatitis from sweat reacting with chemicals in the detergent and fabric softeners used to wash their clothing. In addition, hair dye is both a common irritant *and* an allergen. Always perform a patch test before using a home hair-coloring kit.

Irritant dermatitis may not appear immediately. Sometimes people have been using products consistently for months or years with no reactions, then a reaction suddenly appears. This reaction is not actually "sudden" but a response to a long, built-up intolerance. Finally, your skin announces it's had it. Highly allergenic responses, in comparison, are usually fairly immediate.

Another common cause of irritant or allergic dermatitis is simple. Cosmetic companies may slightly change their formulas without informing the public—which of course they have every right to do. Therefore, even though labels do not say "New and Improved," your skin may recognize that something's different and you'll suddenly begin to break out.

Once you've isolated whatever has triggered the irritation, contact irritant dermatitis can be avoided by discontinuing its use or using a lower percentage of the chemical that triggered the reaction. Existing breakouts can be cleared up by using over-the-counter topical steroid creams, such as Cortaid 10, which are anti-inflammatory.

Perioral Dermatitis

This condition, affecting women in their twenties and thirties, is characterized by patches of mildly itchy or tender, red, pimple-like bumps around the mouth. The skin bordering the lips may be spared while the skin surrounding the mouth, nose, and eyes may be involved. Perioral dermatitis is a variant of rosacea. It usually spontaneously arises, but may be triggered by fluoride in toothpaste or the application of strong fluorinated corticosteroid creams on the face. Treatment includes using a baking soda toothpaste with no color, tartar control, or bleaching agents and avoidance of fluorinated steroid creams. In addition, your dermatologist may prescribe oral tetracycline for a short one- to two-month course and topical agents, such as metronidazole, sulfur, or Elidel, a new nonsteroidal anti-inflammatory cream.

Seborrheic Dermatitis

Seborrheic dermatitis is a dandrufflike condition commonly seen in teen-agers and adults. The actual cause is unknown, but there may be a genetic component—it is often seen in families—and a hormonal component.

Seborrheic dermatitis is the result of an overgrowth of yeast, and it ap-pears as a greasy, pink, scaling rash in the eyebrows, on the sides of the nose, and on the scalp. It may be itchy, and as it worsens, it moves down from the eyebrow area onto the cheeks. Frequently stress-induced, it can appear liter-ally within hours and become better or worse in a very short time. It often flares in winter and is better in summer, with minimal sun exposure.

Because seborrheic dermatitis looks bumpy, red, and scaly, appearing in the mid-face, it is commonly misdiagnosed as either acne or rosacea. And be-cause seborrheic dermatitis often goes hand in hand with acne, especially in teenagers, it's a real recipe for misery.

For facial seborrheic dermatitis, there are many options. Over the counter, you can try a topical sulfur cream, a 1 percent hydrocortisone cream (for a lim-ited time), a topical tar lotion, or ketoconazole cream. Dermatologists can prescribe stronger versions of these creams or Elidel, Protopic, or sodium sul-facetamide.

For seborrheic dermatitis of the scalp, medicated shampoos are the main-stay of treatment. Try Neutrogena Maximum Strength T/Sal Shampoo, con-taining salicylic acid; Proactiv Solution Gentle Formula Anti-Dandruff Shampoo, containing zinc pyrithyrone; and tar-based shampoos, such as Neu-trogena T-Gel or Philip B Anti-Flake Relief Shampoo. Nizoral Shampoo, con-taining ketoconazole, a topical anti-yeast medicine, is available over the counter, and by prescription.

Rotate your medicated shampoos every three to four days and leave the lather in contact with the scalp for at least four to five minutes before rinsing. For example, start with a shampoo with salicylic acid for three to four days, followed by a zinc-based shampoo, then a tar-based shampoo or a ketocona-zole-containing shampoo. This way you will find which shampoo works best. It's fine to shampoo every day if you need to; these shampoos are all relatively gentle. Conditioners may be used on the hair itself, avoiding direct contact with the scalp.

epidermal cysts

You may hear epidermal cysts called infundibular or sebaceous cysts. These terms refer to the saclike growths in the deeper layers of the skin that are filled with a soft, whitish material consisting of keratin, and resembling cottage cheese. Put simply, they resemble gigantic whiteheads and feel like marbles under your skin. Epidermal cysts are created when a hair follicle takes a wrong turn. Instead of forming a hair, for some reason it forms a sac. While epidermal cysts can appear anywhere on the body, most often they occur on the face, chest, back, or behind the ears. People with severe acne often form epidermal cysts.

Because of their deep attachments, these cysts can be removed only surgically. Smaller ones, less than five millimeters in diameter, don't require treatment unless they bother you or are in a place where trauma is likely. For example, if you have epidermal cysts behind the ears and wear glasses, the cysts may be microtraumatized each time you put on or take off your glasses. Eventually these cysts may rupture, causing an infection. Infected cysts are also called boils. They are large and exquisitely painful and can leave scars when they heal. Worse, they can return.

Always alert your dermatologist if you notice an epidermal cyst. They are typically benign, but to be on the safe side, it's best to have them professionally diagnosed. There is no medical reason to remove a benign epidermal cyst. You may want to have one removed if it's driving you crazy, but be aware that the scar may be noticeable, and that in approximately 20 percent of cases, surgeons fail to remove the sac and the cyst returns. If this happens, the entire cyst sac must be surgically removed again.

favre-racouchot syndrome

Favre-Racouchot syndrome is caused by progressive sun damage over the course of many years and is characterized by large comedones (blackheads) around the eyes and on the upper cheeks. It is commonly seen in men and women over the age of fifty, particularly in smokers. Unlike acne, these comedones will not go away on their own. However, treatment with topical retinoids or surgical extraction by a dermatologist is effective. Daily use of sunscreen is a must.

folliculitis

Folliculitis is an inflammation of the hair follicles. It looks like acne but is caused by one of several different bacteria. The red bumps of folliculitis tend to be more deep-seated than acne, felt both above and below the skin, and they usually appear on the arms, chest, buttocks, thighs, and, more rarely, on the face. There are no comedones, and the bumps tend not to be clustered as acne pimples and cysts are. Folliculitis can be itchy and painful at times.

Folliculitis is often suspected as the culprit when acne does not respond to standard treatment. In order to distinguish which bacteria is causing the folliculitis, your dermatologist will take a culture then prescribe appropriate treatment.

Gram-negative folliculitis is responsible for sudden flare-ups in acne or rosacea patients after a long-term course of antibiotics. These patients will experience a sudden onset of pustules around the nose and on the cheeks. Initial flares may respond to a different antibiotic, such as sulfa or ciprofloxacin. Occasionally, a course of Accutane is required.

Pityrosporon folliculitis is triggered by a yeast type of organism. It commonly occurs on the buttocks and is promoted through heat, exercise, and wearing tight-fitting clothing. To prevent it, wear natural fibers, especially cotton underwear, that can breathe. Also, vary your workout routine and be sure to use medicated cleansers and salicylic acid body pads after your workout. As pityrosporon folliculitis is an overgrowth of yeast, treatment with topical and systemic anti-yeast/antifungal medicines, such as Lamisil, Oxistat, and Spectazole, can help.

Pseudomonas folliculitis, or hot tub acne, is a proliferation of itchy pink bumps all over the torso. It's caused by the pseudomonas bacteria, which thrives in hot steamy tubs and Jacuzzis that have been improperly cleaned. It is much more common in home hot tubs than in those in large commercial establishments with better daily maintenance. Frequently, multiple members of a household are affected. Note: A bathroom Jacuzzi will not support the growth of this bacteria, since it's drained after every use.

This rash will resolve spontaneously in three to four weeks. For faster clearing, daily washing with Hibiclens Solution soap (a topical antibacterial cleanser containing chlorhexidine) plus a ten-day course of antibiotics should do the trick.

heat rash, or vacation acne

Take a woman from a North Dakota winter to the beach in Hawaii and sweat glands that are not normally used will suddenly go into overdrive. Top them with an occlusive sunscreen and searing sunburn, and, voilà, heat rash appears in the form of itchy red bumps surfacing from microplugged sweat glands. It can seem as if every square inch of the torso is covered in tiny bumps, ruining a much-needed vacation.

If possible, acclimate gradually when going from cold climates to very hot ones. Also, wear loose-fitting clothing made from natural fibers and use cool, wet towels to stop the skin from overheating. Remember to frequently apply nonocclusive sunscreens containing avobenzone or zinc oxide. And turn on the air conditioners.

Heat rash will resolve on its own. In the meantime, a low-strength over-the-counter hydrocortisone cream or aloe vera gel will ease itching and inflammation. Nonsteroidal anti-inflammatory pills can also be very helpful.

keratosis pilaris

Keratin is a protein material that surrounds the outer root sheath of every hair follicle. Normally, as hair grows up to the surface of the skin, that layer of keratin is shed and renewed. However, with keratosis pilaris, that layer doesn't easily let go; instead it entraps the hair within the follicle. The end result is a buildup of coiled-up dead skin cells and hairs that feel spiky and look like little red cones. Bacteria surround these cones, inflammation results, and the skin feels like sandpaper because every follicle in the region is involved. It's neither painful nor itchy, but because it's bumpy and textured, it invites picking, which makes it worse.

Keratosis pilaris is a common problem for those prone to eczema. It usually appears on the backs of the arms, shoulders, buttocks, the backs of the thighs, and on the cheeks, especially in children. It can be more severe in dry winter months or in arid climates.

Treatment for keratosis pilaris consists of an alpha hydroxy cream (AHA), such as AmLactin or a prescription nonsteroidal cream, such as Elidel, in the morning, and a topical retinoid, such as Retin-A or Tazorac, applied at night. You can also use a loofah type of sponge in the shower, as long as it is cleansed often. This works quite well at smoothing the bumps.

melasma

For information about melasma, see page 209 in chapter 9.

milia

Milia are hard, tiny white bumps, which frequently appear around the eye area. While many people attribute milia to calcium deposits, in reality they are tiny epidermal cysts. (See the previous section on epidermal cysts on page 310.) Some can be caused by heavy, occlusive eye moisturizers.

Milia can appear spontaneously or as a result of previous trauma to the skin. For example, women who have had laser treatments, microdermabrasion, or dermabrasion may wind up with milia once their skin has healed. Though they may look like whiteheads, squeezing does not remove them. They can, however, be lanced and carefully removed by a dermatologist without leaving a scar.

occupational acne

Acnegens are substances that cause acne. Occupational acne appears when people work in environments loaded with acnegens. For example, workers in fast-food restaurants commonly see acne either appear or worsen because the grease in hot, steamy, stress-filled kitchens acts as a comedogenic agent.

Farmers beware: The most potent of all chemical acnegens are dioxins, which are found in herbicides. Dioxins were previously discussed in the section on chloracne (see page 303). Other substances known to cause acne include coal tar and pitch, so road workers and roofers should take proper precautions. Also susceptible are workers in oil refineries, who have regular exposure to petrolatum and its distillates.

As occupational acne is often severe, and since it may be impossible to change jobs, we recommend that you see a dermatologist so an effective, personalized treatment can be created for you.

sebaceous gland hyperplasia

Sebaceous gland hyperplasia tends to appear in people over the age of forty as pinkish-yellow bumps which are lobulated, with small petals at the periphery and a shallow depression in the center.

Sebaceous gland hyperplasia is merely a collection of enlarged oil glands located in the midsection of the face or forehead. It typically occurs in people with oily skin. The bumps created by the enlarged oil glands don't resolve spontaneously and may be mistaken for skin cancer or milia. Cosmetically bothersome, they can be removed with an electric needle or a small surgical excision, if desired.

skin cancer

Skin cancer is often characterized as a pimple that does not heal. Basal carcinomas can resemble cysts or pimples that don't heal. Melanomas are generally black, irregular, flat macules that can appear anywhere on the body. There are rare melanomas that lack brown and black color and look like a red bump that bleeds and fails to resolve. Bleeding of pimples occurs after picking. Bleeding of skin cancer can occur spontaneously or after the lightest touch. In addition, skin cancers are not painful as pimples frequently can be.

Melanomas are the most serious type of skin cancer with a risk rate of one in seventy. They are triggered by genetic predisposition and sun exposure and are more prevalent in fair-skinned individuals with a history of sunburn, although anyone, even those with dark skin, can have one.

An adult acne lesion has a maximum two-month life cycle. If you have a persistent pink or red shiny bump that does not go away after two months, it should be examined and biopsied by a dermatologist, particularly if you're over the age of thirty.

The diagnosis of skin cancer can be tricky, which is why a biopsy may be needed to differentiate between a pimple and cancer. Bear in mind that even if your pimple doesn't heal in two months, the diagnosis will not always be cancer. It is often no more serious than an inflamed cyst. Dermatologists are trained to look through a magnifying glass for extremely subtle, clinical clues, such as translucency, a network of capillaries, and poor definition of border. The biopsied sample will be examined microscopically to arrive at an exact diagnosis.

The treatment for skin cancer is surgical excision, usually done under local anesthesia in the dermatologist's office. For the vast majority of skin cancers, excision will cure it. However, late-stage melanomas often require chemotherapy and radiation and eventually may be fatal. This is why an early diagnosis of melanoma is generally life-saving. So never, ever wait to see a doctor if a pimple persists longer than two months.

steroid acne

Oral Steroid Acne

Corticosteroids, prescribed for a variety of ailments—including asthma, lupus, arthritis, and severe poison oak—can trigger acne outbreaks. Corticosteroid-induced acne often appears as small itchy pimples, especially on the chest.

Anabolic steroids (testosterone), which increase the level of masculinizing hormones, can cause severe cystic acne, with large nodules on the face, chest, and back. It tends to appear abruptly, providing a clue to proper diagnosis.

Treatment for oral steroid acne is to discontinue the use of all steroids, if possible. If not, standard acne treatments, including topical retinoids, benzoyl peroxide, oral antibiotics, and possibly Accutane, should work well.

Topical Steroid Acne

Topical steroid creams used for months to treat eczema, rosacea, or perioral dermatitis can cause acne. Alternatively, people who have done well with topical steroid creams but who suddenly stop using them can see a flare-up of redness and pimples. Treatment with benzoyl peroxide and other topical anti-acne agents usually clears the problem.

Remember, many conditions are associated with or mimic acne. If you ever have any doubts or questions about a skin condition, see a dermatologist rather than self-treat. Identification of acne imitators is not always easy, often requiring the trained eye of an expert for diagnosis and proper treatment.

chapter sixteen

taking care of your skin and body

maintaining healthy, glowing skin is only one part of a healthy lifestyle. Bodies protected from the sun, made fit and strong with regular exercise, nourished by a smart, balanced diet, and well rested by plenty of sleep will heal faster, look better, and live longer.

all about sunscreen

We can never say it enough—sunscreen is a must. The single most effective thing you can do to protect your skin and prevent further aging is to stay clear of harmful radiation.

Throughout the year—winter, spring, summer, fall—sunscreen is a daily necessity for every human, regardless of ethnicity or skin tone. Yet many people, especially those with visible sun damage, feel that since the damage is done, there's no point in using sunscreen. This attitude can be dangerous. It's been documented that no matter what your age, if you start using sunscreen and protective clothing you will have fewer precancerous spots and over time reduce the visible signs of aging.

There is a lot of misinformation conveyed to the public about sunscreens. Through no fault of their own, most people use them improperly. Perhaps they may put it on only once a day, in the morning, or they select sunscreens with ingredients that fail to fully protect them. People have a false sense of security from a bottle of sunscreen claiming eight-hour protection or broad-

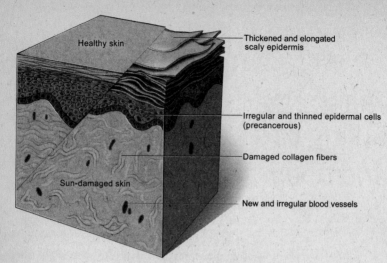

Normal versus sun-damaged skin

spectrum. Unfortunately, not applying the correct sunscreen properly can have serious consequences, beginning with sun damage.

Sun damage, which can lead to precancers and skin cancers, is caused·by two major wavelengths of light: UVA, the aging ray, and UVB, the burning ray.

UVA—The Aging Ray

UVA is a long wavelength of light (320 to 400 nanometers) that penetrates deep into the skin, down to the dermal tissue. It destroys collagen and elastic

UVA CHARACTERISTICS

Active all day
Active all year
Penetrates deeply into the skin
Passes through window glass
Produces brown spots
Promotes cancer, especially melanoma
Promotes melasma
Promotes wrinkles

UVB Characteristics

Most potent between 10 A.M. and 4 P.M.
More potent in summer than in winter
Penetrates superficially into the skin
Initiates cancer
Causes wrinkles

fibers and provokes the pigment-producing melanocytes that cause brown spots (hyperpigmentation) and uneven skin tone. There's further evidence that UVA may be important in the formation of skin cancer, particularly melanoma. UVA is present year-round, from sunup to sundown, rain or shine, in amounts far greater (up to ninety-five times) than UVB. It even penetrates window glass, so be aware of potential damage while driving (or sitting in a sunny office) and protect yourself accordingly.

UVB—The Burning Ray

UVB is a shorter, more intense wavelength (290 to 320 nanometers) that "cooks" the surface of the skin (the epidermis), causing sunburn, destroying cellular DNA, and releasing free radicals. After too much exposure, abnormal skin cells are created. Precancers (actinic keratosis) and skin cancers (basal cell carcinoma, squamous cell carcinoma, melanoma) may result.

What Is Sunscreen?

Sunscreen was invented to block the harmful UVA and UVB rays from penetrating the skin, thereby preventing sun damage, precancers, and skin cancers. There are two types of sunscreen agents: chemical blockers, which absorb ultraviolet light; and physical blockers, which reflect ultraviolet light back into the environment.

UVA chemical blockers include anthranilate, avobenzone (also known as Parsol 1789), and benzophenone. The primary chemical UVB blockers include cinnamate, ensulizole, octinoxate, oxybenzone, Padimate A, Padimate O, and titanium dioxide. Because PABA, an excellent UVB blocker, frequently caused allergic skin reactions, it is no longer used.

The best UVA blockers are avobenzone (also known as Parsol 1789) and zinc oxide (a physical blocker). Since the FDA regulates how sunscreen agents are combined, you will not find both agents in one product. Look for the UVA blockers, either avobenzone or zinc oxide, under "active ingredients" in any tube of sunscreen you use along with the other UVB blockers listed in the preceding paragraph. For the best combined UVA/UVB protection, use an avobenzone or zinc oxide sunscreen with a high SPF for sport or outside activities and one with an SPF of at least 15 for daytime wear. This will offer you the most complete protection from burning and aging possible—and is an absolute must year-round.

How to Apply Sunscreen Effectively

There is no rating scale for UVA chemical blocker products in America. The SPF (sun protection factor) on a product refers only to its ability to block UVB rays. It provides a rough estimate of how long you can remain in the sun without burning. For example, a fair-haired, fair-skinned person will burn in ten minutes in a summer sun at high noon. Using an SPF 15 gives fifteen times additional protection. This equals 150 minutes, or two and a half hours. Not very long, is it? And it's certainly not all day. The key is to reapply frequently, every two hours or less.

Using Sunscreen in Summer Sun and during Outdoor Activities

Most people unwittingly use far less sunscreen than is necessary for adequate protection. Ideally, sunscreen should be applied thirty minutes before any sun exposure. A good habit is to apply it after you brush your teeth in the morning. You need about a teaspoon for your face—and don't forget the front and back of your neck, your ears, chest, and hands and forearms. Reapply it every two hours. You should use up a bottle of sunscreen in a week. If it lasts all summer, you're using it incorrectly. And remember, sunscreen expires, so check the expiration date.

For days at the beach, you'll need about an ounce of sunscreen to cover your entire body. That is one-eighth of an eight-ounce bottle. Remember to reapply it every two hours or after swimming or excessive perspiration. And, since no sunscreen is 100 percent protective, don't view it as a license to bask in the sun longer than you would without it.

One of the most common myths about sunscreen is that there's no reason to use any product containing an SPF higher than 15. This is untrue. Because most people don't apply a thick enough layer of sunscreen in the first place to reach the desired level of 15 or they don't reapply it as frequently, using a high SPF-containing sunscreen increases your chance of adequate protection.

Another myth about sunscreen is that using only a UVB protector with a high SPF (45 and up) will keep you safe. This sunscreen is great against UVB, but it will do little against UVA. So if you use only a UVB-protecting sunscreen, you won't burn if you lie in the sun all day, but you will still suffer unseen skin damage. Remember, UVA penetrates deep into the skin, destroying collagen and elastic fibers and provoking hyperpigmentation and uneven skin tone.

Even if you're using an avobenzone or zinc oxide sunscreen, we recommend avoiding the sun between 10 A.M. and 4 P.M., wearing a broad-brimmed hat (not a baseball cap, since the visor is too narrow), and wearing lightweight, tightly woven clothing to prevent exposure. A company called Solumbra makes lightweight sun-protective clothing and hats containing SPF 30+ incorporated into the fabric to give you additional protection.

Using Sunscreen for All Other Times

Many of our acne patients erroneously avoid sunscreen, believing it will exacerbate blemishes. By nature, sunscreens are oilier than simple moisturizers, because the active sunscreen ingredients are oil-based (occlusive) substances. However, a lotion (oil in water formulation) or a gel will feel less greasy than a cream (water in oil compound). Sunscreen formulations can be light and moisturizing. Alternatively, an occlusive, heavy sunscreen will attract and hold on to heat in your pores, flaring inflammation and possibly causing numerous small red bumps to form. This reaction is not true acne but a condition called miliaria.

When you are following a medicated skin-care treatment for acne, always apply the medicines to the skin first. Let them dry, then put on sunscreen. If you use an additional moisturizer, the order is medicine, moisture, sunscreen. Since so many skin-care products, such as Proactiv Solution, are now dual function, look for sunscreens that are also moisturizers. These products often have the added benefits of antioxidants and vitamins to help stabilize the for-

WHAT TO DO IF YOU GET A SUNBURN

Even the most vigilant of those who protect themselves against the sun sometimes get burned. Here are a few tips to help manage the redness and peeling:

- Take aspirin, which can help stop the swelling from sunburn.
- Take a cool bath with a cup of baking soda added to the water. This will help reduce swelling and pain. For bad blisters, Dome Boro's soaks are soothing, or a paste of baking soda mixed with cold water may be applied.
- Moisturizing may prevent peeling. Pure aloe vera gel is noncomedogenic and soothing. Otherwise, use a moisturizer that you know will not trigger your acne. Now is not the time to try a new product, as it may irritate skin and cause blemishes.
- Try your best not to pick at or pull off the flaky dead skin if you're peeling. This can tear into a deeper layer of skin and potentially cause more damage.
- When the skin is not as tender, gently exfoliate with a gentle buff-puff type of pad or washcloth.
- Benadryl (diphenhydramine, twenty-five milligrams for adults, ten milligrams for children over six) taken three times a day will help relieve itching. Note: Benadryl may cause drowsiness, so take it only when appropriate.
- See your dermatologist if severe swelling occurs or if the sunburn covers a large part of your body.

mulas and perhaps provide some protection of the skin at the cellular level. We recommend the use of these dual-action sunscreen/moisturizers during the day to keep your skin-care routine as streamlined and nonocclusive as possible.

In addition, foundations are now formulated with sunscreens. However, the active ingredient in these foundations is generally titanium dioxide, which does not provide ideal UVA/UVB protection. Don't rely on it. Instead, use these foundations after applying sunscreen. For example, first apply a sunscreen containing avobenzone or zinc oxide to dry skin, then after it has dried apply your foundation. You can also later apply a loose or pressed powder that contains titanium dioxide before going to lunch to freshen makeup and give you an extra layer of protection from the sun.

To keep your sunscreen selection process as simple as possible, we've compiled a list of sunscreens that are safe to use on acne-prone skin.

Sunscreens for Acne-Prone Skin

Alba Botanica Full Spectrum Sun SPF 30

Belladonna Oil Free Sunblock Broad Spectrum SPF 30

Cetaphil Daily Facial Moisturizer SPF 15 with Parsol 1789

Clinique City Block Sheer Oil-Free Daily Face Protector SPF 15

Coppertone Oil Free Faces SPF 30 Hydrating Sunblock

Elemis Vital Face Sunscreen SPF 15

Estée Lauder Sunblock for Face SPF 30

Eucerin Extra Protective Moisture Lotion SPF 30

Korres Sunscreen SPF 15

Lancôme Soleil Sunscreen SPF 15 with Parsol 1789

Neutrogena Oil-Free Sunblock Lotion or Spray SPF 30 or SPF 45

Neutrogena Sensitive Skin Sunblock Lotion SPF 30

Neutrogena Ultra Sheer Dry-Touch Sunblock SPF 30 or SPF 45 with
     Parsol 1789

Olay Complete UV Defense Moisture Lotion SPF 15

Ombrelle Sunscreen Lotion SPF 30

Origins Sunshine State SPF 20

Physicians Formula Sun Shield For Faces Extra Sensitive Skin SPF 15

Physicians Formula Sun Shield For Faces Ultra Light Cream SPF 20

Proactiv Solution Daily Protection Plus SPF 15

Rodan & Fields COMPOUNDS Protect SPF 15

Rodan & Fields RADIANT Protect SPF 15

SkinCeuticals Ultimate UV Defense Sport SPF 45

about moisturizers

Moisturizers coat the dead outer layer of skin (stratum corneum), plumping up the moisture content to make the skin more pliable. The key is to find the right moisturizer to provide maximum hydration without causing new blem-

ABOUT TANNING BOOTHS

Tanning booths are dangerously unsafe for everyone. They may cause more UVA and UVB damage than the sun. This harmful exposure to radiation has been proven to cause cancer and accelerate skin aging. There is never any reason to go to a tanning booth.

ishes. Always look for products that are clearly labeled noncomedogenic. In order to carry that label, products have been laboratory tested and proven not to cause blackheads or whiteheads.

Many fragrances have been desensitized to make them less irritating. If you tend to be sensitive to fragranced products, do a patch test (see page 308 in chapter 15) before applying to acne-prone areas.

Read the label before buying a new product. Ingredients must be listed in descending order of concentration. The first ingredient is usually water (aqua), followed by chemicals and oils or oil substitutes, such as glycerin. Ingredients that appear in the lower half of the ingredient list are usually present in extremely small concentrations and will usually not cause problems. If you tend to react to moisturizers, we recommend that you do a patch test to rule out any irritant or allergic reactions.

There is no one perfect moisturizer for every skin type, and choosing one is a highly selective process. Some women extol the virtues of one moisturizer; others find it overbearing. Some prefer extremely lightweight lotions, while others like creamier formulas. It is often possible to successfully moisturize using a product which is *not* 100 percent oil free; not all oils are comedogenic, and not everyone's skin responds in the same way to them. For example, petroleum products and sunflower oil do not penetrate into the pores. Nor is mineral oil bad, although it has a bad reputation. Actually, many people can tolerate it in an acne formula.

Most moisturizers are emulsions, a mixture of an oil or an oil-like substance and water. By nature, oil and water don't mix, so the trick to making a smooth compound containing both is what's called emulsion chemistry. Different emulsions have different ratios of oil to water.

Water-in-oil emulsions are mostly oil with water added. An ointment is a water-in-oil emulsion, and since the amount of oil far exceeds the amount of water, it will always have a greasy feel to it. Cold-cream cleansers are another example of a water-in-oil emulsion. It's best for those with acne to stay away from these products.

Oil-in-water emulsions are mostly water with oil added. Most lotions and cream moisturizers are formulated this way, and a cream contains more oil than a lotion. Oil-in-water emulsions are great for dry, acne-prone skin.

Oil-free products usually contain glycerin. This is a humectant, which means it holds water in the skin. Other humectants include urea, hyaluronic

What Is a Cosmetic versus a Drug?

The uppermost layer of dead cells on the surface of the skin, the stratum corneum, is an effective shield that protects the skin from the environment. These cells are compacted, tightly bound to each other like shingles on a roof.

Cosmetics do not penetrate the stratum corneum. They cannot enter the living layers of skin (the epidermis and dermis) below. Instead, cosmetics remain on the surface of the skin and may work to prevent water loss from the skin, add moisture, and repair the dead stratum corneum to keep it pliable and moist. A cosmetic can enhance and beautify, but it does not treat a disease. As mandated by the FDA, a cosmetic cannot change the structure and function of the skin. This explains why cosmetic companies make claims such as "*may enhance*" the skin's appearance or "*helps* reduce" the appearance of fine lines. Stronger claims may not be made.

On the other hand, drugs are designed to change the structure and function of the skin to treat disease. Most of the products we have created are medicated, allowing for claims that they treat diseases, such as acne. Sunscreens are drugs. A moisturizer that contains salicylic acid is a drug, too. Any product that contains a drug must list it as an active ingredient in a box and show what percentage of the contents it constitutes. This makes it easier to spot medicated treatments.

Cosmeceuticals are cosmetic products that make quasi-drug claims, such as a moisturizer containing glycolic acid that claims it *may* promote skin-cell turnover. Another example is products containing Vitamin C or retinol that claim they *may* improve wrinkles and boost collagen production. These claims may be true. While there is some science in the medical literature citing ingredients that may improve skin, most claims are theoretical rather than proven. When in doubt, be a savvy consumer. Don't expect to find a miracle wrinkle cream in a jar, and don't believe all the hype. Test them on yourself and see.

acid, and alpha hydroxy acids. Gels often are oil free. Oil-free moisturizers are perfect for those with oily, acne-prone skin.

For sensitive skin, it's best to pick a lightweight moisturizing lotion (oil-in-water emulsion) with a simple formula, one that is fragrance free and with fewer than ten to twelve ingredients listed on the label.

It is important to remember that moisturizers are cosmetics, not drugs, so by law they can't change the structure and function of skin, but they can make your skin feel and look better. We believe you should use what you like and can afford as long as it's not adversely affecting your acne. Ask for samples at cosmetic counters. See how your skin responds. Feel free to experi-

How to Apply Moisturizer

Always apply acne medications first and let them dry before applying a moisturizer. When used in this order, the active ingredients in the acne medications can penetrate into the skin and work effectively.

Use moisturizers sparingly. This means a dime-sized amount. It should be enough to apply a thin coat over the entire surface of the skin where needed. More cream will *not* provide additional moisturizing; indeed, it may clog pores. Apply moisturizer to the face and neck first, then the eye area.

ment, and switch products if you want to. Don't deny yourself the pleasure of choosing a moisturizer that comes in lovely packaging or pampers you. You can also benefit tremendously by using a moisturizer containing acne medicine, such as salicylic acid, or a beta hydroxy or alpha hydroxy acid. This way you can improve your skin's appearance while treating acne. You can try Neutrogena's Multivitamin Acne Treatment or Proactiv Solution Clarifying Night Cream with retinol and salicylic acid.

Acne-Prone Skin

Many people with acne are afraid to use moisturizers on their skin, but this can be a problem for those who have dry skin and acne. The right moisturizer will not make acne worse and it can improve the appearance and texture of your skin. Using the wrong one, however, can trigger cosmetic acne from clogged pores and irritation from the ingredients in the moisturizer. (For more information about cosmetic acne, see page 303 in chapter 15.) Following is a list of moisturizers that are safe to use on acne-prone skin.

Moisturizers for Acne-Prone Skin

Remember that your skin's response to a moisturizer will vary by product. If the use of cream or lotion triggers acne, discontinue it and try something else. Products with an asterisk contain acne-fighting medications such as salicylic acid.

*Aveeno Clear Complexion Daily Moisturizer
Belladonna Botanical Balancer

Belladonna Clarifying Cream
*Biotherm Acnopur Anti-Acne Moisturizing Treatment Gel
Cetaphil Daily Facial Moisturizer SPF 15
Cetaphil Moisturizing Lotion
Chanel Skin Conscience Total Health Moisture Lotion SPF 15
*Clearasil Acne Fighting Facial Moisturizer
*Clearasil Total Control Daily Skin Perfecting Treatment
Clearasil Total Control Intensive Hydrating Moisturizer SPF 10
Clinique Skin Texture Lotion Oil-Free Formula
Cosmence Mission Perfection Daily Purifying Moisture Treatment
Crème de la Mer Lotion
Elemis Absolute Day Cream
Ellen Lange Micro Thera AM Moisturizing Lotion SPF 15
Estée Lauder Verité Calming Fluid
EmerginC Crude Control Hydrating, Protecting, and Balancing Emulsion
Eucerin Daily Control & Care Moisturizer
Eucerin Renewal Alpha Hydroxy Lotion SPF 15
Iman Perfect Response Oil-Free Hydrating Gel
Joey Calm and Correct Gentle Soothing Moisturizer
Joey Pure Pores Tinted Moisturizer SPF 15
Jurlique Viola Cream
Lorac Oil-Free Moisturizer
L'Oréal Pure Zone Oil-Free Moisturizer
Lubriderm Daily UV Lotion
*Neutrogena Multivitamin Acne Treatment
*Neutrogena SkinClearing Moisturizer Daily Face Cream
Olay Oil-Free Active Hydrating Beauty Fluid
Olay Complete Lotion SPF 15
Origins Matte Scientist Oil Controlling Lotion
Peter Thomas Roth Oil-Free Moisturizer
Physicians Formula Oil-Free Moisturizer
Physicians Formula Self-Defense Color Corrective Moisturizing Lotion SPF 15
*Proactiv Solution Clarifying Night Cream
*Proactiv Solution Daily Protection Plus SPF 15
Proactiv Solution Gentle Formula Daytime Lotion
Proactiv Solution Oil Free Moisture SPF 15
Rodan & Fields COMPOUNDS Moisture

Dry Skin

If your skin is dry, as acne-prone skin often is, using a moisturizer is a must to relieve redness and flaking. A therapeutic moisturizer containing an acne medication, such as salicylic acid, and other helpful ingredients, such as alpha hydroxy acids and retinol, will help unplug pores and hydrate the skin.

For those whose acne tends to be concentrated in one area of the face—for instance, the chin—other parts of the face may be drier. When this happens, you may want to use a heavier moisturizer on the dry areas and an oil-free moisturizer on the acne-prone area.

Oily Skin

Oily skin does not need additional moisture. If, however, you live in a dry environment, such as Albuquerque, your skin may become dry and flaky on the surface even when it is still oily underneath. Or sometimes skin becomes dryer in the winter, when there is little moisture in the home and it is bitter cold outside. In these circumstances, a sunscreen containing a lightweight, oil-free moisturizer should help. Exfoliation of the dead skin followed by moisturizing will also brighten your complexion.

Some women with oily skin like to use spritzers, which are cans of sterile water, to mist on their faces when in superdry environments, such as airplanes. Evian is the most well known spritzer. Alchemy also has a Refreshing Floral Mist, which smells wonderful. These sprays will hydrate your skin and leave you feeling relaxed and rejuvenated.

Finally, many cosmetic companies have created mattifying products for those with oily skin. These are shine-reducing moisturizers and powders that absorb oils so that makeup can be applied properly and will remain on your face. Here is a list of mattifying products we recommend. Remember, always patch-test before using on acne-prone skin.

Biotherm Biopur Oil-Free Matte Hydrating Fluid
Clearasil Total Control All-Day Mattifying Moisturizer SPF 10
Ellen Lange Suede Wearable Treatment Mattifying Gel
Estée Lauder Clear Difference Oil-Control Hydrator
Joey Pure Pores Pore Tightener and Filler Serum
Lancôme Hydra Controle Mat Shine-Control Moisturizer

Lancôme T. Controle Instant T-Zone Matifier
Nivea Visage Shine Control Mattifying Fluid
Peter Thomas Roth Max Anti-Shine Mattifying Gel
Proactiv Solution Matte Skin Finish
Proactiv Solution Oil-Free Mattifier with White Tea

Sensitive Skin

Those with truly sensitive skin, such as rosacea sufferers, may need moisturizing. They should look for products that are fragrance free and hypoallergenic, and contain as few ingredients as possible, preferably less than ten to twelve. There is rarely any need to buy products with sensitive-skin claims.

For more information about sensitive skin, see page 274 in chapter 13.

Day Creams and Night Creams

Day creams tend to be light-weight lotions, as many women don't want a greasy look on their skin when they're going about their daily business. They're often formulated with a sunscreen. Night creams are heavier and more occlusive and don't contain sunscreen. In addition, some night creams contain photosensitive ingredients, such as Vitamin C or retinol. These ingredients are deactivated by sun exposure and therefore work most effectively when used at night.

As women age and their skin becomes drier and less pliable, they often seek out a richer night cream. For more information about moisturizing more mature skin, see page 227 in chapter 10.

Eye Creams

Even for those with oily skin, the fragile skin around the eye often requires moisture. Because of the delicacy of this skin, creams created for this area are often thicker and greasier than regular facial moisturizers. This means they can work successfully as moisturizers, but they can also be occlusive. They can also migrate to nearby areas on the cheeks, temples, and forehead, creating acne; and they can promote milia, tiny white cysts under the eye (see page 313 in chapter 15).

Eye creams, such as Crème de la Mer The Eye Balm, Neutrogena Healthy Skin Eye Cream, Proactiv Solution Nourishing Eye Cream, Proactiv Solution Replenishing Eye Serum, and Rodan & Fields COMPOUNDS Moisture Eye, will not cause acne and are not irritating to the delicate skin around the eyes because they have lower doses of active ingredients, such as retinol and salicylic acid. They are also specifically formulated to either hydrate the skin or plump it up to reduce the appearance of wrinkles.

There is no intrinsic need to buy a separate eye cream. It's simply a matter of preference. However, it can be a great idea for women who have acne on their chin or oily areas of their face and dry skin around their eyes. In addition, some women find their regular moisturizers can sting the eye area, whereas eye creams rarely do.

For information about eye makeup remover, see page 354 in chapter 17.

Moisturizing the Neck

Many cosmetic companies have created special creams for the neck. This is not a necessity, as a regular facial moisturizer is sufficient, but they're on the right track. The neck is often a sorely neglected area of the body. In women, the neck does not have as many hair follicles or sebaceous glands as the face, so the skin is much more delicate. It ages poorly. Gravity takes its toll. Sunscreen is forgotten, and the sides and lower neck burn and turn brown with visible red capillaries. The overhanging chin protects the center of the neck from the sun, resulting in a white diamond shape in the middle. Not very attractive!

To avoid this, always moisturize your neck and apply sunscreen on it when you moisturize your face. The neck is usually able to tolerate a heavier moisturizing cream, so you can try richer products on it, such as Crème de la Mer Lotion, Elemis Absolute Day Cream, Clinique Anti-Gravity Firming Lift Cream, and Jurlique Viola Cream. If using a separate neck cream helps you to remember to moisturize your neck, by all means do so.

Moisturizing the Body

Those with acne on the body do not need to moisturize the areas prone to breakouts. For the rest of the body, we recommend a hydrating alpha hydroxy moisturizer, such as Am Lactin. It contains a high concentration of lactic acid, which helps normalize the stratum corneum to prevent flaking and peeling. It doesn't have the most delicious scent in the world, as it's deliberately unfragranced to reduce potential irritation, so we like to add a few drops of pure essential lavender oil to each bottle. Many of our patients also like to use Aveeno Lotion, Cetaphil Cream, Eucerin Lotion, or Vaseline Intensive Care Lotion for very dry areas, such as the elbows and heels.

For maximum hydration, apply body moisturizers when your skin is still damp after a shower.

facials

We love facials, and estheticians who understand problem skin and how to work with it can provide a wonderfully relaxing haven for anyone with acne. They can successfully perform comedone (blackhead) extractions and provide an empathetic ear and soothing treatments. Estheticians who don't understand acne, however, can wreak havoc on your skin and give well-intentioned yet erroneous information about what causes acne and how best to treat it.

The best way to find competent estheticians is through word of mouth. Ask your friends. Also ask about any esthetician's credentials, training, and licensing, as the requirements vary from state to state. Be sure also to ask your dermatologist for recommendations. Many dermatologists have their own facialists on staff, which can be reassuring for patients.

It is safe to have an acne facial once a month. Going more often may cause undue irritation. If you have milia (tiny white cysts around the eyes) or extensive comedones, going once a week for comedone extraction is helpful until the condition is cleared, then maintenance once a month should be sufficient. If comedones persist, it's best to see a dermatologist, who will most likely prescribe Retin-A, Tazorac, Differin, or other retinoids to keep the plugs in the pores from reforming.

We have found that many estheticians do not possess a clear understanding of what prescription retinoids do, and they may unwittingly spread misinformation. Prescription-strength retinoids have been thoroughly studied for over thirty years. They work by normalizing the epidermal layer, increasing cell turnover, and successfully unplugging pores. But they are also deactivated by sun exposure (which is why they should be applied at night) and may increase the skin's sensitivity to the sun. Estheticians often tend to be wary of the use of retinoids, such as Retin-A, because it makes the skin more likely to react during treatments—for which the esthetician is blamed. Always tell your esthetician if you are on any acne medications. Certain procedures, such as waxing, are not advisable while you're being treated with retinoids, and microdermabrasion should be done with caution.

If your skin becomes red or irritated after a facial, your esthetician may have been overzealous. Be sure to bring it to her attention next time. Also, ask what products were used, and if you know you are sensitive to something in particular, say so. In the future, be sure to ask which products will be used and what their active ingredients are—a facial should be a well-deserved pampering experience, not a cause for stress or worry.

body treatments when you have acne

Acupuncture

Chinese medicine is based on the concept of Qi or Chi, best described as the energy of your body. The pathways where the Qi flows are called meridians, and inserting superfine, disposable needles along different points in these meridians will remove energy blockages, lessening pain and helping natural healing.

Acupuncture has not been shown to have any benefit for acne, but it can be wonderful for pain management and the treatment of certain disorders. Many menopausal women have found relief from their symptoms with acupuncture. Qualified acupuncturists undergo rigorous training and are licensed by their state.

Aromatherapy

Aromatherapy is the use of essential oils, distilled from flowers, plants, woods, and herbs, to please the spirit and refresh the body. They are inhaled as vapors, applied to the skin by massage, or poured into a bath.

An experienced aromatherapist can provide an amazing sensory experience—but oil is still oil. When you have acne, avoid oil-based aromatherapy massages (see the following section on Massage Therapy) or facials. Instead, to receive the benefits of aromatherapy, either inhale the oils for their therapeutic benefits or add a few drops to your bath—lavender is particularly soothing, and rosemary and cedar are invigorating. Pure essential oils are extremely concentrated and must never be applied directly to the skin, as they can cause burns and irritation. A few drops of an essential oil added to an unscented lotion or cream will be more than enough for you to reap its benefits. Store oils in dark glass bottles away from sunlight.

Massage Therapy

Massage therapy can be heavenly for aching muscles, especially for athletes, and is definitely one of our favorite stress-busters. Those with body acne, however, need to be concerned about the massage oils used by the therapist, as many of them are heavy and occlusive. They may feel wonderful, but they can leave an aftermath of pimples.

A deep-tissue massage without oil or cream does not feel as luscious as a massage with them, so speak to your therapist before the massage begins. You may want to bring your own noncomedogenic moisturizer, such as Cetaphil Moisturizing Lotion or Cream. Many massage therapists today are aware of the skin sensitivity of their clients and will be happy to work with you. Many already use nonocclusive lotions or oils.

Saunas and Steam Baths

Heat can soothe tired muscles and be a terrific stress-reducer. Saunas use intense, dry heat; steam baths use intense, wet heat. Both cause bodies to work up a good sweat, flushing the skin and releasing impurities. Always take a cool shower after a hot heat treatment, and be sure to drink plenty of water and take it easy before returning to your daily activities. A good time to apply acne medications is following a sauna or steam bath, once your skin is thoroughly dry.

Note: Those with rosacea should avoid saunas and steam baths because the flush/blush response to the heat will exacerbate your condition.

exercise

Exercise cannot improve acne, but it is a must for your health and well-being. One reason for the growing epidemic of obesity in this country is the lack of exercise. Healthy bodies need healthy workouts.

Exercising properly means working up a sweat, though, so acne sufferers need to be careful about what they wear and how they cleanse afterward. Acne may be worsened by tight-fitting clothing, ill-fitting sports equipment, makeup, and not washing after exercise. (For more information, see page 292 in chapter 14.) Here are some general rules to follow in order to exercise without aggravating your acne.

Clothing

Those with body acne should look for garments that wick moisture away from the body. Wear lightweight loose-fitting cotton or microfiber workout gear. A bonus to wearing cotton is that it allows the skin to breathe, and if it's loose it's less prone to create friction and aggravate acne. Many synthetics, such as Lycra or nylon, can trap heat and moisture against the skin, creating a fertile breeding ground for the *p. acnes* bacteria, which causes breakouts.

Equipment

Friction from sports equipment is known to cause acne (see page 176 in chapter 8). We see many high school football players with a distinctive pattern of acne from ill-fitting helmets and shoulder pads each season. If a helmet slides around on your forehead, try lining it with a layer of soft, washable cotton fabric, which you should wash after every workout. (Old cotton T-shirts work great.) If you surf or dive, make sure wetsuits fit properly, especially under the arms. In addition, clean and dry all sports equipment after using to prevent acne-aggravating bacteria from invading.

Makeup

Although sometimes difficult for those used to wearing foundation and concealer, it is always best to try to wear as little makeup as possible during exercise. Products with a noncomedogenic (not pore-clogging) label have been tested under controlled laboratory conditions—which usually do not include heavy sweating. Therefore, a product such as a foundation that is noncomedogenic in normal, daily use may become comedogenic when the user exercises. Wash as soon as possible after working out; when your skin is dry, apply your acne medication, then your makeup.

Wash after Exercising

Sweat on its own doesn't cause acne, but heavy perspiration can cause even noncomedogenic products to clog pores or cause irritation. Always try to shower immediately after a workout, using a medicated, exfoliating cleanser. Do not scrub with a back brush or loofah, as they can unduly harm the skin. If a shower is not possible, change from wet clothes as quickly as possible. Dry your skin by blotting gently with a clean, dry towel, then wipe down acne-prone areas with salicylic acid cleansing pads, such as Proactiv Solution Clear-Zone Body Pads. Keep them tucked in your gym bag or purse so they're always handy.

nutrition

In chapter 1, we discussed the myths that sugar, chocolate, and fried foods cause acne. There is a another theory, one arguing that acne vulgaris is a disease of Western civilization, where the traditional diet high in refined carbohydrates permanently boosts insulin, elevates growth hormone levels, stimulates the sebaceous secretions that produce acne, and ultimately leads to inflammation and the breakdown of the body. On the other hand, a recent study published in the *Journal of the American Medical Association* stated that "Diet plays no role in acne treatment in most patients . . . even large amounts of certain foods have not clinically exacerbated acne." We think far more research needs to be done before sweeping conclusions may be drawn about the effect of diet upon acne.

In the meantime, we'll tell you what we've learned about acne and diet: To propose that the inflammation of acne can be stopped if you eliminate all carbohydrates from your diet is just too simple. First, realize that acne is a complicated process occurring in genetically predisposed individuals and is triggered by hormones, stress, climate, and mechanical irritation. Second, if carbohydrates were the source of acne, it would follow that overweight people, who consume large quantities of carbohydrates every day, should all have acne—which, of course, they don't. We've seen many patients who've been on no-carbohydrate or very low-carbohydrate diets for weight loss or who have carefully regulated their diets to monitor their blood sugar levels or for anti-inflammatory benefits—yet they continue to have acne. The message from the authors of restrictive fad diets is often "Change your diet and your acne goes away." Yet even when our patients had the discipline to stick to these diets, their acne remained unchanged. Worse, they blamed themselves. This is disturbing to us, as it takes us right back to the myth that acne is your fault. The truth is, acne is *not* your fault.

We believe in the tried and true for acne treatment, and we also believe that the tried and true works for nutrition. Use common sense. Knowing that chocolate doesn't cause acne is not a license to binge on chocolate truffles. Eating a sensible, balanced diet will serve you best in the long run. Fad diets may work for rapid weight loss, but they rarely work for permanent mainte- nance of that weight loss, as they impose a ridiculously restrictive lifestyle. (If they did work, bookstore shelves would not be lined with hundreds of diet books and obesity would not be one of the leading causes of illness and death in America.)

We both do our utmost to eat a healthy diet of unprocessed foods, which may be easier for us than for some, as we live in California, where fresh, or- ganic food is easy to find. With so many families burdened with stress, work, and school commitments, however, there often is little time to cook properly. Unfortunately, supermarket prepackaged, processed foods and restaurant fast food are usually laden with salt, sugar, and dangerous hydrogenated (trans) fats. Avoid them as much as possible. Instead, eat simple foods, such as steamed vegetables, broiled chicken or fish, and whole grains—all are easy to prepare.

Certain foods, especially those containing iodides, *can* trigger acne in sus- ceptible individuals. Macrobiotic diets are not recommended for anyone with acne. You should also avoid a steady diet of seaweed, shellfish, sushi, and sea salt (look for salt without added iodine).

Avoiding fish and seafood to prevent acne is contrary to the advice given in the book *The Acne Prescription,* by Dr. Nicholas Perricone. In this book, Dr. Perri- cone states that an "anti-inflammatory" diet is one of the essential parts of his treatment philosophy, and he encourages readers to consume large quan- tities of fish, most notably salmon, for its anti-inflammatory properties and high levels of essential fatty acids and to regulate blood sugar levels. We do not agree with this approach to acne treatment, and we believe that excessive consumption of fish may be detrimental to the health of many people.

"While it is beneficial to eat fish on a regular basis, it is not advisable for children, teenagers, and women of childbearing age to consume large quantities of certain fish," says Dr. Jacqueline Moline, a specialist in environmental and occupational medicine at the Mount Sinai Hospital School of Medicine in New York. "Recent studies show that farmed salmon may contain dangerously high levels of polychlorinated biphenyls [PCBs], which is linked to breast cancer, and other toxicants, including dioxin. Certain fish, such as tuna, kingfish, swordfish, mackerel, seabass, halibut, and shark, may contain high levels of mercury and should not by consumed more than once a week. Children, teenagers, and women of childbearing age should consume these fish less than once a month. Further information on fish advisories can be obtained through your state department of health websites."

Furthermore, according to Dr. Jane Hightower, internist and mercury toxics expert at California Pacific Medical Center, San Francisco, mercury has dangerous effects on the nervous system and will cause brain damage, autism, and mental retardation in a fetus. Mild elevations of mercury in adults will double the risk of heart attack. In addition to avoiding a steady diet of fish, here are some more tips for eating, not only to avoid acne flare-ups but for better health:

- Prepare large amounts of your favorite meals and freeze them in serving-size portions for later use.
- Replace refined foods, such as white flour, with whole grains. For example, cut down on white bread, pasta made with white flour, and desserts. Sugar is high in calories and has little nutritional value. Whole grains are far more filling and provide necessary, appetite-zapping fiber.
- Drink water. Eight cups a day is recommended for flushing toxins out of your body and reducing hunger.
- Avoid any foods with partially hydrogenated fats.
- Never supersize anything! A three- to four-ounce portion of steak, chicken, or fish is the size of your palm. A cup of cooked rice or pasta is the size of your fist.
- Avoid stimulants, such as coffee or other caffeinated beverages. If you love

coffee or tea, indulge in the morning and switch to decaffeinated drinks later in the day.

- Green tea has anti-inflammatory benefits. Try drinking it instead of coffee or black tea. Green tea has lower levels of caffeine, and it's delicious and refreshing when iced.
- Sugared drinks have no nutritional value and provide excess calories. Fruit juice is also laden with sugar calories. Artificially sweetened drinks often contain phosphorus, which can interfere with the absorption of calcium needed for strong bones and elevate blood sugar. It's best to avoid all these sweet drinks and stick to water.
- Limit alcohol consumption to one drink a day.
- Eat hormone-free foods. That means milk and dairy products, poultry, and beef that are certified organic and hormone-free or kosher.
- Use salt sparingly. Taste food before blithely sprinkling it on.
- Never skip breakfast.
- Make lunch the biggest meal of the day. This way, calories will be burned throughout the day.
- Keep healthy snacks available at home and work.
- Stay off the scale. Weighing yourself regularly causes stress. Weigh yourself no more than once a month.
- Don't beat yourself up if you eat a candy bar now and then.

supplements

As with diets, controversies are constant about what vitamins and minerals are necessary for optimal health. It has been said that the only people who truly benefit from vitamins are the manufacturers earning vast profits from consumers who think that if one pill is good, a handful must be better. Supplements are one of the most misunderstood and controversial aspects of good nutrition. For example, the American Cancer Society does not recommend supplements, because the best source of nutrients will always be food. Yet how many of us eat a truly balanced and nutritious diet every day?

Our bodies must have the RDA (recommended daily allowance) for most vitamins and minerals in order to have an effective metabolism, convert fat and carbohydrates into energy, and construct body tissues. Vitamins and minerals have no calories and therefore do not provide energy by themselves. In fact, megadoses (three or more times higher than the RDA) of water-soluble vitamins, such as C and B-12, are excreted, which means you may have very expensive urine. In addition, the fat-soluble vitamins A, E, and K are stored in the body and can be toxic in large doses, causing severe liver or kidney damage. As with cosmetics, do your homework about supplements. Be a sensible, smart consumer.

One of the keywords when considering supplements is "antioxidant." When your body uses oxygen, cells naturally form by-products, called free radicals, that can damage cells and contribute to the aging process. Antioxidants neutralize free radicals. Vitamins A, C, and E all contain antioxidants.

The best sources of antioxidant vitamins are the following foods:

Vitamin A—Beta-Carotene

Broccoli, cantaloupe, egg yolks, fortified grains, fortified milk, liver, low-fat dairy products, mangoes, peaches, pumpkin, squash, tomatoes, and yams

Vitamin C

Bell peppers, broccoli, cantaloupe, citrus fruits and juices, collard greens, kale, kiwi, papaya, raw cabbage, spinach, and strawberries

Vitamin E

Apricots, broccoli, fish, fish oils, fortified cereals, nuts, seeds, shrimp, vegetable oils, and whole grains

Since most of us don't get our RDA of vitamins and minerals through our diet, we recommend the daily nutritional supplement levels in the table below. If you can find a multivitamin that contains the levels of vitamins and minerals listed in the table, additional supplements are not needed for healthy skin.

sleep

Few of us get enough of the refreshing sleep we need. A body suffering from chronic sleep deprivation will not have the resources to build a strong immune system. While a robust immune system won't prevent

Vitamins and Minerals	Function
biotin 2.5 milligrams	strong hair and nails
calcium chews, which are easily absorbed by the body 500 milligrams once or twice daily	strong, healthy bones
folic acid 400 micrograms	stress reliever
multivitamin	necessary for overall bodily functions
niacin 100 milligrams	stress reliever
selenium 100 micrograms	antioxidant
*Vitamin A 5,000 to 10,000 international units (do not exceed this dosage)	antioxidant
Vitamin B$_1$ (thiamin) 100 milligrams	stress reliever
Vitamin B$_2$ (riboflavin) 100 milligrams	stress reliever
Vitamin B$_6$ 100 milligrams	stress reliever
Vitamin B$_{12}$ 100 micrograms	stress reliever
Vitamin F (linoleic acid) 1 teaspoon to 1 tablespoon of flaxseed oil. Do not use this oil for cooking. Try it in a salad or as a straight dose.	acne patients are often deficient in Vitamin F
† zinc 15 to 30 milligrams, mild to moderate acne; 100 milligrams, severe acne	anti-inflammatory

* Vitamin A has been proven helpful for acne in a dosage of 20,000 units daily for three months. Use is then discontinued for at least three months. Discuss this possibility with your dermatologist before self-treating, as high doses can damage the liver.

† Zinc doses above 30 milligrams can cause nausea, so take it with meals.

acne, it can help fight infection and reduce stress so pimples clear up more quickly.

For those of us who are already overburdened in this stressful world, being able to relax in order to go to sleep is often a near-impossible task. Refer to the tips on page 101 in chapter 4 for nighttime stress-busters and try these tips as well:

- Try to sleep on a regular schedule.
- Avoid drinking any beverages with caffeine after noontime. If this doesn't help, avoid caffeine altogether. Read labels, as caffeine is often added to drinks that you least expect to contain it.
- Avoid alcohol. It is metabolized as sugar by the body, so it is also a stimulant. Don't drink within four hours of bedtime.
- Exercise in the morning or afternoon. Try to let at least three to four hours elapse between exercise and bedtime.
- Do something relaxing in the hour or so before getting into bed. Arguments, overexcitement, hours at the computer, and bill-paying will rev you up, not calm you down.
- A light bedtime snack (without sugar) is okay. Avoid eating a full, heavy meal.
- Hot beverages, such as decaffeinated teas, are soothing and relaxing. Try one before bed.
- Trade massages with your loved one.
- Make your bedroom a haven—clear out the clutter and move the computer to another room. It's tough to sleep in a room with the nagging concerns of your day surrounding you. Also choose soothing colors for walls and bedding.

A healthy body is certainly reflected in your skin. Sun protection, daily exercise, smart nutrition, and adequate sleep contribute to a sense of well-being, both physically and emotionally, resulting in a glowing complexion and a greater ability to manage stress. These good habits, while not a cure for acne, will help you reap health benefits in the long run.

chapter seventeen
makeup that works

"Every morning for the past ten years I have skillfully covered up each blemish whether I was going to the store or going to the prom. The most ridiculous time I put makeup on was before going to physical training at my Army post. After running, my soldiers would often notice I was sweating makeup. It was very frustrating. I didn't want to look 'glamorous' going for a run. I simply wanted to look presentable. And I couldn't do that without concealer."

—Joanna, age twenty-six

"Makeup was a protective shield for me. I got to where I was extremely good at hiding my acne, and people never dreamed it was as bad as it was. I didn't answer the door if I didn't have makeup on when people came over. My mother would lie to my dates and keep them in the living room if all my makeup wasn't on yet."

—Adrianna, age eighteen

for women with acne, properly applied makeup can be a lifesaver. Used improperly, though, it can look like a mask, accentuating the breakouts and causing more embarrassment and shame. Many of our patients tell us they spend hours in the bathroom every morning, desperate to cover each pimple, then spend additional time during the day checking and rechecking, adding more concealer and powder, all the while constantly worrying about their appearance. Their stress levels are palpable. For them, makeup is a necessary shield to hide their complexions from the curious eyes of the world.

Many teens and adult women, have never been taught how to apply makeup properly. No one told them that if skin is not properly hydrated, the foundation will look streaky, and the powder will cake. Comfortable with what they know, they often use the same products and colors for years, even as their appearance and lifestyles evolve.

There's no need to stay in a makeup rut simply because you have acne, since formulations improve and styles evolve. The thick, cloying, pore-clogging foundations used decades ago no longer exist. With the availability of quality products today, using makeup can be a tremendous amount of fun, and buying a new lipstick or experimenting with color can be an instant pick-me-up when your skin is getting you down.

Choosing makeup is an individual decision and should be based on your skin tone and taste in colors. In terms of comedogenicity, you need to be wary not so much of individual ingredients but how products are formulated. Some products may, for instance, contain ingredients, such as mineral oil or petrolatum, that can be acne triggers, but in such minimal concentration that they do not confer comedogenicity to the product. Look for the label noncomedogenic or nonacnegenic to feel confident that your acne won't worsen with makeup application. And, always patch-test new products first if you know you are sensitive to specific ingredients (see page 308 in chapter 15).

We believe in a minimal approach to makeup. The fewer products with the least amount of ingredients you put on your skin, the better. This will not only keep acne at bay but help streamline your makeup routine and the time necessary to perform it. For this purpose we have created dual-function, medicated makeup that provides healing as well as full coverage. And even with a minimal approach, you can play around with whatever colors and formulations work for you and try new products and textures.

Once your acne is healed, you will be liberated from needing to use makeup as a camouflage and can enjoy using it to enhance your natural beauty. "I can't express how great it is to not run away from people who come to my house unannounced, when I don't have any makeup on," Lynette, age thirty, told us. "I even had to be very careful about my makeup getting smeared by my kids, and I kept them at arm's length from my face. Now they rub up against me and I roll around with them, and it's just thrilling! And when I do wear makeup now, it's all about making myself look better, not as a shield to hide behind."

Following are some of the best tips about makeup application we've learned from professional makeup artists. The products listed are available at drugstores, department stores, or company websites. Remember, have fun with your makeup—let it be a life-enhancing experience, not an obsessive chore.

before you start

- Always begin with a clean, dry face. The correct order for successful makeup application is medication, moisture, sunscreen, makeup. Try using dual-function products, such as a moisturizing sunscreen, to lessen the number of products on your face. Remember, always let your medicated products dry completely before applying anything else.

- Never use medicated cleansers containing benzoyl peroxide, salicylic acid, or sulfur on the eye area, as they can be intensely irritating.

- When in doubt, make sure your makeup is noncomedogenic or nonacnegenic. These terms indicate that the product has been tested and shown not to promote acne.

- It's often best to apply foundation and powder to skin that has been primed with some form of moisturizer. Otherwise, foundation and powder can cake and be uneven in appearance. For those with extremely oily skin, a mattifying lotion (see the list on page 328 in chapter 16) will help set makeup so it doesn't streak.

- It's easy to smear mascara during application, which you then have to remove from the skin. If this happens often, particularly if you have long lashes, try applying your eye makeup and mascara before your other products. This way, if mascara smears by the side of your eyes or onto your cheeks, you won't have to reapply your concealer or foundation. This is especially important when you're using medicated products first.

- Makeup varies in different lighting. For instance, if you work in an office with fluorescent lighting, it will look different from the way it does in your bathroom. For a more even and natural look, apply makeup in natural light. Sitting near a window and using a hand mirror works well.

- More is not better, especially for those with severe acne. The temptation is to keep reapplying concealer or powder during the day, but this can often have the opposite effect, drawing attention to the pimples as well as adding potentially acnegenic ingredients to the area.

- Makeup migrates into the pores. For those with acne, medicated makeups containing salicylic acid or benzoyl peroxide allow this migration to benefit your complexion by healing and preventing acne.

- Makeup also rubs off. To limit this, keep your hands away from your face whenever possible. We know this can be extremely difficult, but if you keep rubbing the makeup off, you'll want to keep reapplying it, which sets up a vicious circle of overuse and irritation.

- "If you have extremely oily skin that causes your makeup to streak after several hours, place a piece of cellophane tape over the streaks and pull it off," suggests Melissa Greene, a makeup artist in Brooklyn, New York. "It sounds crazy, but it works. This will pull off the oil and leave your makeup intact. You can also try blotting papers, such as Proactiv Solution Oil Blotter Sheets or Lancôme Matte Finish Shine-Control Blotting Sheets."

- Don't be afraid of color, but if you have a lot of acne, it's best to highlight only one area of your face at a time. If you like dramatic eyes, go for subtle lips, and vice versa. Keep your cheeks neutral. And if your face tends toward redness, stay away from the red, pink, and purple families for shadows and blush, as they can appear to intensify it.

- Makeup formulations are all different. Experiment until you find the best colors and textures for your skin. Note: Nearly all brands accept returns if a product causes irritation.

- Never share makeup, especially mascara and eye shadows. This can cause infection and contamination.

- Applying makeup is an acquired skill, one that is often crucial for women with acne. A makeup lesson from a professional makeup artist who understands acne can be illuminating and save you hundreds of dollars by steering you away from the products that might not work best for you. Being taught how to apply makeup properly will also help cut down the time it takes to put on makeup, an asset to anyone already overburdened with work, school, and family commitments.

brushes

Choosing the Right Brush

The most important tool in your makeup arsenal is a concealer brush. Synthetic bristles aren't as tight as natural ones, so they are better for concealer brushes. Bristles for other brushes can be either synthetic or natural as long as they are fairly soft. You can use a bigger, longhandled brush at home and put a smaller one in your makeup bag.

Some women like to apply foundation with a brush or small sponge. Small brushes are also better for applying eye shadow, as they are softer and easier to clean than tiny foam applicators.

Care and Cleaning of Brushes

Brushes must be cleaned often, at least two to three times a week. "Use a very small drop of gentle dishwashing liquid, such as Dawn, directly on the brush," says Melissa Greene. "Rinse it well, then squeeze out the excess water until there are no more suds. Lay it flat to dry, with the bristles hanging over the edge of the sink."

You can also wash brushes by rubbing the bristles against a bar of unscented Dove soap and rinsing until water runs clear. If you use sponges, wash after every use. It's easier and more hygienic to use disposable ones.

Be conscientious about cleaning your brushes. They will be laden with bacteria, dead skin, and dust unless washed properly. The last thing you want to do is trade one skin problem for another.

color correctors

Acne often causes redness, as does rosacea. Regular foundations are not formulated to correct this, but you can easily do so yourself with a green color corrector. Applying a light layer of a green corrector—no matter what your skin tone, from the palest to the darkest—will help neutralize the redness. Apply regular foundation after the color corrector.

Following is a list of color correctors we recommend. Be sure to patch-test any new color corrector first to make sure it doesn't trigger your acne.

Face Matte Foundation in Mint
Face—The Great Face Color Corrector Kit
Physicians Formula Beauty Spiral—Lime
Physicians Formula Gentle Cover Concealer Stick—Green
Physicians Formula Concealer Twins
Urban Decay Urban Camouflage 3-in-1 Concealer
Origins Light Makes Right Color Corrector

makeup primers

Most makeup artists swear by an underbase, or makeup primer, for those with acne. It is applied over moisturizers and under the foundation. If your skin is fairly clear, it can be used as a foundation replacement or alone as an oil-free moisturizer. "Makeup primers have no acnegenic agents in them, and they feel comforting, especially when your skin is rough and irritated, so they're really soothing for those with acne," says Jill Goldberg, a makeup artist at the Paul LaBreque Hair Salon in New York.

Makeup primers can work wonderfully to minimize shallow scars and allow you to use much less foundation. You'll find that foundation can then be applied evenly and will stay true longer. "When you use a primer," Ms. Goldberg adds, "your foundation can then be used in a minimal way to even out skin tone, which is actually what it's designed to do. You can then use your concealer to conceal."

Following is a list of makeup primers we recommend. Be sure to patch-test any new makeup primer first, without foundation, to make sure it doesn't trigger your acne.

Nars Makeup Primer
Philosophy Clear Makeup (This kit includes The Present, a skin perfector underbase, a clear powder for topical shine reduction, and a neutral eye pencil.)
Proactiv Solution Makeup Primer
Smashbox Photo Finish Foundation Primer
Vincent Longo Water Canvas Base Primer

foundations

The most important product you will be wearing is foundation. Beauty editors are fond of saying "Buy the best foundation you can afford, spending less on eye colors and lipstick." That doesn't mean that only expensive foundations work to adequately cover acne; however, it is important to buy the best noncomedogenic foundation for you.

Hilary Clark, a makeup artist in San Francisco, says that "there are two common mistakes made when applying foundation. The first is using too much, which makes you seem to have a mask on. More makeup will not necessarily give you more coverage. The second is having the wrong color foundation. Few women truly need a pink-based foundation. Foundation with a yellow base will work much better to downplay redness."

The foundation should always match your skin tone, which can be difficult unless you have it custom-blended. An easy alternative is to sample foundation on your cheek and on your neck, then go outside. Checking the color in daylight will give you an accurate reflection of how well it matches your skin tone. If you plan to use a color corrector, first apply a dab of it in the test area so you can tell how well the foundation will blend over the color corrector and your skin.

Some foundations now come in unique cream-to-powder formulations—they feel creamy when applied, then dry to a matte finish. Oil-free formulas usually work best for oily skin. Read labels carefully. Look for foundations containing silicone (dimethicone or cyclomethicone), which has no effect on acne and gives an even application.

Following is a list of foundations we recommend. Be sure to patch-test any new foundation to make sure it doesn't trigger your acne.

Almay Nearly Naked Touch-Pad Liquid Makeup
Almay Skin Smoothing Foundation with Kinetin
Biotherm Sense Matte Hydro-Matifying Foundation
Bobbi Brown Oil-Free Even Finish Foundation
Chanel Double Perfection Fluide Matte Reflecting Makeup (for very oily skin)
Chanel Teint Fluide Universel Multi-Vitamin Natural Makeup
Clé de Peau Cream Foundation
Estée Lauder Double Wear Stay-in-Place Foundation
Joey Pure Pores Pore Minimizer Foundation
Lancôme Adaptive All-Day Skin Balancing Makeup
Laura Mercier Foundation
Lorac Oil-Free Foundation
L'Oréal Air Wear Breathable Long-Wearing Foundation
Neutrogena Healthy Skin Oil-Free Liquid Makeup
Neutrogena Skin Clearing Oil-Free Makeup (with salicylic acid)
Origins Nude and Improved Bare-Face Makeup
Prescriptives 100% Oil-Free Matte Finish Foundation
Proactiv Solution Sheer Finish Compact Foundation (with salicylic acid)

Sacha Dual-Action Powder Foundation
Stila Complete Coverage Foundation
Urban Decay Liquid Surreal Skin

concealers

Concealers are thicker than foundation and are designed to be used sparingly. A concealer that is labeled for use near the eyes should always be used in that area. Your foundation should not be applied near the eye, as it may be irritating to the eye itself.

As with foundation, concealers should match your skin tone as closely as possible. Always test a concealer under the foundation you plan to use so you can accurately assess how it looks, and be sure to test in it in daylight. Concealer that is too light or too pink or applied with too heavy a hand will make pimples more noticeable. Instead, always use a concealer that is yellow-based to cover blemishes, as this will help counteract redness.

How to Use Concealer to Cover a Pimple

The makeup artist Jill Goldberg has devised a system for concealing acne blemishes, which can often be hard to disguise, especially if they are bumpy.

- Always use a small, synthetic bristle brush meant for concealer. Your fingers are too broad.
- Be as gentle as possible.
- Use only a very tiny amount of concealer.
- Work quickly.
- Never dab concealer directly onto the middle of pimples and cysts—this is what makes them look cakey, with red edges.

For Unbroken Small Comedones

- Work from the inside out.
- Start from the top of the base of the comedone.
- Lightly fan out the concealer.
- Feather out to blend into foundation.

For Open Comedones, Such as Blackheads and Whiteheads

- Work from the outside in.
- Dot concealer along the outside of the pimple.
- Work it in, gently over the pimple.
- Feather out excess to blend in.

Following is a list of concealers we recommend. It is not necessary to patch-test concealer before use. Concealers with a ** contain medication such as salicylic acid or sulfur to help fight acne.

Alchemy Medic Blemish Treatment Concealer
Bobbi Brown Creamy Concealer Kit
Clinique Continuous Coverage Concealer
Dermablend Quick Fix
Face Concealer
Joey Calm and Correct Concealer for the Face
**Joey Pure Pores Hide & Heal
Kevyn Aucoin Beauty The Skin Enhancer
Kiora Corrector Palette
**Neutrogena Skin Clearing Oil-Free Concealer
Physicians Formula Wanderful Wand Brightening Cream Concealer
Prescriptives Camouflage Kit
Prescriptives Concealing Wand—Red Corrector
**Proactiv Solution Concealer Plus
YSL Touche Eclat

powders

Powder "sets" foundation and concealer and helps keep them from disappearing or streaking. It gives a polished look and absorbs oil, making it a must for those with oily skin. Powders may also be worn by themselves without underlying foundation. Some loose powders can even achieve the effect of foundation by absorbing oil and concealing redness. If worn alone, powders must always be applied over a moisturizer, as they'll streak otherwise.

Try to match the color of the powder to your skin tone as closely as you possibly can. Powder that is too light will look fake and ashy, and too dark will accentuate redness.

Many powders are now extremely lightweight. Women with acne often reapply powder often during the day, so it's best to stick to sheer formulas—your foundation and concealer will be doing the heavier duties. You'll want to apply loose powder with a brush. Pressed powder can be applied with a brush, cotton pad, sponge, or a puff.

Following is a list of powders we recommend. It is not necessary to patch-test powders before use.

Bare Escentuals Loose Foundation
Estée Lauder Equalizer Loose Powder
Joey Pure Pores Finishing Powder
Lancôme Matte Finish Shine-Control Sheer Pressed Powder
L'Oréal Feel Naturale Ultrafine Light Softening Powder
L'Oréal Ideal Balance Pressed Powder
MAC Sheer Pressed Powder
Nars Pressed Powder
Neutrogena SkinClearing Oil-Free Pressed Powder (with salicylic acid)
Proactiv Solution Sheer Finish Loose Powder
Proactiv Solution Sheer Finish Pressed Powder
YSL Pressed Powder

blushes

Blushes tend to be overused by many women, whether they have acne or not. Blushes should always be applied with a subtle hand and blended carefully with a large, soft brush. Cream blushes are more likely to have comedogenic ingredients, so powder or gel blushes are best. Avoid bright red or pink hues, as these will only intensify redness. Also, some red dyes and many blue dyes are highly comedogenic. Carmine is not.

If your face tends toward redness, stick to neutral tones and those with a gold, honey, or bronze base. Peach tones are also good. Note: Blush shades should only be two to three shades darker than your own skin, as you want to appear naturally flushed, not embarrassed!

Apply only a very small amount of blush in the apple of your cheek; too much looks artificial. Use a large brush to lightly circle the area. Blend so there is no obvious demarcation between blush color and foundation.

Some makeup artists like to use sheer bronzers instead of blushes. Their brown-yellow hues can help counteract redness. If you want to try a bronzer, go for a very sheer formula, such as Nars Laguna, that has no orange undertones. This can be particularly effective for those with rosacea, who tend toward redness in the cheeks and don't need red applied to the face.

Following is a list of blushes and bronzers we recommend. Acne reactions are rare, but if you're worried, do a patch test of blushes or bronzers before use.

Alchemy Complexion Gel
Bare Escentuals Bare Minerals Blush
Bobbi Brown Bronzing Powder
Clarins Bronzing Duo in Bright Sun or Morning Sun
Clinique Blushwear
Dior Terra Bella Sun Powder
Estée Lauder Cool Bronze Loose Powder
Face Bronzer
Joey Chiseled Cheeks
Lancôme Star Bronzer Bronzing Powder Compact
L'Oréal Feel Naturale Powder Blush
Nars Laguna Bronzing Powder
Revlon All-Over Bronzing Powder
Sacha Matte Blush-On
Urban Decay Afterglow Powder Blush

eyeliners and eye shadows

Subtle eye color can make even small eyes appear larger and draw attention away from acne-prone areas of the face. For a polished, professional look, stick to neutrals, perhaps with a slightly darker eyeliner. Eye pencils are easier to control and less likely to smudge. Colors that work well for eye shadows will be any outside of the bright pink, red, and purple hues, but if you like lilac, for example, you can try it as long as it is toned down with a yellow base. Gold, beige, and bronze work well for all skin tones.

Using an eye shadow primer will keep colors from fading and sliding off the skin. You can try Paula Dorf Eye Primer or Smashbox Lip and Lid Primer. If your skin is very oily (or wrinkled), be sure to use a primer, and avoid cream shadows and liners, as they tend to migrate into creases and around the eyes.

The creamier the texture, the more oil there is in the formulation. Alternatively, pressed-powder shadows will absorb oil.

Glittery effects in eye shadow are usually derived from mica, a common mineral that can sometimes cause irritation, so save them for parties or special evenings out. Anything with excess shine, glitter, or iridescence is best avoided until acne is healed. A hint of shimmer is much more effective.

Following is a list of eyeliners and eye shadows we recommend. It is not necessary to patch-test eyeliners and eye shadows before use.

Almay Bright Eyes Eyeliners
Almay Eye Shadow Palettes
Bare Escentuals Bare Minerals Liner Shadow
Bobbi Brown Eye Shadow
Chanel Ombre Unique Crème Illuminating Eyeshadow
Clarins Soft Shimmer Eye Color
Cover Girl Eye Enhancers
Dior Duostyl DoubleStick Eyeshadow and Liner
Dior 5-Colour Eyeshadow Compact
Estée Lauder Pure Color Eye Shadow Duos
Face Matte Eye Shadow
MAC Cream Color Base
MAC Wet/Dry Powder Eye Liner
Maybelline Cool Effect Shadow/Liner
Neutrogena Shimmer Sheers
Origins Slipcover—Color For Eyes
Prescriptives Powder Eye Pencil
Revlon ColorStay Eyeshadow

mascaras

Mascara adds bulk, color, and the illusion of lengthening to lashes and is an indispensable element to most makeup wardrobes. For women who don't like to use a lot of color on their faces, a quick swipe with a mascara brush can instantly open up the eyes. It's best to stick with nonwaterproof mascaras, which can easily be removed with a gentle cleanser. Waterproof mascaras are difficult to remove without oil, which can lead to clogged pores.

To use mascara, apply one coat to the top lashes, then let it dry thoroughly.

EYE MAKEUP REMOVERS

Eye makeup, especially mascara, must be removed every day. Otherwise, small amounts can remain around the eye area and even cascade down the cheeks, creating acne on the cheeks, temples, and forehead.

Water-based shadows and mascaras do not require a special eye makeup remover. In fact, most gentle cleansers, such as Cetaphil Gentle Skin Cleanser or Rodan & Fields COMPOUNDS Gentle Wash, work effectively to remove makeup without stinging. If you do like to use a separate eye makeup remover, remember to always wash your face after using it to rinse away any remainder on the skin. Avoid using toilet paper or washcloths in the eye area, though, as they may be too rough for this tender skin.

Mascaras labeled waterproof or long-lasting contain waxes that cannot be dissolved with soap; they require an oil-based remover, such as Vaseline or products containing mineral oil, which is occlusive and not advisable for acne-prone skin. Oily eye makeup removers can also promote milia, tiny white cysts under the eyes. We recommend you stick to water-based mascaras and nonoily makeup removers instead.

Following is a list of eye makeup removers we recommend:

Almay Gently Clean Non-Oily Face Makeup Remover Pads
Almay Non-Oily Eye Makeup Remover
Aveda Pure Comfort Eye Makeup Remover
Clinique Rinse-Off Eye Makeup Solvent
Maybelline Expert Eyes 100% Oil-Free Eye Makeup Remover
Prescriptives Quick Remover For Eyes
Proactiv Solution Makeup Removing Cloths

You can then apply a coat to the lower lashes, if desired. Let dry before repeating. Using an eyelash curler before applying mascara can add to the appearance of bulk and curling of the lashes, so you may be able to use less mascara, lessening the chance for it to smear.

Mascara can easily become contaminated with bacteria, which can cause eye infections. Never share mascara. And be sure to throw mascara out after two to three months, or sooner if it appears to be drying or has a noticeable odor.

Following is a list of mascaras we recommend. It is not necessary to patch-test mascara before use.

Almay One Coat Mascara
BeneFit A Plush Mascara
Clarins Pure Curl or Pure Volume Mascara
Cover Girl Super Thick Lash Mascara
Estée Lauder More Than Mascara
Lancôme Magîcils Color On Splash Off Mascara
Maybelline Great Lash
Paula Dorf Mascara
Revlon Lash Fantasy
Sephora Mascara

lipsticks

If you have pimples around the mouth, you might want to reconsider the products you use on your lips. Lipsticks and glosses are greasy by nature, with high concentrations of petroleum, wax, and other comedogenic substances. Lips themselves cannot break out, but the skin around them is susceptible. The greater the shine and stickiness of the lipstick or gloss, the greater the potential for pore-clogging. Creams and glosses have the most oil. Look for slightly matte or moisturizing formulas instead. Flat matte and frost lipsticks however, are often very drying.

If you like lip liner, use it first—either in a neutral shade or one exactly matching your lipstick. Keep the point sharp. Applying lip liner to the entire lip will provide a base for lipstick to remain on longer and keep it from migrating to nearby skin. You can also use gel blush or cheek blush stains to tint your lips in place of lip liner. They may be worn alone or as a base for lipstick, allowing the color to last longer and look very natural.

If skin is red or irritated, stay away from bright reds, pinks, and violets. Pink-brown or pink-gold shades work better.

Following is a list of lipsticks and lip liners we recommend. It is not necessary to patch-test lipsticks or liners before use.

Alchemy Refreshing Lip Gel
Almay Pure Tints Protective Lip Care
Almay Stay Smooth Anti-Chap Lipliner
Aveda Uruku Lip/Eye Liner
Bare Escentuals Lipstick

HYDRATING ACCUTANE-DRIED LIPS

One of the most common side effects of Accutane is extremely dry lips. As lips themselves do not contain hair follicles or oil glands, products that contain occlusive moisturizing agents will help combat chapping. Lipsticks tend to be hydrating, but stay away from matte or frost lipstick formulas, as they tend to be drying. Using sheer formulas with a slight tint of color works well. Try Alchemy's Refreshing Lip Gels or Nuxe's honey-based tinted balms, which are soothing yet long lasting.

When you use lip balms, try to limit application to the lips themselves; they are not designed to be applied to the skin, since they clog pores. You may want to use a lipstick brush for accurate application.

Following is a list of hydrating lip treatments we recommend:

Alchemy Medic Emergency Mouth Treatment
Alchemy Refreshing Lip Gel
Bag Balm Ointment
Black Up Lip Care Kit
Blistex Lip Balm
Burt's Bees Lip Balm
Clarins Moisture Replenishing Lip Balm
Clé de Peau Lip Treatment
Elizabeth Arden 8-Hour Cream
Eucerin Cream
Jurlique Lip Care Balm
Karite Lips
Nivea Lip Care Repair
Nuxe Lip Balm
Philosophy Kiss Me Lip Ointment
Vaseline Lip Therapy

Bobbi Brown Lip Stain
Chanel Hydracaresse Hydra-Treatment Lipstick
Clarins Rouge Eclat Lipstick
Clinique Chubby Stick
Estée Lauder Pure Color Velvet Lipstick
Joey Opti-Brite Lipstick Swirl
Lancôme Rouge Absolu Crème
Laura Mercier Lipstick
MAC Satin Lipstick

MAC Sheer Lipstick
Neutrogena Lipcolor
Prescriptives Soft Suede Lipstick
Revlon Absolutely Fabulous Lipcream
Vincent Longo Lipstick
YSL Lip Markers

makeup for skin of color

There are now lines of makeup for women of color, who've often been frustrated by the lack of skin-matching foundations and concealers available. These are created with yellow or olive bases, often in oil-free formulations, and come in a wide variety of hues to match the varied skin tones of African-American, Asian, and Hispanic skin. The colors of the shadows, lipsticks, and blushes tend to be highly pigmented and also yellow-based, which makes experimentation very enjoyable.

African-American Skin

Black Up

Oil-Free Fluid Foundation
Stick Foundation
Concealer/Anti-Dark Circles
Two-Way Powder Cake
Blush
Eyeshadow Palette
Eye and Lip Liner
Long Hold Lipstick

Fashion Fair

Oil-Free Crème to Powder Perfect Finish Foundation
Perfect Finish Crème Makeup
Cover Stick Concealer
Fragrance-Free Oil-Control Pressed Powder
Translucent Pressed Powder

Iman

I-Stick Foundation
Perfect Response Oil Blotting Pressed Powder

I-Conceal Concealer
I-Blush
I-Shadow
I-Lips

Asian Skin

Zhen

Dual Powder Foundation
Matte Foundation
Oil Blotting Papers
Tinted Moisturizer with SPF 15
Concealer—Brush Pen
Mosaic Bronzing Powder
Runway Colors Shadow Compact
Lip Silks Moisture Lipstick

Hispanic Skin

Zalia

Oil-Free Foundation Liquid
Foundation Stick Concealer
Color Blend Powder Blush
Mascara
Matte Eyeshadow
Cream Lipstick

After clearing your acne with the Rodan and Fields Approach, you will no longer need makeup to conceal and disguise imperfections. Instead, you will discover and enjoy the art of using makeup to enhance your own natural beauty!

glossary

Acne Excoriée des Jeunes Filles Compulsive picking of acne lesions, which often leaves incurable, disfiguring scars and holes in the face.

Acne Vulgaris Medical name for acne, an inflammatory skin disease occurring around the hair follicle and oil glands. The variety of lesions includes blackheads, whiteheads, pimples, pustules, nodules, and cysts. Acne is triggered by hormones in genetically susceptible individuals, resulting in a process of a plugged pore, entrapped oil inside the follicle, bacterial invasion and proliferation, and the body's response with inflammation.

Aloe Vera A hydrating agent with cooling, calming qualities.

Alpha Hydroxy Acid A fruit acid derived from fruit, milk, or sugar with exfoliating properties. It sweeps away dead skin cells while tightening and refining pores.

Androgen A masculinizing hormone found in both men and women, which increases in production during puberty. When this happens, it stimulates oil production (sebum) in hair follicles, leading to acne.

Antiandrogens Any substance that inhibits the body's production of androgens.

Antibiotics Medications that control acne by curbing the body's production of the p. acnes bacteria and decreasing inflammation. They are prescribed in either topical (creams, gels, pads, and lotions applied directly to the skin) or oral form.

Antioxidant A substance that soaks up free radicals, which are destructive molecules that damage cells.

Arnica A naturally occurring botanical that may help heal bruises and reduce redness and swelling.

Avobenzone (Parsol 1789) Chemical blocker of UVA light from the sun, used in sunscreen.

Azelaic Acid Synthetic agent with antiacne capabilities.

Benzoyl Peroxide An antimicrobial and oxidizing acne medication that works by removing p. acnes bacteria and aids in unplugging pores and reducing oil production.

Blackhead (Open Comedo) A plugged follicle that reaches the skin's surface and ruptures. The plug's dark appearance is not from dirt but a buildup of melanin, the skin's dark pigment, and oxidized oil.

Blue Light Therapy Part of the rainbow of visible light (410 nanometers) emitted by a light source from a machine in a doctor's office. It works by sterilizing the skin for a short period of time; in doing so, it may remove acne bacteria and temporarily improve acne when used in conjunction with traditional topical acne medications.

Broad-Spectrum Sunscreen Sunscreen that blocks the effects of UVA and UVB radiation from the sun.

Chamomile   Plant with skin-calming qualities.

Collagen   Protein fibers in the skin's second layer, the dermis.

Comedogenic   Causing clogged pores.

Comedone   Plug (or clog) in a hair follicle, which results when dead skin cells are trapped and compacted by oil.

Comedone Extractor   Instrument used to remove the contents of comedones.

Cortisol   Produced by the adrenal glands in response to stress, cortisol is a hormone that stimulates the sebaceous glands, triggering the production of extra oil. This increases the incidence of comedones, causing acne breakouts.

Cortisone   Drug with anti-inflammatory properties.

Cosmetic Acne (Acne Cosmetica)   A condition resembling acne vulgaris that is characterized by small pink or red bumps and local inflammation of the skin. It is triggered by comedogenic (containing pore-blocking ingredients) cosmetics and skin care products.

Cysts   Large, painful, solid bumps formed within hair follicles located deep within the skin. Cysts can become big enough to protrude from the face.

Dermatitis   Skin condition characterized by a rapidly spreading red rash that may be itchy, swollen, and blistered.

Dermatologic Surgery   Surgery to repair or improve the function or cosmetic appearance of skin tissue, most notably for scars. Methods include chemical peels for skin color, texture, and tone; cryosurgery for precancers, excisional surgery for cysts, moles, and skin cancers; and injection surgery for keloid scars.

Dermis   The second layer of the skin, which serves as a foundation for the epidermis and makes up the principal mass of the skin.

Epidermis   The skin's outer layer, consisting of corneocytes (the outermost layer of dead skin cells), melanocytes (which produce melanin, the substance that gives your skin its color), and Langerhan cells (which work with the immune system to help fight off disease).

Epithelial   Referring to the cells of the skin's outer layer, the epidermis.

Estrogen   One of the naturally occurring feminizing hormones responsible for regulating the menstrual cycle and causing female secondary sex characteristics.

Exfoliation   The regular removal of dead skin cells from the epidermis, revealing fresher skin. It occurs naturally. Because this process becomes sluggish over time, it can be achieved manually with scrubs or chemically with glycolic acid, alpha hydroxy acids, or other substances.

Follicles   Also called pores, these tiny holes house the fine hairs that cover our faces and bodies. Oil glands at the base of each follicle produce sebum, which travels up the hair shaft and out onto the surface of the skin to provide necessary lubrication.

Glycolic Acid   An effective exfoliant, it renews skin by dissolving dead skin cells and deep-cleaning pores.

Green Tea   A plant with antioxidant properties.

Hormones   Chemical substances that govern the processes of the human body. For example, androgens, the hormones that cause physical maturation during puberty, stimulate the body's production of oil, which can result in acne.

Hydroquinone The only FDA-approved skin lightener, it has a bleaching action on excessive, clumped, abnormal melanin (dark pigment) in the skin.

Hyperpigmentation Increased pigment in the skin that may result from hormones, skin injury, or sun exposure.

Inflammatory Causing inflammation (swelling). With acne, the word inflammatory is usually used to describe lesions that are inflamed by chemical reactions or bacteria in clogged follicles.

Isopropyl Alcohol A common ingredient of many facial toners, isopropyl alcohol is a strong astringent that can strip the skin of necessary oils, causing dryness and irritation.

Isotretinoin (Accutane) Oral medication used to treat severe inflammatory acne. It works by reducing sebum production in pores.

Keloid A scar resulting from excess collagen, which forms into a lumpy fibrous mass.

Keratin An insoluble protein that is the primary component of skin, hair, nails, and tooth enamel.

Keratinocytes Epidermal cells.

Kojic Acid An herbal skin-brightening agent.

Laser Therapy Skin treatment that uses specific wavelengths of light to remove the *p. acnes* bacteria on the skin. Also used to treat blood vessels and scars and for hair removal.

Lentigines Also known as freckles, liver spots, or brown spots, they are caused by chronic and acute sun exposure.

Lesion Any kind of wound or sore on the skin from injury or disease.

Melanin Color granules found in melanocytes, which manifest themselves as the general color of brown or dark spots (lentigines) on the skin.

Melanocytes Cells producing melanosomes, which in turn produce the melanin that contains the pigment in skin.

Melasma (Chloasma) Often known as the mask of pregnancy, these are localized brown patches on the forehead, cheeks, and upper lip caused by hormones and sun exposure. Melasma can be persistent and difficult to treat.

Menopause The natural cessation of menstruation as a result of aging. A woman is clinically termed menopausal after one year with no menstruation.

Microcomedo The first stage of comedo formation; a comedo so small that it can be seen only with a microscope.

Microdermabrasion An intensive treatment for deeply penetrating pore-cleansing and skin-cell exfoliation.

Milia Tiny white cysts found mainly in the area around the eyes that may appear spontaneously or as a result of either previous skin injury or use of occlusive skin care products.

Miliaria Small red bumps on the skin formed as a result of exposure to the sun and heat while wearing occlusive sunscreen.

Niacinamide A physiologically active form of niacin (B_3), that may regulate sebum and improve skin texture and reduce redness.

Nodules Large, painful, inflamed, pus-filled lesions lodged deep within the skin. They may become big enough to protrude from the face.

Noncomedogenic Skin-care products that have been tested and proven not to clog pores.

Occlusive Skin-care products containing pore-clogging ingredients.

Oral Contraceptives Birth control pills, containing some combination of estrogen and progesterone, often prescribed for hormonally triggered acne, especially in women with irregular menstrual cycles.

Papules Pimples that appear as small, firm pink bumps on the skin.

Perimenopause The years before menopause when feminizing hormone levels drop and menstrual cycles become irregular. Perimenopause usually begins between thirty-five and fifty.

Pilosebaceous Gland Glands found in the skin. Pilo means hair and sebaceous refers to the sebaceous, or oil, gland. Acne is a disease of the pilosebaceous gland.

Pimple An inflamed red bump on the skin, most commonly as papules or pustules.

Pores (see also Follicles) Tiny holes that house the fine hairs that cover our faces and bodies. Oil glands at the base of each follicle produce sebum, which travels up the hair shaft and out onto the surface of the skin to provide necessary lubrication.

Postinflammatory Hyperpigmentation Pink-to-brown color in the skin that occurs after a wound or pimple heals. Not permanent scars, they often take weeks, perhaps months, to fade.

Progesterone One of the feminizing hormones responsible for regulating the menstrual cycle and causing female secondary sex characteristics.

Proprionibacterium Acnes (p. acnes) Bacteria on the skin that causes the inflammation seen as pimples. *P. acnes* naturally occurs on all skin types as part of the skin's natural sebum maintenance system.

Pseudofolliculitis Barbae (Curly Hair Disease) Acne-like breakouts usually called shaving bumps. As hairs begin to grow back after shaving, waxing, or plucking, they become trapped inside the follicle, causing irritation and swelling.

Puberty The time of life when a child begins the process of physical maturation and becomes capable of sexual reproduction. Onset is usually in the early teens and is accompanied by a large increase in hormone production, often leading to acne.

Pustules Small, round acne lesions that are clearly inflamed and contain pus. The most common type of pimple, they may appear red at the base, with a yellowish or whitish center.

Radio-Frequency Treatment (Thermage) A heat-energy treatment that penetrates deeply into the skin, shrinking both scars and oil glands. It may also tighten collagen.

Retinoids Chemically related to Vitamin A, retinoids regulate growth of epithelial cells, aid in the reduction of comedones, and encourage normal skin-cell sloughing and renewal.

Rhinophyma The most severe form of rosacea, it results in an enlarged nose from enlarged oil glands and overgrowth of collagen.

Rosacea Acne-like skin condition characterized by a flush/blush reaction of skin, usually on the face and neck. Rosacea is often accompanied by central face acne.

Salicylic Acid A mild acid that works as a keratolytic agent, encouraging the sloughing of dead skin cells by stimulating the peeling of the top layer of skin and the opening of plugged follicles. Also known as beta hydroxy acid.

Sebaceous Glands Oil-producing glands at the base of every sebaceous hair follicle (or pore). Found in the greatest density on the face, neck, back, and chest, these follicles may be the sites of acne lesions.

Sebum Oil, fatty acids, and wax naturally produced by sebaceous glands and expelled up through the hair shaft and onto the skin to keep it soft and pliable.

Sloughing Part of the skin's natural renewal process, sloughing is the act of shedding dead skin cells to make room for new ones.

Spironolactone A mild diuretic with antiandrogen properties. Used in combination with oral contraceptives to treat acne and some forms of hair loss in adult women.

Stratum Corneum The top dead layer of skin above the epidermis that acts as a physical barrier between the lower living levels of skin cells and the outside.

Sulfur A naturally occurring element that absorbs excess skin oils and heals blemishes while cooling and calming redness and inflammation.

Testosterone A naturally occurring male hormone responsible for the induction and maintenance of secondary male sexual characteristics.

Tretinoin Synthetic Vitamin A, tretinoin is the active ingredient in retinoids, which help renew skin-cell turnover and unplug pores.

Triclosan A limited-spectrum topical antibacterial agent found in soaps and leave-on hand purifiers.

UVA Light A long wavelength (320 to 400 nanometers) of ultraviolet light that deeply penetrates the skin, affecting both the epidermis and dermis. UVA causes skin tanning, brown-spot formation, and skin wrinkling and is also believed to play an important role in melanoma (skin cancer).

UVB Light A wavelength (290 to 320 nanometers) of ultraviolet light that affects primarily the epidermis. UVB light causes sunburn and suntan and is linked to skin cancer formation and skin aging changes.

Vasodilators Foods or medications that cause the blood vessels to dilate (open up), resulting in temporary or permanent redness.

Whitehead (Closed Comedo) Clogged pores that are closed by skin cells that have grown over the surface opening of the pore, trapping the plug (comedo) beneath the skin. Whiteheads usually appear on the skin as small, whitish bumps.

Zinc Oxide FDA-approved sunscreen ingredient that physically blocks the penetration of UVA and UVB radiation.

index

Page numbers in *italics* refer to illustrations.